Medical Armageddon

VOLS. III AND IV

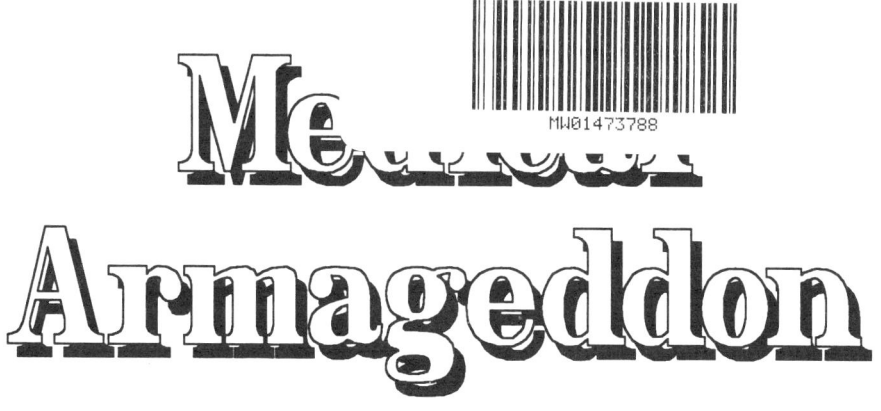

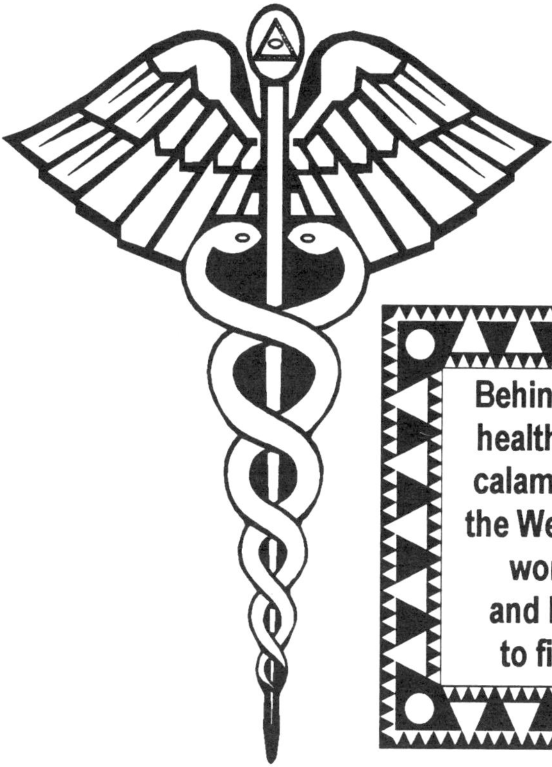

Behind the healthcare calamity of the Western world and how to fix it

Michael L. Culbert DSc

*COPYRIGHT © 1995,
C and C Communications*

Neither this book nor any part may be reproduced in any form or by any means, electronic or mechanical, including photocopying, microfilming and recording, or by any information retrieval system, without written permission in writing from the publisher.

**C AND C COMMUNICATIONS
San Diego, California**

First Printing: February 1995

LIBRARY OF CONGRESS CATALOGUE CARD NUMBER 94-69293

ISBN: 0-9636487-2-1 (Book Two; Vols. III & IV)
ISBN 0-9636487-3-x (set of two books)

PRINTED IN THE UNITED STATES OF AMERICA

ACKNOWLEDGMENTS

The author cannot possibly name all the contributors -- by word, deed or thought -- who in some way helped make the *Medical Armageddon* series a reality, so he admits guilt in omitting many of them.

He will forever be indebted to the scientific inspiration of Dr. Robert Bradford, founder-president of the Bradford Research Institutes, American Biologics, and the Committee for Freedom of Choice in Medicine, Inc., as well as to the innovative staff of the American Biologics-Mexico SA Medical Center, Tijuana, with whom he has long been associated.

He is also indebted to attorney (and medic) William Moore Jr., for originating the concepts of the "allopathic industrial complex" and the phrases "cancer con" and "heart hustle" while, over the years, providing background information and guiding ideas for medical reform. A continuing contributor in terms of ideas and historical background has been the frequently embattled California physician Bruce Halstead MD, a long-time vice president of the Committee.

So many other physicians, researchers, data-gatherers, and other writers and authors have contributed directly or indirectly to the author's efforts that he feels chagrined to note that mentioning them all would be too cumbersome and he simply expresses his heartfelt gratitude to them all.

The constantly-altered manuscript, of course, would never have been ready for presentation in any form without the faithful, plodding efforts of his computer-oriented companion and colleague, Dante I. Camino, and proof-reading help from Bernardino S. Juat Jr.

San Diego, California
Winter 1994/1995

"... and behold, a pale horse, and its rider's name was Death, and Hades followed him; and they were given power over a fourth of the earth, to kill with sword and with famine and with pestilence..."

REVELATION 6:8

INTRODUCTION TO THE
MEDICAL ARMAGEDDON SERIES

The 15-section *Medical Armageddon* series (with Appendices) was originally conceived as a single book detailing the problems of American healthcare delivery -- but in its years of research and preparation it became apparent that the subject was too vast to be conveniently contained in a single volume of easily readable type.

Michael L. Culbert DSc, chairman emeritus and a former president of the Committee for Freedom of Choice in Medicine Inc. and the author or co-author of 15 prior books in the areas of metabolic therapy and medical politics and economics, hence opted to make the full *Medical Armageddon* exposé available as a four-volume, two-book series.

The prevailing theme throughout is the following:

The original healing thought-construct (or *paradigm*, a favorite word throughout this series) on the planet was *holistic* in nature. But through twists and turns in history, as this series explains, the dominant Western healing model became *allopathic medicine*, the treatment of symptoms by contraries, which conveniently matched the needs of an expanding global pharmaceutical empire.

The allopathic paradigm in earlier times effectively neutralized its competitors in the medical marketplace -- and even, in American English, co-opted the very terms "medicine," "doctor" and "physician" to such a degree that the general public is almost wholly unaware that *other* schools of medical thought, each legitimate and with sufficient historic pedigree, exist.

A large part of the neutralizing of its opposition by allopathy involved the worldwide drug interests which, in turn, have sprung from an interlock of major industrial/governmental endeavors whose planetary power staggers the imagination. Allopathic medicine in the United States and, by implication, most of the Western world, has become state-mandated medicine. The current American medical model may be more definable as *fascist* medicine than any other.

The advent of what the author calls throughout the Allopathic Industrial Complex (AIC) or "The Club" would not be of great importance to the human family if it were delivering value in kind. However, as this series graphically portrays, the AIC has been virtually powerless in the face of the great chronic, *man-made* diseases of the modern era, which now stand poised to wipe out, first, the Western gene pool and, thereafter, the remainder of the population. Not only has allopathic medicine shown itself essentially incapable of stemming cancer, AIDS, cardiovascular conditions, immunological and environmental disorders of all kinds as well as the growing legion of geriatric and pediatric diseases, it has often been a large part of the problem in their development and spread.

At the same time, state-sanctioned fascist medicine, in a country which thinks of itself as the "land of the free, the home of the brave," has ruthlessly suppressed medical innovation and outside-the-AIC-pale medical research. This series pinpoints the tip-of-the-iceberg extreme cases in which the policing powers of the AIC have been brought to bear against individual physicians, researchers, healers and whole industries (healthfoods, for example) who or which pose a conceptual or economic threat to the Allopathic Industrial Complex.

Yet it is among some of this suppressed or overlooked research, and among many suppressed and persecuted medical innovators, that the *only* medical hope for the survival of the human race is to be found. The general population, sensing this on an intuitive level, is hence beginning to abandon the allopathic paradigm in droves and to seek so-called "alternative," "unconventional," "unorthodox" substances, techniques and therapies in an all-out bid to save their lives and health -- the New Medicine. The AIC, responding in kind, on the one hand is attempting to co-opt or absorb what it can of the New Medicine while protecting its vested interests and slowing down medical progress as deftly as possible.

The author argues that the evolution of the New Medicine for the 21st century is increasingly the rediscovery of the holistic paradigm in healing and its coupling with modern-era advances in diagnostics and therapeutic application -- *integrative medicine.* Protocols of the same are already visible, are saving lives and are reducing suffering even while many of their developers, creators, heroes and heroines remain viciously assailed, hounded, persecuted and prosecuted by venal elements of the AIC.

The 15 sections (plus Appendices) of this series are:

I. FEDSTAPO (The Incredible Story of Health-Freedoms Suppression in America.)

II. AN AMERICAN CHAMBER OF HORRORS (Modern Medicine as a Threat to our Health.)

III. MILKING AND BILKING THE SYSTEM (Greed and Gouging Nourish the Medical Money Machine.)

IV. ERROR BY CONSENSUS: THE RISE OF 'SCIENTIFIC MEDICINE'

V. THE PERPETUATION OF ERROR: VICTORY OF THE

ALLOPATHIC PARADIGM

VI. THE INSTITUTIONALIZATION OF ERROR: THE COMING OF THE ALLOPATHIC INDUSTRIAL COMPLEX

VII. THE AMA: ORGANIZED ALLOPATHY, THE DRUG INDUSTRY, AND THE FIGHT AGAINST 'QUACKERY'

VIII. THE DRUG INDUSTRY: RIDING THE RECESSION-PROOF GRAVY TRAIN

IX. THE FDA: STORM TROOPERS FOR THE DRUG TRUST (How a Good Idea Went Wrong)

X. HEART HUSTLE: SCHEMES, SCAMS AND BIG BUCKS IN THE CARDIOVASCULAR INDUSTRY

XI. CANCER CON: OF MICE, MEN, MONEY AND MALIGNANCY

XII. APRICOT POWER: LAETRILE AS THE MARINE CORPS OF THE 'ALTERNATIVE' REVOLUTION

XIII. AIDScam and CFSide: IMMUNE DYSREGULATION -- END OF HUMANITY OR END OF ALLOPATHY?

XIV. FOOD, SUPPLEMENTS AND THE 'ALTERNATIVE' REVOLUTION: THE AMERICAN MEDICAL PARADIGM BEGINS A GRUDGING SHIFT

XV. TOWARD THE MEDICINE OF THE 21ST CENTURY: A NEW PARADIGM IN HEALING EMERGES

APPENDICES

A: Solving the healthcare crisis while rescuing liberty

B: The Committee for Freedom of Choice in Medicine, Inc.
        plan for healthcare reform
        Addendum re/federal/state conspiracies
against physicians, the healthfood industry, and related matters

C: Model state-level legislation for medical freedom of choice

D: RESOURCES
        Selected bibliography

        Organizations

INDEX

Dedicated to the memory of

Gylah Bess Culbert

1910-1995

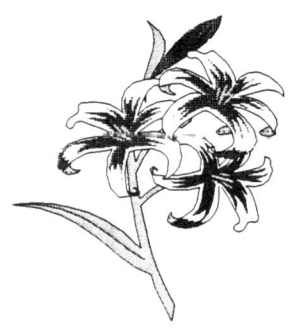

VOLUME III

X. HEART HUSTLE: Schemes, scams and big bucks in the cardiovascular industry   325

Killer number one: 'heart disease' — Mysteries in the victories — The trouble(s) with angiograms — Of cabbages and things — 'Ballooning' profits, dilating for dollars — When in doubt, prescribe a drug — The cholesterol conundrums — A torpedo attack in the *Atlantic* — Cholesterol is a many-splintered thing — The fight over fat — Enter the triglycerides — Bringing home the groceries — The exercise/diet teeter-totters — The EDTA chelation saga — Joining the 'alternative' revolution — The dietary heart of the matter

XI. CANCER CON: Of mice, men, money and malignancy   371

The unkindest cuts — The falsest premises — An endless carnage — A ministry of misinformation — Some modest gains — Malignant truth-twisting — Lies, damned lies, and statistics — Shaking up The Club — The big business of Cancer Inc. — And more test traps — The roots of illogic — Treatment worse than the disease — From microbes to viruses to genes — A litany of failure and disaster — Belling the cat — Word games and cognitive dissonance — Keeping abreast of a scandal — More worthless tests — The great PSA caper — And now, drugs as preventives! — The carcinogen-of-the-month club — The radiation holocaust — 'security' and coverup —Suffer the little animals — The ACS: propaganda central — Some rays of hope — Diet and malignancy — For 'control' rather than 'cure' — More tigers in the jungle

XII. APRICOT POWER: Laetrile as the Marine Corps of the 'alternative' revolution   433

An apricot kernel shakes things up — The issue: freedom of choice — Laetrile captures 24 states — Uniting Left and Right — An ancient background — Proofs from epidemiology — Cancer as a nutritional deficiency — John Beard and the trophoblasts — Cancer Inc.'s war on 'unprovens' — The beginnings: Coley, Warburg, Gerson — The campaign against Glyoxylide — Taking on Harry Hoxsey — Dr. Ivy and Krebiozen — Fitzgerald lets a cat out of the bag — Enter Dr. Dean Burk — A newspaper editor gets hooked — The laetrile juggernaut — The 'great laetrile smuggling trial' — A revolt starts in Alaska — The Establishment counterattack — Attempted KO: the 'laetrile clinical trial' — Laetrile's real victories

XIII. AIDScam and CFSide: Immune dysregulation — end of humanity or end of allopathy? 471

AIDS as apocalypse — Common sense vs. panic — Making the facts fit the theory — Enter the 'co-factors'— Cancer Inc, joins AIDS Inc. — AIDS in Africa: horror and hoopla — An oriental conundrum — HIV: the ever-lengthening incubation — HHV-6: riddle within an enigma — Conspiracy theories arise — An African swine fever connection? — The sorry saga of AZT — AIDS theory: failing on all fronts — Hope from the unortho-docs — The syphilis connection — Positivity in negativity? — Enter CFS, the crippler — AIDS, CFS: parts of one syndrome? — More diseases of civilization — Sentinels of calamity — The holistic challenge

XIV. FOOD, WATER, SUPPLEMENTS AND THE 'ALTERNATIVE' REVOLUTION: The American medical paradigm begins a grudging shift 539

Dawn breaks in Virginia — Behind the paradigm shift — 'Quackbusters' attack — The squelching of nutrition — The medical esoterics — Clues from the veterinarians — Terror at the tap — Topsoil terror — Uncovering a coverup — A carbohydrate calamity — Problem one: the food business — Making the dietary connection — The oxidology revolution — The Club co-opts — The pill-popping medics — Cancer Inc. does an about-face — The dam bursts

XV. TOWARD THE MEDICINE OF THE 21ST CENTURY: A new paradigm in healing emerges 579

New medicine — or extinction — Genetics as a last gasp — Oxygen therapy returns —Co-opting live cell therapy — Rise of the 'X factor' — PNI says it all — Holism comes west — Of subtle energy, *prana* and *qi* — Homeopathy triumphant — Everything is energy — Biophysics, magnets and oxidology — Rediscovering Tesla, Reich, Rife, Priore, *et al.* — Toward the final link

X
HEART HUSTLE:
Schemes, scams and big bucks in the cardiovascular industry

"The moment one has offered an original explanation for a phenomenon which seems satisfactory, at that moment affection for his intellectual child springs into existence and, as the explanation grows into a definite theory, his parental affections cluster about his offspring and it grows more and more dear to him . . . there springs up unwittingly a pressing of the theory to make it fit the facts and a pressing of the facts to make them fit the theory."
— **George V. Mann PhD**

"The evidence shows that high fat consumption, when accompanied by plenty of the essential nutrients that all cells need, does not *cause atherosclerosis or heart disease."*
— **Dr. Roger J. Williams**

"The use of the term invasive *is right-on. Somebody is going to be invaded and it isn't going to be the doctor. People who have seen these [*balloon-wielding*] mavericks in action claim the slickest ones can stick a catheter into a groin and wind it around inside the body until it finds a wallet."*
— **Charles T. McGee MD**

". . . A program that may have begun in sincere but misguided zeal for the public good became intertwined with greed. The world was learning how much money could be made scaring people about cholesterol."
— **Thomas J. Moore**

Killer number one: 'heart disease'

By any measure, the combination of conditions lumped together as "heart disease" (heart and circulatory disorders, coronary artery disease, arteriosclerosis, peripheral vascular disease, heart attack, stroke, congestive heart failure, etc.) still constitutes the major killer in American medicine, as it does in most of the Western world:

About a million Americans die every year of some form of heart disease, about a half of them from heart attacks. In the early 1990s the American Heart Association (AHA) estimated cardiovascular deaths as 43 percent of *all* fatalities, with one American dying of a heart-related condition every 34 seconds.[1]

Worldwide, heart disorders cause almost a fourth of *all* deaths, or about 12 million per year.[1a]

Even so, in terms of the chronic disease plague sweeping the Western world, heart/ circulatory disease has seemingly been the single brightest light — for, at least in terms of fatalities, death rates from heart attack and stroke have been declining for years, a positive trend in disease-survival statistics which would constitute some kind of social triumph were it not eclipsed by the relentless rise in cancer deaths, the spreading AIDS pandemic, the rapidly advancing immunological disorders rampant in the "civilized" world and the fact that heart and circulatory diseases themselves continue to rise in incidence.

It is difficult to estimate the true numbers of individuals who have slowly developing fatty buildups of blood vessels (atherosclerosis) which may not be reflected as true hardening of the arteries (arteriosclerosis) for years or decades, just as it is difficult to assess how many Americans truly have "the silent killer," high blood pressure, whose hypertension also may not be detected for decades, if ever. If both diabetes and its far more prevalent predecessor condition, hypoglycemia, are added to the picture — with diabetes considered contributory to heart disease — then it is a good estimate that at least a low majority of Americans have a pre-heart disease condition which, if left unchecked should they not expire due to something else, will become "heart disease."

Data from the AHA, Health Care Financing Administration, American Health Information Management Association and the World Health Organization confirmed in 1992 that by 1988 the US cardiovascular disease death rate had continued to show impressive declines — myocardial infarctions (heart attacks) had dropped from 226.4 per 100,000 population in 1950 to 120.1 per 100,000 that year. As of 1992, it was projected that about 70 million Americans had some form of cardiovascular disease and that the combination of disorders was costing about $109 billion both in health services and lost productivity.[2]

A year later, with fewer actual cases, the nation's heart disease bill was set at about $117 billion (1993 estimate). This included $75 billion for hospital and nursing home services, $18 billion for physician and nurse services (as apart from institutional costs), $7 billion in drugs, and an estimated $17 billion in lost productivity.[3] Congestive heart failure, afflicting 3 million Americans, was estimated to cost $60 billion a year to treat.[3a] By 1994, the cost of approximately 400,000 coronary bypasses, 300,000 balloon angioplasties, 58,000 repairs to damaged heart valves, and 2,000 transplants of healthy hearts into patients whose own hearts were considered irreparable was an estimated $50 billion per year, or almost 6 percent of the "healthcare delivery" tab.[3b]

What all these figures add up to are boosts in overall healthcare cost inflation, mammoth profits for the Allopathic Industrial Complex (AIC), a considerable drag on the economy — and, yes, unquestionably, at least some lives saved.

Mysteries in the victories

Clearly, the medical and governmental orthodoxy has not known what to make of declining deaths from "heart disease" because so many mysteries lurk in the statistics:

An AHA science writers' seminar was told in 1993 that "about half of all deaths from heart disease are sudden and unexpected, regardless of the underlying disease. Thus, 50 percent of all deaths due to atherosclerosis (fatty buildup of the coronary arteries) are sudden, as are 50 percent of deaths due to degeneration of the heart muscle, or to cardiac enlargement in patients with high blood pressure."[4]

This was a roundabout way of saying that despite a multi-billion-dollar annual campaign based on the cholesterol hypothesis of heart disease causation and the multi-billion-dollar industry in heart disease diagnostic devices and techniques, which frequently turned in erroneous or misleading figures, including nationwide efforts to count cholesterol in as many citizens of all ages as could be induced into a mobile lab for such purposes, the actual precipitating reasons for heart fatalities were *unknown* in perhaps as many as 50 percent of cases.

By some other reliable estimates the commonly accepted risk factors for coronary artery disease — excess saturated fats and cholesterol, cigarette smoking, diabetes, high blood pressure, inadequate exercise, obesity, emotional stress, alleged genetic predispositions — are not present in 40 percent of people who die of heart attacks.[5]

In the meantime, the development and application of synthetic compounds (drugs) to be used against heart disease and stroke have continued to constitute a growth industry of extremely profitable dimensions, and the heart-diagnosis, heart-treatment devices and techniques element of "healthcare delivery" are alive and well even if it cannot be demonstrated that, overall, they do very much good.

In the 1990s, while the combination public-private effort to curb the nation's number-one killer seemed to be paying off, it became obvious to observers, statisticians and social critics that the figures were declining primarily because of what people were doing themselves.

They were indeed smoking less (cigarette smoking being broadly accepted as a major risk factor for heart disease), they were exercising more (although, oddly enough, research on physical exertion as a block to heart disease was surprisingly thin in conclusive results), they had drastically altered their eating habits — and they were consuming vitamin pills and other dietary supplements in ever-growing numbers.

What was not clear in the 1990s was just how, let alone if, the change in dietary habits (fewer animal fats and animal proteins, more fruits and vegetables, fewer refined carbohydrates "junk foods") alone accounted for the decline and if so which foods or combinations were doing the trick. Even so, the change in dietary habits promoted by any number of food faddists, nutritionists and a hodgepodge of reasonably scientific studies did indeed correlate with overall declines in heart-disease fatalities.

The heart disease death-rate decline has provided the Allopathic Industrial Complex (AIC) with a propaganda victory that seems justified as long as one does not look too closely.

First, as has been suggested, death from heart attack seems to occur whether or not diagnosis of the disease has been made, or made correctly — an incredible result indeed following years of multi-billion-dollar investments in high-technology diagnostics.

The trouble(s) with angiograms

The gold standard heart-disease diagnostic for years has been the coronary angiogram — or arteriogram — insertion of a catheter up the aorta just above the heart, injection of a dye-like tracing material into the heart arteries, and observation of this material by X-ray.

While many medical critics and even some cardiologists have long wondered about just how accurate, useful or necessary a procedure the angiogram (first introduced in 1963) is, by 1992 the facts were beginning to come in:

A *Journal of the American Medical Assn. (JAMA)* reported[6] that nearly half of all coronary angiograms were either unnecessary or could have been postponed. But why do so? The 1992 estimates were that one million angiograms were being performed that year at a cost of about $5,000 each — that is, a roughly $5 billion industry in angiograms all by themselves.

Even though cardiologists had embraced the coronary angiogram (angiograph) — allowing them, for the first time, to see minute obstructions in the main arteries of the heart as a kind of road map — serious doubts had been raised within a decade of the launching of the test:

Major studies in 1974,[7] 1976,[8] 1979[9] and 1984[10] found huge swings in interpretations of the test. One analysis (1984) was quite specific:

*The physiologic effects of the majority of coronary obstructions cannot be determined accurately by conventional angiographic approaches. The results of these studies should be profoundly disturbing to all physicians who have relied on the coronary arteriogram to provide accurate information regarding the physiologic consequences of individual coronary stenosis (*obstruction.*)*[11]

Yet, the fact that most of these tests were published in the "learned" journals failed to make much of a dent in their widespread use — and the medical media (that is, reporters and commentators wined and dined by medical orthodoxy) simply failed to pick up what amounted to a major story: a primary heart-disease diagnostic tool is inaccurate at best, a scam at worst.

And of course there is the corollary problem that the diagnostic technique may be dangerous in and of itself — since, as of 1993, it was known that for every thousand angiograms performed, about one person dies from a complication related to the angiogram. Even a possibly fatal heart rhythm may be sparked simply by the presence of the dye-like tracing substance in the artery.[12]

The coronary angiogram is not the only expensive diagnostic toy which has come under a cloud of suspicion.

In 1991, a San Francisco Veterans Administration (VA) hospital study found[13] that a heart-scan technique utilizing drugs and radioactive isotopes (estimated to be performed on 500,000 patients a year at an annual cost of $500 million and costing between $700 and $1500 per test) was probably "useful" only a third of the time, "questionable" another third, and "not warranted" another third. Yet it had become a "standard presurgical test" since the Food and Drug Administration (FDA), the corrupted arbiter of "safety" and "efficacy" in medical diagnostics and therapeutics, had approved it earlier that year.

The controversy over diagnostics (whether they are useful, accurate or necessary, let alone their contribution to the total costs of healthcare in the United States) immediately dovetails with the controversy over therapeutics.

Of cabbages and things

The major heart disease therapies have consisted of the resurrected coronary bypass procedure, the insertion of inflatable balloons in blood vessels (balloon angioplasties — also called by the prodigiously cumbersome term PTCA, or percutaneous transluminal coronary angioplasty), and a shelf full of expensive drugs variously aimed at lowering cholesterol (this based on the notion — ever more in doubt — that cholesterol is the major contributor to heart disease), combatting irregular heartbeat (arrhythmia), dissolving clots, opening blocked vessels (vasodilators) and/or "channel blockers," each of which has constituted a spinoff mini-cardiovascular industry — and/or, for maintenance, inserting battery-driven heart stimulators (Pacemakers), another mini-industry.

Hyped to the public with virtually the same intensity and lack of balancing commentary as the coronary arteriogram and the need to assess cholesterol levels, the coronary bypass had, by the 1980s, become a multi-billion-dollar moneymaker all by itself, the Cadillac surgical procedure of cardiovascular medicine, the technique to which most advanced "coronary" patients were turned over in the belief that they were soon to be in the best medical hands possible. And in some advanced cases the procedure truly saved lives.

The regular coronary artery bypass graft surgery (perhaps puckishly referred to from its acronym CABG as "cabbage") consists of removing veins from elsewhere in the body (usually the legs), connecting one end of the vein to a fresh blood supply from the aorta and connecting the other end to a blocked or obstructed artery at a point somewhere beyond the blockage — hence the term "bypass."

It is essential to realize that heart disease fatality rates were already falling consistently before the advent of the "cabbage" or, quickly thereafter, the balloon angioplasty, so that cardiovascular surgeons taking much credit for helping reduce heart disease deaths because of these expensive procedures are on a par with the promoters of certain vaccinations who take credit for the reduction in the incidence of an infection through the immunization process *after* the infection or disease is beginning to die out on its own.

Medicine loves high technology — and cardiovascular medicine positively fell in love with the coronary artery bypass graft approach (cabbage). Some 75,000 of the surgeries were done in 1975. This number increased to 230,000 in 1987, 392,000 in 1990, 407,000 in 1991, and slipped to 331,000 in 1993.[14,15,15a,15b] Since the technique, including a "heart-lung" machine to stop and re-start the heart, may cost anywhere from $25,000 to $50,000 and several may be done in one patient, the dimensions of the "cabbage" business are considerable. The total hospital bill for CABG operations in 1993 was set at $13.5 billion.[15c]

Medical critic Charles McGee MD noted in 1993 that "the operating surgeon may charge between $3,000 and $6,000 for a cabbage. Multiply that by over 200 cabbages per year and it begins to add up to a respectable income. It is common for successful cabbage surgeons to bank over $1.5 million a year."[16]

Clearly, such techniques are for more affluent societies, whether they are paid for privately, through group private insurance plans or by the public. McGee observed that the incidence of coronary bypasses is 75 percent less in Europe, where medicine in general is far less expensive, and also far less in America's government-run Veterans Administration (VA) hospitals, where doctors are paid a salary.

But what did "qualified experts," by the 1990s, really think of the CABG?

In July 1992, the American Heart Assn. publication *Circulation* released results of an 18-year survey of about 700 veterans and found that whatever benefits there might be for the "cabbage" fade within five years and disappear within 11. The authors were primarily interested in the procedure's effects on stable *angina pectoris*, a severe heart disease-connected chest pain which some other studies had long suggested might be minimized by the complex surgery.[17]

In 1991, the *Journal of the American Medical Assn. (JAMA)*, observing fatality statistics from bypasses, reported[18] that heart disease patients may be up to four times more likely to die from a "cabbage" by one surgeon than by another, and that fatality levels varied from hospital to hospital. Hospital death rates for the bypass varied from 3.1 percent to 6.3 percent; the rate among surgeons caromed between 1.9 percent and 9.2 percent.

But such fairly tepid studies were actually old-hat:

A Veterans Administration study in 1977 had found[19] that the 11-year survivals of coronary byass patients as contrasted with those who had been managed "medically" (essentially, by drugs) showed a statistically insignificant difference of 58 percent for the former against 57 percent for the latter. This was the first comparison study on the subject, and while it allegedly shocked cardiologists it did not dim establishment enthusiasm for the procedure.

In the Coronary Artery Surgery Study (CASS), released in 1990, a 10-year followup showed that the survival rate was 82 percent among those who had had the operation vs. 79 percent for those "medically" managed.[20]

As early as 1978, Dr. Henry McIntosh of Baylor College of Medicine's Methodist Hospital provided one of the first followup critiques of the CABG. According to his 10-year review:

> . . . *Available data in the literature do not*

indicate that myocardial infarctions, arrhythmias, or congestive heart failure will be prevented, or that life will be prolonged in the vast majority of patients.[21]

McGee noted that following publication of this first major negative criticism of the coronary bypass "McIntosh was forced to leave his position at Baylor."[22]

'Ballooning' profits, dilating for dollars

When cardiological experts are not deviating blood flow around a blocked artery they often turn to, or suggest, the alternative to the coronary bypass — the balloon angioplasty, introduced in the 1970s. This was a mechanical application of the theory of stretching or widening (dilating) arteries — in this case through insertion of a small balloon.

In 1990, cardiologists performed about 285,000 balloon angioplasties as contrasted with between 380,000 and 392,000 coronary bypasses, and some of these procedures were done on the same patients. About 303,000 were done in 1991.[23,24] About $6.5 billion was spent on angioplasties in 1993.[24a]

But the "heart balloon," while less expensive ($16,000 and up) than the bypass, comes with risks. It was reported in 1988[25] that about 1 percent of angioplasty patients died, 4.3 percent suffered heart attacks, 3.4 percent required emergency surgery, and that in about a third of cases the blocked arteries reopened through the procedure would close again in several months and need to be reopened again. Earlier, Harvard Medical School had warned that "a coronary artery may be torn during the procedure, or a clot can form in the dilated area."[26]

(The 1994 annual meeting of the American Heart Assn. was told that between bypasses and angioplasties about 16,000 patients were dying annually.[26a])

The problem of keeping artificially widened clogged coronary arteries open led to a flurry of interest in Europe and the United States for the "intravenous stent." This was a tiny tube formed of woven stainless-steel mesh designed to be inserted into a previously clogged artery after it had been reopened by surgery or after a balloon angioplasty had been performed.

The approach was first tested in Europe in 1988, but by 1991 it had become clear that "stent" patients were not faring any better than patients who had not received it. This led one American heart specialist to comment on this and similar artery-opening devices that

> *... (the process) has resembled the mating of elephants — carried out on a high level ... with much noise and trumpeting, with the results not evident for two years and the product not perfect.*[27]

Even the perhaps more promising laser recanalization (LR) technique (a catheter with a laser beam which burns out a hole in arterial deposits), which may often accompany a balloon angioplasty, is, according to one study,[28] only indicated in 10 to 15 percent of patients with blocked arteries, primarily due to age considerations.

We have already seen (*III*) that inserting battery-driven Pacemakers, at about $9,000 per implant, may be unnecessary or questionable in upwards of 50 percent of cases (in some surveys), but electronic technology as applied to faltering hearts keeps on ticking:

In 1993 the FDA approved a cigarette case-sized "defibrillator," an abdomen implant which sends "mild electrical impulses" to the heart both to prevent cardiac arrest and correct abnormally fast heart rhythms. The retail cost: $18,200.[29]

The allopathic fraternity, aware of cost differentials, continually debates whether the cabbage or the PTCA (balloon angioplasty) is "better," and all the data are not in.

But some are. A review of the first 2½ years of a 10-year comparative trial in the United Kingdom of one thousand randomized angina patients to determine long-term effects of one procedure against the other measured non-fatal heart attacks as the "primary endpoint." In data reported in 1994, or at 2½ years, the heart attack rates were 8.6 percent for the cabbage and

9.8 percent for balloons — or, as Robert Henderson MD, cardiologist of Manchester's Wynthenshaw Hospital, put it: ". . . The data suggest that the risk of death or MI [myocardial infarction] is the same whichever treatment strategy you use."[29a]

And in another 1994 study — this on 200,000 Medicare patients who had suffered a heart attack in 1987 — it was found that some 25 percent of bypasses, angioplasties and catheterizations on older patients could be eliminated at a substantial cost savings with a negligible impact on mortality — simply because they do not do much good. Said Harvard's Dr. Mark McClellan, lead author of the report: "Virtually all medical technologies are useful in some patients. The question is, where do you draw the line?"[29b]

The same year, more studies, which contrasted cabbages with balloon angioplasties, added fuel to the fire, sometimes cloaking the controversy in considerable medical gobbledegook:

An Emory University-University of Washington survey of 132 individuals randomly assigned to various treatment groups found[29c] that neither the coronary bypass nor balloon angioplasty differed "significantly with respect to the occurrence of the composite primary endpoint" and that "consequently, the selection of one procedure over the other should be guided by patients' preferences regarding the quality of life and the possible need for subsequent procedures."

The "primary endpoint" was "a composite of death, Q-wave myocardial infarction, and a large ischemic defect identified on thallium scanning at three years." The translation of all this seemed to be that since the pathological and/or mortal outcomes were essentially the same with either approach the best advice to patients should be, "take your pick."

To be sure, at the same time a German study[29d] confirmed improvements in chest pain (angina) with both approaches, yet summarized negatively that "in order to achieve similar clinical outcomes, the patients treated with PTCA (angioplasties) were more likely to require further intervention and antianginal drugs, whereas the patients treated with CABG (coronary bypass) were more likely to sustain an acute myocardial infarction at the time of the procedure." A tepid endorsement of both procedures?

When in doubt, prescribe a drug

When cardiological orthodoxy is not "bypassing" arteries with veins removed from one part of the body and "harvested" elsewhere, or inflating clogged arteries with balloons or inserting various electrical devices into the body to stimulate or normalize flagging hearts, it is relying on ever-more-expensive synthetic compounds (drugs).

These are prescribed to combat high blood pressure (hypertension), considered a strong contributor to heart disease and estimated to afflict somewhere between 60 to 70 million Americans who spend more than $11 billion annually on this condition alone; or to lower cholesterol, a naturally occurring fatty substance which cardiology believes is the biggest single culprit in overall heart disease; or to combat irregular heartbeat (arrhythmia); or to break up clots in the circulatory system, since the latter can lead directly to fatalities; or as "calcium channel blockers"; or to help control other aspects of the multiplicity of conditions and pathologies which directly or indirectly are involved in "heart disease."

Each class of drugs constitutes a spinoff or mini-industry on its own, and, of course, each has fallen under critical review and suspicion.

In her masterful roundup of medical ignorance, Jane Heimlich noted[30] both that "doctors don't know what causes 90 percent of high blood pressure" (itself an astounding reality, given the multi-billion-dollar, long-term research investment of medical and governmental orthodoxy in trying to find out) and that non-drug approaches to hypertension have been overlooked or ignored. However, so panicked are hypertensives over their mystery condition, and so generally successful are certain high blood pressure drugs at keeping the "numbers" down that increasing numbers of Americans are now lifelong consumers of drugs without which, they truly believe — or have been made to believe by their doctors — they cannot survive. And, though this may be true in some cases, various lines of research have confirmed the ability to treat high blood pressure without drugs and/or for patients to be able to go off the drugs.[31,32,33]

As early as 1979, the National Heart, Lung and Blood Institute's Hypertension Detection and Followup Program found[34] that death rates among hypertensives could be reduced by almost 20 percent *without* drug treatment.

Then, the cleverly acronymed MRFIT (for Multiple Risk Factor Intervention Trial) found[35] in a one-year study on coronary heart disease prevention that patients who had been treated intensively with thiazide diuretics (the classic standby of high blood pressure treatment and aimed at ridding the body of excess fluids and salts) had *higher* death rates than those who either took other drugs or no drugs at all. This led to speculation that such drugs might themselves be toxic — but their use continued.

Other studies have shown that lowering blood pressure with diuretics may indeed reduce the risk of stroke — the most feared endpoint of hypertension — but does not prevent heart attacks. Also, noted Heimlich,[36] such drugs can cause biochemical changes which increase susceptibility to heart attacks. Part of the problem, she added, is that diuretics have long been known to stimulate increases of blood sugar and uric acid which can exacerbate diabetes and gout.

That is, the classic drugs used to treat high blood pressure, a presumed key role player in overall "heart disease," may actually enhance the chances *for* "heart disease" and may be toxic in and of themselves.

In the late 1980s, the dangers in drugs developed to treat irregular heartbeat (arrhythmias) came to light, particularly with the flaps over Riker Laboratories' Tambocor and Bristol Laboratories' Enkaid, FDA-approved modalities both (*IX*), since a National Heart, Lung, and Blood Institute clinical trial had shown that they *increased* the risk of heart attack and death among the 200,000 or so Americans estimated to have the problem.[37]

"Calcium channel blockers," another class of drugs, have hardly fared any better.

Once the latest popular breakthroughs, it now seems clear that such products may help the patient feel better after a heart attack or a round of severe angina pain, but they will not save the patient's life.

A trio of US investigators concluded the above in 1989 after reviewing 28 controlled studies involving 19,000 patients. Their data, in the *British Medical Journal,* found both that channel blockers not only failed to protect cardiac patients against a heart attack or death but that "the data suggest a somewhat higher probability of harm than benefit."[38]

Here, then, was an umpteenth demonstration of the classical medical dilemma in which the cure may be worse than the disease.

In spring 1994, trials sponsored (even) by drug companies of the common anticoagulant drug heparin were halted because of what *The New York Times* called "an unexpectedly high risk of paralyzing and fatal strokes."[38a]

The surprise finding in three studies concerning a common heart-attack drug was that high doses of it are unacceptably dangerous. A similar risk of strokes was found among individuals receiving hirudin.[38b]

We mention elsewhere (*VIII*) the turf wars in the development and marketing of clot-dissolving drugs, during which, by 1993, the vastly more expensive T-PA (tissue plasminogen activator), at roughly $2,200 per treatment, had slightly edged out the much cheaper ($200 to $300 per treatment) streptokinase for first place.

The 2½-year, $65 million study (largely financed by biotech giant Genentech, T-PA's producer) of 40,000 patients in 15 countries seemed at best a pyrrhic victory for T-PA, with health economists noting that when all was said and done treatment with T-PA rather than streptokinase would cost about $200,000 for each life saved. Since only about 20 percent of heart patients are treated with either drug (both of which must be injected within the first few hours of a heart attack to be effective), the question nagged: is it worth it?[39]

The answer may have been a qualified "yes," if results of a multi-university-monitored National Registry of Myocardial Infarction study announced in late 1994 means much — they showed a decline in hospital heart-related deaths coinciding with increased use of blood clot-dissolving drugs. The registry, though, was said to have been funded by Genentech.[39a]

In 1991, American heart specialists were up in arms over a Finnish study criticized for its low numbers (though 1,222 patients followed over 15 years hardly qualifies as unduly low) that men who used drugs to lower cholesterol or high blood pressure died more often from *heart disease*, violence, accidents and suicide than did men who did nothing to cut the risk.[40]

This was followed in 1994 by soul-searching questions among physicians as to the wisdom of prescribing "hypolipidemic" drugs, especially for the elderly, when there seems to be an increased risk of both cancer and possible cancer-promotion by such drugs in "seniors."

Noted physicians Stephen B. Hulley and Thomas B. Newman: "Treatment of cholesterol may produce harmful effects specific to older age. Adverse drug reactions become more common as drugs are used in combination and have less predictable excretion patterns."

They feared that "the most important harm is the possibility that cholesterol-lowering intervention could actually increase, rather than decrease, the overall death rate." Adding to the basic mysteries:

> *In elderly people, this inverse association extends over a wider range of cholesterol levels, and in women* total mortality rates appear to be lower in those with high blood cholesterol than those with moderate levels *[author's emphasis.] We do not understand the causal basis for this finding, and until we do, it is not safe to assume that lowering*

blood cholesterol in the elderly will have a net beneficial effect. A larger concern is the separate body of evidence revealing increased mortality from cancers and injuries in primary prevention trials of middle-aged men [author's emphasis].[40a]

(In what the ever-creative drug industry might consider to be a "save" following such bad news, the 1994 meeting of the American Heart Assn. (AHA) was informed of a large Scandinavian study of the cholesterol-lowering drug simvastatin (Zocor), described as a "powerful" compound: in a five-year followup it was said to have "sharply" reduced the risk of death in people who had earlier been treated for heart attacks and angina pain. The data showed that the "need" for either a CABG or an angioplasty was thus lower in the treated group. However interesting the results (and there was no evidence the drug actually helps people live longer, nor are its long-term effects known about), the study on 4,444 men and women at 94 hospitals was financed by . . . Merck & Co., a heavy hitter in cholesterol drug development.[40b])

As the *Wall Street Journal* noted, the results also set the stage for a major market battle between Merck and Bristol-Myers Squibb, which claimed similar results with a competing drug, Pravachol.[40c]

The above are elements of a gathering accumulation of data and observations from wary researchers beginning to question the central premises of American orthodoxy in "heart disease" — that the excess of cholesterol is the major contributor to the problem, and that drugs to lower cholesterol therefore represent the best approach to solving it.

The great cholesterol conundrums

In fact, the cholesterol mania is probably the biggest false premise in cardiology, and has so colored this subdivision of the medical arts that it is roughly akin to the central, probably false, premise in oncology (*XI*) which holds that there are 300 or more separately caused kinds of cancerous tumors each requiring its own special treatment.

The passion over cholesterol in the 1970s-1990s led to confusion on a mass scale, as housewives were told first one thing and then another about the dangers of cholesterol-laden foods, what adequate cholesterol levels were or are, and, right along with the cholesterol concern, which kinds of fats (saturated, unsaturated, polyunsaturated) should be used or not used in the diet, and which cooking oils had how much of which.

In the meantime, as the cardiology industry and government joined forces to alert the public to the presumed dangers of excess cholesterol, let alone of fatty diets — forgetting that the American diet has *always* been fatty and that American "heart disease" was essentially an unknown entity before 1878 — food producers and processors also were driven into an intense round of labeling and re-labeling products to make sure that the correct amounts of cholesterol and other fats were noted. The situation reached *reductio ad absurdum* in the 1980s/1990s as distibutors of foods which by their very nature could *never contain* any cholesterol began affixing on their products labels stating "does not contain cholesterol," an activity roughly akin to a paper clip manufacturer affirming that his product "absolutely contains no sugar."

The assumption that cholesterol is the central villain in heart disease (more culpable, indeed, than genetic predispositions, cigarette smoking, high blood pressure and diabetes, all known contributors thereto) was naturally, inexorably matched by the scramble to develop synthetic compounds (drugs) aimed at *lowering* cholesterol. Indeed, to excuse this whole series of unfortunate linear thoughts, the AIC orthodoxy needed to come up with a whole new disease — *hypercholesterolemia* (too much cholesterol) — as a rationale. (This may be different from the genetically influenced "familial hypercholesterolemia," which allegedly "runs in families.") Finding that civilized (rather than primitive) societies were afflicted with this disease was the semantical equivalent, at an earlier time when the benzodiazepines were drugs of choice as tranquilizers and sedatives, of believing that people had somehow been born with a Valium deficiency.

There is probably no area of medicine as fraught with contradiction, controversy, 180-degree-angle turns in concepts and outright confusion as the cholesterol theory of heart disease which, did it not have such potentially lethal and life-altering dimensions, would better be dismissed as a highly expensive comic opera.

In setting the stage for the cholesterol wars, two background realities should be made clear:

1. There are obvious connections between heart disease and the dietary practices of the "civilized" West. Since high-fat foods, *among other dietary things*, are factors in such connections, and since a measurable primary blood fat is in fact cholesterol, it does not require too great a leap of faith to assume, even inappropriately, as it may turn out, that there is some link between cholesterol and heart disease. Unfortunately, what seems to have happened is that the leap of faith was a jump to the wrong conclusion — or at least mostly so.

2. Cholesterol is an absolutely essential body compound, comprising a high concentration of normal brain tissue and serving as a basic building material for the manufacture of cortisone, sex hormones, Vitamin D and other essential body substances. *Too little* cholesterol could result in what medicine oftens calls a "negative outcome" — death.

The cholesterol theory — as part of the broader lipid (blood fat) theory — developed through research over time which seemed to show that certain groups of people who consumed large amounts of "saturated" (hard) fats also had higher rates of cholesterol and higher rates of "heart disease." It was known that cholesterol is a major contributor — but not the only one — to the buildup of materials which clog the circulatory system and which thus might lead to heart attack, stroke and other calamities. The corollary reality was that animal fats are high in cholesterol (which is of animal origin anyway), and that high-animal fat diets lead to higher cholesterol levels which lead to heart problems.

The trouble with this seemingly logical sequence of events is, as usual, in the multiple exceptions thereto. As Charles T. McGee MD and other researchers have pointed out, there are numerous *primitive* societies whose food patterns were or are high in saturated fats but among whose members heart disease is rare or unknown. There are examples of countries where fat consumption went down — but "heart disease" went up.[41,42]

As we shall see (*XIV*) no small part of these odd disparities may very well have to do not with how much but rather what *kind* of fat in general, and cholesterol in particular, is being consumed. "Primitives" are apt to be consuming "natural" rather than industrially altered "oxidized" cholesterol — a very likely crucial distinction.

More strikingly, information in the late 1980s and 1990s developed which increasingly showed that heart disease might exist in people without noticeable elevations in cholesterol, that some very high-risk (from a cholesterol point of view) individuals were without heart disease — and, more astonishingly, that despite widespread efforts to lower cholesterol through dietary manipulation, levels often mostly remained about the same in the broadest sectors of the population.[43]

In other words, the combined research on dietary fats as related to cholesterol as related to atherosclerosis/arteriosclerosis (the buildup of fatty composite tissue in blood vessels leading eventually to hardening of the arteries) as related to "heart disease" is only somewhat better than thin and, at the very least, confusing.

But it has led to wholesale attacks on parts of the food-processing industry (by any measure a major contributor, albeit unknowingly, to the plague of Western chronic disease), particularly meat and dairy products producers. It has stimulated flipflops in domestic decision-making as to whether butter (saturated fat) is worse or ultimately better than margarine ("plastic" fat to some extent) and which kind of cooking oil to use, or how many eggs — if any — should be eaten.

A torpedo attack in the **Atlantic**

Although voices of dissent cropped up occasionally as the United States fell prey to a veritable frenzy of cholesterol-counting and label-changing, a roundhouse attack on the new national enterprise of reducing the fatty substance was not effectively mounted until 1989, when science writer Thomas J. Moore published *Heart Failure*,[44] with a preliminary chapter hitting the pages of the *Atlantic Monthly*[45] with the force of a well-guided torpedo.

In essence, reported Moore, the decades-long, multi-billion-dollar national campaign against high cholesterol was in fact an over-funded, hype-ridden exercise which had swollen the profits of drug manufacturers and even certain food processors while failing to show any real improvements in the longevity of "heart disease"-conscious Americans. Moore was instantly backed by a small group of heart specialists, and roundly assailed by the cardiologically orthodox.

Moore assessed years of studies and statistics on the cholesterol approach:

— *Lower* cholesterol levels may be related to *higher risks* for both cancer and stroke. (Not much later, it would also be found that lower cholesterol levels often also accompanied the development of AIDS conditions).

— The surest way to lower cholesterol, assuming such is a worthwhile activity, is to take alcoholic drinks — an observation backed, throughout the 1990s, by several lines of unrelated research.

— Neither long-term safety nor the ability to prevent heart attacks had been demonstrated for either of the major FDA-approved cholesterol-lowering drugs at the time (cholestyramine and lovastatin), and "if experience with animals is included, the potential long-and short-time hazards of lovastatin include heart attacks, cancer, stroke, liver damage, cataracts and severe muscle pain and damage."

— The promotion of lovastatin had turned into an industry itself, with Merck reporting in 1988 that 350,000 people were already taking the drug on a constant basis and an estimate of the profits from cholestryamine for some five million people estimated at about $10 billion per year.

— The National Cholesterol Education Program (NCEP), at the time underway full-bore in hospitals, schools, television stations, health fairs and in mobile cholesterol-checking vans, was at the time estimated to be costing between $10 to $20 billion a year.

Moore traced the evolution of the national preoccupation with cholesterol levels from 1951, described the extensive studies and federal involvement of the National Heart, Lung and Blood Institute and such private organizations as the American Heart Assn. in programs which attempted to show that dietary change could lower levels of the essential fatty acid substance and that somehow this would be a good thing to do.[46]

But long-term studies such as the ongoing Framingham Heart Study, the Heart-Diet Pilot Program, MRFIT, the Coronary Primary Prevention Trial (CPPT) and the Coronary Drug Project had mostly failed to connect dietary change with alterations in cholesterol levels or cholesterol-lowering drugs with the prevention of heart disease and the extension of life.

The data did not demolish the statistical connection between the so-called "bad" form of cholesterol — LDL (low-density lipoprotein) — and elevated heart disease risks for younger and middle-aged people: they simply failed to show, he analyzed, much relevance one way or the other for older Americans in whom "heart disease" risks were presumably higher.

Moore reported that 1988 had been the pivotal year when "the heart institute acquired powerful new allies." He wrote:

The American Medical Association, a major drug manufacturer and two huge drug companies joined forces to "declare war on cholesterol." The public-relations and advertising campaign began to reach the public early this year [1989] and included national and local television programs, special magazine features, cereal-box advertisements, books, videocassettes, brochures, discount coupons, and posters.

Although the effort appeared to be a public-service campaign, it was in reality a business scheme to sell products and physicians' services . . .

The drug company Merck Sharpe & Dohme was already aggressively marketing its new cholesterol-lowering drug, lovastatin, under the name Mevacor. Kellogg was preparing to launch a new oat-bran cereal (Common Sense), and American Home Products to promote a cooking-oil spray (Pam) that, like almost every other vegetable oil, contains no cholesterol.

The National Cholesterol Education Program guidelines suggested that treatment should not begin without a complete physical, a patient history, and a laboratory workup. This was not lost on the AMA, which noted pointedly that screening programs had found that "as many as 25% of the participants either have no personal physician, or have not seen their doctor within the past five years."

Thus a progam that may have begun in sincere but misguided zeal for the public good became intertwined with greed. The world was learning how much money could be made scaring people about cholesterol. And the mainstream organizations were being joined by thousands of less responsible profiteers offering miracle treatments, wonder diets, instant cholesterol checkups, and a variety of other services and goods whose effects were non-existent, unproved or hazardous.[48]

Moore hardly had the last word. The cholesterol-fighting industry and national campaign, costing well over $20 billion dollars a year by the 1990s, relentlessly produced new evidence to attempt to link cholesterol with "heart disease," and some of which research certainly did suggest such connections — that is, it showed strong correlations between heart problems and dietary factors, among which high fat consumption seemed to be a major element.

We will suggest that such studies may have been focused, at least in part, on the wrong thing or things, primarily because of "paradigm capture" (attitudinal bias to support a pre-held conclusion — in this case, prove cholesterol to be the villain at all costs).

Cholesterol is a many-splintered thing

In American medical semantical manipulation — an intricate problem in an essentially free, rather than an authoritarian, society — shifts in premises and attitudes are only hinted at, and come slowly, as if the social-collective mental terrain should first be irrigated with new words and thoughts. Hence the semantical (as well as scientific) cholesterol capers:

The puzzled American public was first informed that cholesterol *itself* was the suspect villain, and standard blood chemistry tests would indeed spit out gross numbers indicating levels of the substance. A "high" — assessment of which tended to vary over the years — was contrasted with a "low" in terms of total cholesterol.

Just when this quantification exercise was more or less understood by doctors and patients alike, it started surfacing that actually it wasn't total cholesterol overall that made the difference — it was the contrasting amounts of the "bad" cholesterol, or LDL (low-density lipoprotein), and the "good" cholesterol (HDL — high-density lipoprotein). Then we learned there was VLDL (*very* low-density lipoprotein). And it was found there were at least two LDLs — "native" LDL and "oxidized" LDL. And there is even an *IDL* — intermediate-density lipoprotein.

This gradually-induced attitude shift stirred confusion over counts, numbers, products and labels. Was a food dangerous because of "total" cholesterol? Was a blood test which did not discriminate between the two major cholesterols worth anything? Should one give up beefsteaks and Big Macs because of the first set of numbers or the second? Puzzlement galore.

In 1993, two new dimensions expanded the cholesterol conundrum:

• A UCLA study indicated that actually HDL is not totally a "good" cholesterol after all, but that there is — among its five subdivisions — a "bad" version of it, and that tests might have to be refined in order to distinguish between various forms of HDL, quite aside from the established need to distinguish between LDL and HDL.[48]

• Stanford and Cambridge University studies, as well as the observations of some independent researchers, found how a recently described mysterious form of cholesterol called Lp(a) — lipoprotein (a) — might clog arteries. This research suggested that Lp(a) could permit cells that make up arterial walls to proliferate unchecked — hence accounting, at least in part, for "occluded" arteries.[49a]

(Both Vitamin C champions Linus Pauling PhD and Matthias Rath MD, a Hamburg University heart specialist, were primary groundbreakers in advancing the Lp(a) cholesterol theory, and both asserted that the best nutritional route to arterial/circulatory health is Vitamin C.

(Rath, particularly, has outlined how Vitamins C and E and the amino acids lysine and proline constitute the more natural ways to prevent and reverse atherosclerosis.[49b] Such research not only continues to strengthen the case for ascorbic acid [Vitamin C] in overall health but to vindicate the decades-old notions of the pioneering Shute brothers in advancing Vitamin E for heart health in general.

(Too, as Rath has pointed out,[49c] the Vitamin C deficiency connection to heart disease is *not* new:

(— In 1941, Canadian cardiologist J.C. Patterson reported that more than 80 percent of his heart disease patients had an ascorbate deficiency as a significant risk factor.

(— In 1948, American physicians R.W. Trimmer and C.J.

Lundy reported that 70 percent of their coronary artery disease patients had very low Vitamin C serum levels.

(It should be emphasized that the Shute brothers were viciously assailed by US-led Western medicine for their views of Vitamin E at an earlier time, just as Pauling, Stone and the Vitamin C champions were later when insisting that ascorbates played a role in health in general, cancer, the common cold, and arterial disease prevention in particular.)

Further confusing the issue, several studies suggested that the widespread bacterium *Chlamydia pneumoniae* might be playing a very big role in everything from atherosclerosis (since Finnish studies suggested it might be a "causative agent" in 60 to 70 percent of cases) to clogged arteries in general to heart attacks.[50]

To say nothning of increasing evidence linking elevated levels of the amino acid homocysteine to hardening of the arteries, with a claim made that some 21 percent of Americans have such higher levels and that they correlate to threefold higher heart disease risks.[50a]

And, further, some research has suggested that — as certain areterial blockages "resemble" cancerous tumors — they might arise from the uncontrolled growth of smooth-muscle cells in arteries injured by plaques (or even by angioplasties). Enough blockages turned up the presence of mutated p53 genes (as in cancer) and even of cytomegalovirus (CMV), a virus among whose many negative aspects seems to be involvement in heart disease, to somehow implicate the latter two elements in arterial problems.[50b]

Total cholesterol? LDL but not HDL? A version of HDL? IDL? Lipoprotein (a)? Any or all of the above plus chlamydia? Homocysteine? Gene p53? CMV? Was "medical science" truly closer in the 1990s to unraveling the cause or causes of occluded arteries, coronary artery disease and heart attack? (Let alone of hypertension?)

As early as 1981, foreign blood fat (lipid) experts were questioning both whether cholesterol or dietary fat in general caused atherosclerosis or if elevated cholesterol levels were related to higher death rates.[51]

Typical of their opinions was that of Peter Skrabanek, professor of community health, Trinity College, Dublin, who argued that

> *Lowering cholesterol does not lower overall mortality. None of these studies have shown people live any longer. It is a fascinating sociological phenomenon that some experts, in the face of massive evidence to the contrary, have come up with recommendations based on wishful thinking and dogmatic beliefs. They are guilty of unethical behavior.*[52]

In 1984, the Lipid Research Clinics Coronary Primary Prevention Trial was said to have the first hard evidence that a cholesterol-lowering drug, cholestyramine, was associated with a lower rate of heart attacks. This study has been subjected to criticism for statistical prestidigitation, but perhaps the most important parallel element to come out of it was the startling reality that in this survey of 3,806 men at "high risk" for a heart attack there were three times more deaths from suicide, homicide and trauma in the drug-treated group than in the control group. When this difference was taken into account, the difference in death rates essentially vanished.[53] This, and other studies, have led some to wonder whether certain heart disease drugs might be causally related to violence.

McGee has also described[54] how the so-called Consensus Development Conference of "cholesterol experts" meeting in Bethesda MD in December of that year (1984) was actually rigged to promote the cholesterol hypothesis in advance of the meeting.

The past president of the American Heart Assn. (AHA) in 1990 greeted a recently published study in the *New England Journal of Medicine* as "the smoking pistol" while the director of the National Heart, Lung and Blood Institute called it research which would "knock down the critics of the cholesterol hypothesis."[55]

What stimulated the glee was a 10-year followup study on 863 patients which seemed to show that by lowering blood cholesterol levels the need for invasive procedures against "heart disease" could be greatly reduced, and that lowering cholesterol seemed to be connected to a reduction of plaque in the arteries and thus a reduced risk of heart attack. It was said that this study of people with normally functioning hearts — and not all of the elements of whose lifestyles were taken into account — should "put everything to rest except die-hard critics whom nothing will satisfy."[56]

The fight over fat

But the critics kept right on coming. In the Summer 1992 *The Choice*, we reported on the following recent studies:

— While dieting is good, it is not good enough to have much of a cholesterol-lowering effect and, in some people, may do more harm than good. (*Stanford University*)

— "Several large studies" in the US and Europe indicated that although lowering cholesterol reduced the risk of fatal heart attacks, "through mechanisms that scientists do not understand, the decrease in deaths from heart attacks has been offset by an increased risk of death from suicides, violence and accidents." (*Los Angeles Times*)

— Experiments in monkeys showed that lowering cholesterol reduces levels of the brain "neurotransmitter" serotonin. Low levels of serotonin in humans had previously been linked to an increased risk of suicide and aggressive behavior. (*Same*)

— Dietary manipulation by changing from (ostensibly high-cholesterol) saturated fats to unsaturated fats "can cause more health problems than it solves." (*New England Journal of Medicine*)

Dr. Hyman Engleberg, internist at Cedars-Sinai Medical Center, set the issue squarely:

> *These studies knock into a cocked hat the whole proposition that every American should lower*

cholesterol levels. People who have had a heart attack, stroke or a very bad early history have everything to gain than to lose by lowering their cholesterol, but for a healthy population, they have as much to lose as to gain.[57]

But the campaign droned on, with the cardiological/federal establishments arguing that everybody should be aware of his cholesterol levels — with some groups even arguing that this awareness should begin at age 2! Such ideas, of course, provided a virtually open-ended market for cholesterol tests and, in an anticipated millions of cases, the lifelong need for drugs.

In 1992, two impressively large reports hit the cholesterol hypothesis with what should have been a mortal blow.

First, a report in the *British Medical Journal* evaluated 22 studies in which efforts had been made to see if lowering blood cholesterol rates would mean a concomitant fall in heart attack deaths. In roughly half the studies death rates rose — in the other half they fell. The author stressed that since 1970 only articles backing the cholesterol hypothesis had been cited in medical references. He added:

Lowering serum cholesterol concentrations does not reduce mortality and is unlikely to prevent coronary heart disease. Claims of the opposite are based on preferential citation of supportive trials.[58]

But that was Great Britain.

In the USA, the AHA journal *Circulation* released a huge review (525,737 men and 124,814 women in the United States, Japan, Europe and Israel). The general conclusion: dropping cholesterol levels might have little value for healthy people, low-cholesterol diets for healthy children could be dangerous, and cholesterol levels in women in general had little connection with death rates.

Though the 13 authors of the 19 studies admitted uncertainty as to how to evaluate the raw data, they nonetheless pointed out that in men the only groups who died more often were those whose cholesterol levels were either very high or very low. For the other 64 percent, there was simply no meaningful correlation between levels of the substance and death rates.[59]

At the same time, a growing number of heart experts were questioning the recent recommendations that low-fat diets be implemented for all children two and over. Dr. Thomas B. Newman, University of California-San Francisco, found such recommendations to be a "national scandal."[60]

In 1993, the *Journal of the American Medical Assn. (JAMA)* argued[61] that national guidelines calling for screening of the nation's 80 million young adults could cost the country billions of dollars a year and end up doing more harm than good to those screened.

There simply is no justification for routine cholesterol tests before age 35 in men and 45 in women, the authors argued. The study pointed out that the long-term effects of cholesterol-lowering drugs were not known and that studies touting the benefits of lowering cholesterol levels were tipped more toward the middle-to-old age bracket than any other. Leaders of the Heart, Lung and Blood Institute and the NCEP program were "appalled" at the information.

Also in 1993, yet another study, this by the National Health and Nutrition Survey, tracking 13,000 Americans between 20 to 74, found[62] that average blood cholesterol levels as well as heart disease deaths in general had declined over the prior 12 years, again suggesting a possible relationship between the two. The survey had the benign effect, at least, of arguing for dietary change, weight loss and exercise as treatments of choice for those with high cholesterol.

What may be one of the last few nails being pounded into the coffin of the cholesterol theory of heart disease was a four-year survey of 997 patients studied by Yale and University of Connecticut cardiologists and released in late 1994:

This review of cholesterol levels, coronary heart disease mortality and morbidity, and indeed "all-cause" mortality, led to a firm conclusion:

Our findings do not support the hypothesis

that hypercholesterolemia or low HDL-C are important risk factors for all-cause mortality, coronary heart disease mortality, or hospitalization for myocardial infarction or unstable angina in this cohort of persons older than 70 years.[62a]

The question remained: how important are they for persons *younger* than 70 years?

By the 1990s, Merck's lovastatin (Mevacor) had become the top cholesterol-lowering drug and had captured 50 percent of the market in this class of drugs. Yet, as Moore had speculated in the *Atlantic Monthly* from animal-study data, Mevacor's principal adverse reaction is liver damage, reported to occur in some 1.9 percent of its users. Liver function tests were recommended at monthly intervals and then periodically.[63]

The trouble with cholesterol-lowering medications, as is so often the case with other drugs, has been that their effects are temporary. Cholesterol-drug treatment only, then, has usually meant that suspension of the drug means the return of higher cholesterol levels. The result is, as usual, the option of lifelong use of the medication.

By the 1990s, the total costs of taking cholesterol-reducing drugs along with lab tests and doctor visits was estimated at $3,000 per year per patient the first year, then $2,000 annually forever. Hence, it was not unexpected for Merck to announce wholesale profits of lovastatin at $1 billion annually.[64]

Enter the triglycerides

Just as the cholesterol-counts-most school of American cardiovascular thought seemed sufficiently riddled with contradictions to lead any honest researcher to look elsewhere for blood-fat connections to heart disease, the matter of "the other" major lipid, triglyceride, entered the picture.

The American Heart Association's annual meeting in November 1991 was spiced with hints that maybe the cardiovascular establishment might have it if not all wrong then quite a bit wrong by its concern over the ever-more-dismembered cholesterol (that is, HDL, LDL, VLDL, other lipoproteins, subdivisions and particles of the same).

It was pointed out that triglycerides are important as heart-disease risk factors particularly when combined with high levels of certain cholesterols. And a review of the voluminous and ongoing Framingham Heart Study noted that people with high triglyceride levels have the highest blood-sugar levels — and twice the risk of developing diabetes as people with normal triglyceride levels. This becomes doubly important since it is broadly assumed that diabetes itself is an important risk factor for heart disease.[65]

In January 1992, Helsinki University's Dr. M. Heiki Frick reported[66] that people with *normal* cholesterol levels but with high triglycerides were four times as likely to suffer heart attacks and might wrongly be given a clean bill of health by cholesterol-conscious doctors.

In 1994, a US team showed that even when drug therapy agressively lowered LDL cholesterol, triglycerides continued to contribute to the growth of heart vessel blockages.[65a]

Bringing home the groceries

Lurking behind such research are of course several spectres — including the fact that, assuming fats of one kind or another are indeed linked to heart disease, which seems a fair assumption, a multi-billion-dollar industry has been looking at the wrong one or ones and at the very least developing potentially damaging drugs to be used against these wrong targets.

This would be a common error in allopathic thinking — the wrong cause of a condition is attacked by the wrong weapon, while attempting to prevent the condition in the first place remains a vaguely understandable concept.

(The earliest pharmaceutical attempt to find a drug way to treat atherosclerosis dangled from the same false linear logic. In the early 1960s, as Dr. Edward L. Lambert noted,[67] researchers who realized that patients who died prematurely of heart attacks usually had increased amounts of cholesterol in their blood [though increased amounts of whatever else were not clarified], and assuming a diet low in animal fats would reduce cholesterol, but also aware that it was difficult to get meat-happy Americans to change their diets, looked for the typical "quick fix" to do the trick. What they came up with was the William S. Merrell Company's drug triparanol.

(The FDA, naturally, approved the drug — on the basis of animal tests and a single clinical [human] trial. Thousands of patients received the drug, but a thousand of them developed cataracts from doing so. After it was later found the drug had little effect in reducing atherosclerosis, it was removed from the market. That is to say, American patients were *presumed* to have a disease — too much cholesterol — and they were given a drug to treat the "disease." But many of them developed a *real* condition from taking the drug. Another bright moment in allopathic logic).

What is in play in all the above considerations is the fact that, for the Allopathic Industrial Complex (AIC), heart disease is *big business*, no sin in and of itself, but that very business provides an impetus for the industry and its subsidiaries *not* to look for cheaper, better approaches — including the best one of all, of course, which would be prevention of heart disease as an overall aspect of promotive health. This is not to say that many cardiologists, researchers and physicians are *not* legitimately interested in finding ways to prevent heart disease — it simply means that the economic mechanism favors expensive drugs and high technology in diagnostics and therapeutics, as is true in virtually all other areas of allopathic medicine. Treatment, not prevention, "brings home the groceries."

The parallel reality is that standard medical (that is, allopathic) thinking as it involves heart disease is simplistic in that it looks for that "quick fix" — a single orderly solution to a complicated medical problem. The allopathic paradigm (*IV*) needs "things to treat" and treatments. It is allopathic in essence to see a breakdown of the heart/circulatory system as a mechanical breakdown which needs, in essence, a plumbing job.

Something needs to be re-routed, or widened, or cut or burned out. Yet, as in every other area of medicine, clues and information abound that heart disease calamities are mostly if not entirely preventable (as many heart specialists themselves are beginning to sense, and as some have argued), and that dietary and other lifestyle factors are pre-eminent in its prevention. We discuss the nutritional/metabolic/alternative therapy revolution both in this section and elsewhere (*XIV*) as it applies to heart problems and health promotion in general.

Because, in the heart disease subdivision of the AIC, there are sufficient existing data available, should anyone seek them out, not only to establish the utility of nutrients against heart/circulatory problems and for overall cardiovascular health (notably diet programs, very much including the challenging one put together by Dean Ornish MD in seemingly outright defiance of the heart disease industry) and enough information on nutritional aspects (deficiencies/excesses) in *all* disease states for even the minimally curious to wonder why such things are not more generally known about.

The exercise/diet teeter-totters

By the mid-1990s it was also becoming increasingly evident that two of the pillars of non-drug heart disease prevention — over-exercising and over-dieting — not only could not be relied upon to cut meaningfully into heart disease statistics but might also be making the problem worse.

A 45-hospital, 1,228 heart attack-survivor study conducted by Boston's Deaconess Hospital stressed that out-of-shape individuals who suddenly undertake strenuous activity face 100 times the risk of a heart attack, particularly if they never exercise at all. Analysts claimed this meant that about 4 percent — or 60,000 — heart attacks in any given year were provoked by a sudden outburst of strenuous activity (splitting firewood, moving the furniture, suddenly exercising). The risk was said to be less for those who worked out regularly, but even those who exercised five times a week doubled their risk of a heart attack if they suddenly did something strenuous beyond the usual workout.[67a]

And several studies showed that "yo-yo" dieting — making intermittent efforts to "eat right" followed by gaps in the program — and/or constantly trying diets showed a higher correlation to heart disease and diabetes than never dieting at all (!)

In what epidemiologist Steven N. Blair described to the American Heart Association as a "paradox", results of a study of 12,025 Harvard University graduates also showed that men who kept their weight steady — even if overweight — had less risk of heart disease than men with very fluctuating weights.[67b]

Out of such studies come increasing emphasis on prudence rather than faddism — suggestions that rational eating habits (more fruits and vegetables, fewer fats) rather than crash diets, and reasonable exercise rather than sudden involvement in extreme physical activity — equate with better coronary health.

The EDTA chelation saga

And, incredibly, within the precincts of allopathic thought there exists in heart disease prevention and management a time-honored, well-tested technique which deals mechanically with the very problem which orthodox cardiology insists is at the root of so much cardiovascular distress — the "occluded" blood vessel.

And, also incredibly, this technique or procedure, about which thousands of research articles have appeared worldwide in appropriately "peer-reviewed" medical literature, and which is currently practiced by a thousand or more credentialed US medical practitioners, is virtually unknown to the American medical consumer whether he assiduously views television news programs and reads news magazines and newspapers or not. This technique or procedure has already saved hundreds of thousands of lives, is itself essentially non-toxic and only minimally "invasive" and — at the real root of its being unknown to the public at large — is far less expensive than standard surgical and drug therapies in heart disease. Too, its proponents would add, it is all that much more effective.

The fact the American public is basically oblivious to it and that heart disease victims are routinely not even informed about it, while some of its most credentialed and otherwise allopathically educated proponents have usually been unable to publish about it in "learned journals," is a casebook example of the AIC at work, and of how all parts of the AIC can coalesce to jam the information-processing apparatus even of an ostensibly free society.

The technique/procedure in question is chelation therapy — usually meaning EDTA chelation therapy — and, to compound the irony, it is largely a product of American research and original application whose central element, EDTA itself, is both a recognized treatment for lead poisoning and a preservative widely used in medicine.

For proponents and researchers it is the best, if not the only, way to unclog blood vessels, the best way to return flexibility to the rubbery system of capillaries, veins and arteries through which the body's life-sustaining blood is pumped from its master organ, the heart. And, it seems to have many positive ancillary effects as well.

It is not the province of this book to elucidate the technique in detail. This has been done by a battery of both credentialed researchers and lay medical writers. (The author includes himself in the latter category as co-author with the late Harold Harper MD, one of chelation therapy's pioneers, of a 1977 book on this subject,[68] and journalistic treatment of it in another.[69]) In the modern era, significant contributions in the United States to the chelation literature have been made by Drs. Harper, E.W. McDonagh, Bruce W. Halstead, Garry F. Gordon, Elmer Cranton, Morton Walker, Richard Casdorph, and James P. Carter and such informed lay medical writers as Harold and Arline Brecher and Jane Heimlich, among the more prominent.

Chelation therapy (from the Greek word "chela," meaning "claw"), is the administration of a substance (usually intravenously, although natural "chelators," as in certain vitamins and other nutrients consumed orally, exert some of the same action) which has the ability to rid the body of heavy metals and minerals, substances usually thought of as toxic, and decidedly so when they are in excess. The primary substance used is the synthetic amino acid ethylene-diamine-tetraacetic acid (EDTA), known under other names, and similar compounds.

The way in which EDTA and similar compounds "bind to" toxic metals or minerals involves a knowledge of physics. The empirical reality is that such "binding" occurs, and the result is that certain heavy, potentially toxic metals and minerals may be made soluble so they may be excreted through the kidneys, depending on the integrity of the same and other factors. Because some necessary minerals may also be removed in the process, a standard EDTA "drip" includes replacement minerals.

While synthesized in Germany in 1931, it was an American — Dr. Norman E. Clarke Sr. MD, cardiologist at Providence Hospital, Detroit — who discovered the multiple uses of the compound ranging well beyond its utility in curing lead poisoning.

There is some conflicting information about the early days of EDTA chelation therapy, including the scattered research on it which produced anything negative (and which is parroted today by the medical establishment), since scores of papers were published at home and abroad (primarily during the 1950s) favorable as to its effectiveness against several conditions, particularly arteriosclerosis. Indeed, as late as 1970 even the FDA referred to calcium EDTA or disodium EDTA this way:

This drug is possibly effective in occlusive vascular disorders and the treatment of pathologic conditions to which calcium tissue deposits of hypercalcemia may contribute ...[70]

As late as the early 1960s, Abbott Laboratories' "package insert" for EDTA contained arteriosclerosis as an "indication" for its use.

But it was also in the early 1960s that the Food, Drug, and Cosmetic Act was once again amended, with the FDA securing the power to oversee both the "safety" and "efficacy" of drugs — an event which vastly expanded FDA clout and also allowed the federal agency to be used as a weapon by gigantic companies to block competitors (*IX*). It was also time for Abbott's patent on EDTA to run out. To attempt to re-license an "old drug" for a new purpose meant in effect investing millions of dollars in a generic drug it could not control. For this and other reasons, EDTA was left — in terms of its demonstrated utility in various forms of heart disease — in a kind of regulatory limbo.

Worse for the compound, though, it represented a monumental challenge to the rapidly developing heart disease industry — an essentially far-less-expensive alternative to complicated, expensive surgery and medications.

But research concerning its use went on throughout the world. Dr. Clarke was hailed as a chelation pioneer in the Soviet Union, which elevated EDTA chelation therapy to the second most common treatment for artery disease. It became the preferred method of heart disease treatment in Communist-era Czechoslovakia and throughout many countries was administered successfully against all kinds of blood vessel diseases, gangrene, stroke, senility, diabetes, kidney disorders and other degenerative conditions. Our own research group found that it seemed to "potentiate" another form of US-"unapproved" medicine — "live cell" or "cellular" therapy.

While research went on around the world, with the ultimate publication of literally thousands of articles in scientific and medical journals extolling the multiple benefits of EDTA, the US heart disease industry was growing by leaps and bounds. Just as, at about the same time, the cancer industry was not about to be sidetracked by laetrile, megavitamins or any other nutritional form of treatment, the heart disease industry looked askance at the use of an old, potentially inexpensive compound cutting into the growing surgical/heart drug business.

Joining the 'alternative' revolution

Worse, for the American medical orthodoxy, EDTA chelation therapy largely fell into the hands of medical mavericks who began to utilize multifactorial nutritional protocols against degenerative disease. Shunned as an outsider, it now became part of American outlaw medicine, at least in the eyes of the AMA, FDA and the American Heart Assn. (AHA). It became that most despicable of medical entities in the USA — an "alternative" medicine. It thus fell under the same kind of legal/judicial attack that all other aspects of "alternative" therapy faced in the United States.

Yet unlike so many of these, EDTA chelation therapy was among the best-documented, most provable of therapies both domestically and around the world. An organization of allopathically trained American physicians who believed in and practiced EDTA chelation therapy was formed. The organization developed more research and protocols for use of the compound and fought for its acceptance and authorization. Even so, EDTA ran up against the same sorts of stone walls the AIC hurled against non-toxic cancer treatments.

By 1993, it could be reported that over the years EDTA chelation therapy had had a tremendous track record for safety and that some 500,000 Americans had been treated with it over the years with no reported fatalities as long as the protocol advanced by the chelating doctors' group, now called the American College for the Advancement of Medicine (ACAM), was used.[71]

The lengthy battle of EDTA chelation therapy for recognition in the United States, particularly well described by such modern-day writers as the Brechers,[72] and Drs. McGee and James Carter,[73] has followed a path similar to that of laetrile against cancer. It has been subjected to media and institutional bias and literally rigged or bias-riddled research aimed at finding it "unproven," and was the only item listed as "quackery" by the FDA's publication *FDA Consumer* which we are aware of that ever won both a retraction and an apology from the agency publication.

While more than a thousand American physicians practice EDTA chelation therapy, most of the publications in which they are forced to report their research and successes are not "cross-indexed" into medical computer banks. Articles favorable to or simply open-minded about chelation hence appear in "alternative" and foreign medical journals. The mainstream American public simply does not know, in the main, that this relatively simple approach to numerous heart and circulatory problems, costing so little in comparison with "accepted" procedures, exists.

Chelation therapy, while officially "unapproved" at the federal level, has been officially sanctioned by several states, and in others has been "legalized" by court action. But at this writing securing public and private medical insurance coverage for the technique ranges from the difficult to the impossible — another key way in which "unwanted" therapies are harassed in the United States.

Because of its cold-shouldering by US orthodoxy and its necessary flirtation with "unorthodoxy," EDTA chelation therapy has won a distinctive place in "alternative" treatments and thus will form part of the medicine of the future.

Not always successful by itself as a single modality (as so few things are when arrayed against multifactorial degenerative diseases), EDTA chelation therapy takes its place within individualized, integrated protocols along with diet, detoxification and nutritional support as an extremely valuable therapeutic tool.

In the meantime, its struggle for recognition and vindication against the massed forces of the AIC epitomizes what the fight for medical freedom of choice in America is all about.

The dietary heart of the matter

And, also in the meantime, the new dimensions in the therapy and management of cardiovascular calamities — in totality the major medical threat to "civilization" as we know it — point to *promotive health* as a guidepost for the 21st century.

Within promotive health is the fullscale retooling of eating habits and dietary programs (see *XIV*) as they relate to the promotion of health overall and the prevention of chronic disease in general.

Even in a world of chemically tampered-with foods it is already within our grasp to identify those dietary elements which help lead to cardiovascular good health.

Among the more recent developments have been those which strongly point to the so-called "Mediterranean diet" as among the heart-healthiest of the Western world.

In June 1994, the Lyon Diet Heart Study (Michel de Lorgeril *et al.*) concluded from a study of patients who had had initial heart attacks that a "Mediterranean diet" seemed to be more efficient than presently used diets in the secondary prevention of coronary events and death."[74]

The strongest correlative feature in such a diet, the study noted, was the high presence therein of alpha-linolenic acid, an essential *fatty* acid which — again, as metabolic and other outside-the-pale medics and researchers had long argued — is useful in overall cardiovascular health (and may also contribute to better immunological health). But as the authors were quick to note, the diet — being high in vegetables and fruits together with olive oil — is also high in antioxidants, which are increasingly coming into their own as protective against chronic diseases.(*XIV*)

In the Lyon study, rapeseed margarine substituted for olive oil and was the chief source of alpha-linolenic acid. The study, assessed *The Lancet*, "raises the question of whether [alpha-linolenic acid] could have effects similar to those of eicosapentaenoic acid [*another fatty acid long suspected of overall health benefits*] and other long-chain n-3 fatty acids derived from fish." Moreover

> ... *[I]f high intakes of [alpha-linolenic acid] are as effective as oily fish in reducing the risk of coronary heart disease, there are considerable implications for preventive strategies, since it is easier to substitute vegetable oils rich in [alpha-linolenic acid] for other sources of dietary fat than to increase consumption of oily fish on a mass scale. Few vegetable oils contain much [alpha-linolenic acid], the most readily available in western countries being soya oil and rapeseed oil* ...[75]

The Lyon study followed by about five years the earlier

"diet and reinfarction trial" (DART), in which eating only "oily" fish was associated with a 29 percent reduction in total mortality in the first two years following an initial heart attack.[76]

The Lyon study preceded a 1994 report by Boston University School of Medicine which noted that advice then in place which touted the advantages of a low-fat diet was off-base — at least insofar as certain essential fatty acids are concerned — and in so doing again vindicated the beliefs and practices of many metabolic therapists.

The Boston research pointed out that a major risk factor in atherosclerosis is an insufficiency of the EFAs (essential fatty acids) linoleic and linolenic acid. Since they cannot be manufactured by the human body they need to be consumed from outside sources — particularly soybeans, green leafy vegetables and various nuts and seeds in which they are plentiful.

Linoleic acid, an "omega-6" fatty acid, is particularly abundant in safflower oil, corn oil, cottonseed oil and soybean oil. Linolenic acid, as found in fish oils, also is prominent in soybean and canola oils, flaxseed and purslane.

All of which may explain why a 10-year, 24-country, 55-population study by epidemiologist Dr. Yukio Yamori and colleagues at Kyoto University found that the low incidence of heart disease in Japan (and among selected other populations) is likely the result of the seafood-rich diet of its residents. "Oily" fish, shrimps and octopus, the researchers found, contain substances which may prevent the clogging of arteries.[78]

In 1993, the Dutch "Zutphen Elderly Study" found yet another factor — flavonoids — as useful in reducing the risk of death from coronary heart disease in elderly men.[79]

Flavonoids also fall within the ever-broadening confines of the "antioxidants" and are present in vegetables, fruits and such beverages as tea and wine. They are known to inhibit the oxidation process of the so-called "bad" cholesterol, LDL, at least in the test tube.

By fall 1994 information on vitamin supplements as being useful in preventing heart disease continued to be noticeable in studies and surveys both large and small.

At the Second International Conference on Antioxidant Vitamins in Disease Prevention in Berlin, Canadian researchers, reporting on a seven-year followup of 2,226 men aged 45 to 76, showed that those who used vitamin supplements — particularly Vitamin E — were less likely to develop or die from heart disease than those who did not. Laval University epidemiologist Francois Meyer's work showed that vitamin pill-popping men have about a fifth the risk of developing heart disease than those who are not.[80]

At about the same time, North Carolina School of Medicine research showed that carotenids — the colorful compounds which make spinach green and squash yellow and of which beta-carotene is the best-known member — was associated with 36 percent fewer heart attacks and deaths over 13 years than in men with lower carotenid levels.[81]

All such research is pointing, one seemingly trivial study at a time, as the allopathic thought-process tediously struggles to see the forest rather than the trees, to the overriding importance of proper diet not only in enhancing overall cardiovascular health but helping enhance health in general.

In this general view, more fish, fish oils, and certain vegetable oils, together with a diet high in fruits and vegetables, would seem to be rational eating options. Together with the "poor people's diet," emphasizing less animal fat and protein, no or fewer refined carbohydrates and stimulants, we are nearing the metabolically logical dietary program.

That such a diet correlates increasingly with the absence of advanced chronic disease — and hence the reliance on drastic measures to manage the same — helps explain the lukewarm enthusiasm for such research on the part of significant sectors of the AIC.

The continuing tragedy is that while so many billions of research dollars have been pumped into the AIC for diagnostics and drug development against the human-created diseases of civilization, so little has gone into adequate nutritional science which, more than any other factor, would provide ironclad evidence of how to prevent or at least mitigate them.

References

1. American Heart Assn., January 1993.
1a. Haney, DQ, The Associated Press, Nov. 17, 1994.
2. American Heart Assn., January 1992.
3. *The Choice*, XIX: 1, 1993.
3a. The Associated Press, January 1994.
3b. Ubell, Earl, "When is heart surgery really called for?" *Parade*, March 13, 1994.
4. *Ibid.*
5. McGee, CT, *Heart Frauds*. Coeur d' Alene ID: MediPress, 1993.
6. *J. Am. Med. Assn.*, Nov. 11, 1992.
7. Grodin, CM, *Circulation* 49, 1974.
8. Zir, LM, *et al., Circulation* 53, 1976.
9. *Medical World News*, Dec. 24, 1979.
10. White, CW, *et al., New Eng. J. Med.* 310, 1984.
11. Cited in McGee, *op. cit.*
12. McGee, *op. cit.*
13. *The Choice*, XVII: 3,4, 1991.
14. McGee, *op. cit.*
15. *The Choice*, XVIII: 2, 1992.
15a. The Associated Press, Jan. 18, 1984.
15b. de Lisser, Eleena, "Number of major cardiac surgeries was nearly flat in 1993, survey finds." *Wall Street Journal*, Oct. 3, 1994.
15c. *Ibid.*
16. McGee, *op. cit.*
17. *The Choice*, XVIII: 2, 1992.
18. *J. Am. Med. Assn.*, August 1991.
19. *New Eng. J. Med.* 311, 1977.
20. Alderman, EL, *et al., Circulation* 82, 1990.
21. McIntosh, HD, *et al., Circulation* 57, 1978.
22. McGee, *op. cit.*
23. Natl. Center for Health Statistics and Commission of Professional Hospital Activities, Washington DC, 1992.
24. *The Choice*, XVIII: 2, 1992.
24a. de Lisser, Eleena, *op. cit.*
25. "New caution on the heart balloon," *US News & World Report*, July 25, 1988.
26. "Hearts and balloons," *Harvard Medical School Health Letter*, November 1986.
26a. Raeburn, Paul, *The Associated Press*, Nov. 16, 1994.
27. *The Choice*, XVII: 1, 1991.
28. Seeger, JM, *et al.*, "Initial results of laser recanalization in lower extremity arterial reconstruction." *J. Vasc. Surg.* 1, 1989.
29. *The Choice*, XIX: 2, 1993.
29a. Goldsmith, MF, "Once again, CABG vs. PTCA — trial results today." *J. Am. Med. Assn.*, Jan. 26, 1994.
29b. Winslow, Ron, *The Wall Street Journal*, Sept. 21, 1994. Also: McClellan, Mark, *et al.*, J. Am. Med. Ass'n. Sept. 21, 1994.
29c. King, SB, *et al.*, "A randomized trial comparing coronary angioplasty with coronary bypass surgery." *New Eng. J. Med.*, Oct. 20, 1994.
29d. Hamm, CW, *et al.*, "A randomized study of coronary angioplasty compared with bypass surgery in patients with symptomatic multivessel coronary disease." *New Eng. J. Med.* Oct. 20, 1994.
30. Heimlich, Jane, *What Your Doctor Won't Tell You*. New York: HarperCollins, 1990.
31. Heimlich, *op. cit.*
32. Langford, HG, *et al.*, "Dietary therapy slows the return of hypertension after stopping prolonged medication." *J. Am. Med. J.*, Feb. 1, 1985.
33. Stamler, Rose, *et al.*, "Nutritional therapy for high blood pressure." *J. Am. Med. J.*, March 20, 1987.
34. "Five-year findings of the hypertension detection and follow-up program." *J. Am. Med. J.*, Dec. 7, 1979.
35. "Multiple risk factor intervention trial." *J. Am. Med. J.*, Sept,. 24, 1982.
36. Heimlich, *op. cit.*
37. *Ibid.*
38. *The Choice*, XVI: 1, 1990.
38a. Altman, LK, *The New York Times*, Oct. 17, 1994.
38b. *Circulation*, October 1994.
39. *The Choice*, XIX: 2, 1993.
39a. Bishop, JE, "Drugs to dissolve blood clots save lives, study shows." *Wall Street Journal*, Nov. 16, 1994.
40. *The Choice*, XVII: 3,4, 1991.

40a. Hulley, SB, and Newman,TB, "Cholesterol in the elderly: is it important?" *J. Am. Med. Assn.*, Nov. 2, 1994.
40b. Haney, *loc. cit.*
40c. Bishop, JE, "Class of anticholesterol drugs cuts risk of death, researchers find." *Wall Street Journal*, Nov. 17, 1994.
41. McGee, *op. cit.*
42. *Medical World News*, June 7, 1982.
43. McGee, *op. cit.*
44. Moore, TJ, *Heart Failure*. New York: Random House, 1989.
45. Moore, TJ, "The cholesterol myth." *Atlantic Monthly*, September 1989.
46. *Ibid.*
47. *Ibid.*
48. *The Choice*, XIX: 2, 1993.
49. *Ibid.*
49a. Schaefer, EJ, *et al.*, "Lipoprotein (a) levels and risk of coronary heart disease in men." *J. Am. Med. Assn,*. April 6, 1991.
49b. Rath, Matthias, *Eradicating Heart Disease*. San Francisco CA: Health Now, 1993.
49c. Rath, Matthias, "Vitamin C deficiency: the primary cause of cardiovascular disease." *Body & Soul*, IX: 2, 1994.
50. The Associated Press, May 1993, cited in *The Choice*, XIX: 2, 1993.
50a. Lee, Arthur, in *Proc. Natl. Aca. Sci.*, cited in *USA Today*, July 5, 1994.
50b. Speir, Edith, *Science*, July 15, 1994, and cited in *USA Today*, July 15, 1994.
51. McGee, *op. cit.*
52. Brisson, GJ, *Lipids in Human Nutrition*. Englewood NJ: JK Burgess, 1982.
53. Moore, TJ, "The cholesterol myth." *Op. cit.*
54. McGee, *op. cit.*
55. *The New York Times,*, cited in *The Choice*, XVI: 4, 1990.
56. *Ibid.*
57. *The Choice*, XVIII:2, 1992.
58. Ravenskov, U, *Brit. Med. J.* 305, 1992.
59. Jacobs, D, *et al.*, and Huller, SB, editorial, *Circulation* 86, 1992.
60. San Jose *Mercury News*, cited in *The Choice*, XVIII:3, 1992.
61. Hulley, SB, *et. al.*, *J. Am. Med. Assn.*, March 17, 1993.
62. *J. Am. Med. Assn.*, cited in *The Choice*, XIX: 2, 1993.
62a. Krumholz, HM, "Lack of association between cholesterol and coronary heart disease mortality and morbidity and all-cause mortality in persons older than 70 years." *J. Am. Med. Assn.*, Nov. 2, 1994.
63. McGee, *op. cit.*
64. *Ibid.*
65. *The Choice*, XVIII: 1, 1992.
65a. Hodis, HN, *et al.*, *Circulation*, July 1994.
66. *Ibid.*
67. Lambert, EC, *Modern Medical Mistakes*. Bloomington IN: Indiana University Press, 1978.
67a. The Associated Press/*New Eng. J. Med.* December 1993.
67b. The Associated Press, March 20, 1994.
68. Harper, Harold, and Culbert, ML, *How You Can Beat the Killer Diseases*. New Rochelle NY: Arlington House, 1977.
69. Culbert, ML, *What The Medical Establishment Won't Tell You that Could Save Your Life*. Norfolk VA: Donning, 1983.
70. McDonagh, EW, *Chelation Can Cure*. Kansas City MO: Platinum Pen, 1983.
71. McGee, *op. cit.*
72. Brecher, A, and Brecher, H, *Forty Something Forever*. Herndon VA: Healthsavers Press, 1992.
73. Carter, JP, *Racketeering in Medicine*. Norfolk VA: Hampton Roads, 1992.
74. de Lorgeril, *et al.*, "Mediterranean alpha-linolenic acid-rich diet in secondary prevention of coronary heart disease." *Lancet*, June 11, 1994.
75. "Commentary," *Lancet*, June 11, 1994.
76. Burr, ML, *et al.*, "Effects of changes in fat, fish and fibre intakes on death and myocardial reinfarction: diet and reinfarction trial (DART)." *Lancet ii*, 1989.
77. Siguel, EN, and Lerman, RH, *Metabolism*, September 1994, cited in Brody, JE, *The New York Times*, Aug. 24, 1994.
78. Scott, Susan, "Healthy ocean fisheries healthy for human hearts." Honolulu *Star Bulletin*, June 13, 1994.
79. Hertog, MGL, *et al.*, "Dietary antioxidant flavonoids and risk of coronary heart disease: the Zutphen Elderly Study." *Lancet*, Oct. 23, 1993.
80. "Vitamins might help to fight heart disease." *Orange County Register*, Oct. 8, 1994.
81. Morris, Dexter, *J. Am. Med. Assn.*, Nov. 9, 1994.

XI
CANCER CON: Of mice, men, money and malignancy

"Although it is shielded from the public by high-minded pronouncements and scientific jargon, the cancer establishment is afflicted with a mental and moral malaise. It is more interested in maintaining the status quo than in finding the answers to the cancer riddle, and will defend that status quo against all comers. Its struggle to retain credibility and power may well last decades and cost millions of lives, unless the source of its funding — the taxpaying public — demands reform."
— **Gerald B. Dermer PhD** (*The Immortal Cell*), **1994**

"In the end, any claim of major success against cancer must be reconciled with this figure [a graph showing climbing US cancer death rates between 1950-1990]. *I do not think such reconciliation is possible and again conclude, as I did seven years ago, that our decades of war against cancer have been a qualified failure."*
— **Epidemiologist/biostatistician Dr. John C. Bailar III, 1993**

"Millions of people no longer automatically believe what the leaders of the cancer establishment tell them. They are resisting the introduction of carcinogens into the environment; demanding alternative forms of therapy; suing companies; signing petitions; writing, picketing, and protesting. Scientists and doctors are pursuing independent avenues of research . . . Given the current impasse in the war on cancer, it is most likely that [this rebellion] *will gain strength and spread. Eventually it may play a decisive role in bringing the war on cancer to a successful conclusion."*
— **Ralph W. Moss PhD** (*The Cancer Industry*), **1991**

"This 'cancer establishment' pushes highly toxic and expensive drugs, patented by major pharmaceutical firms which also have close links to cancer centers. Is it any wonder they refuse to investigate innovative approaches developed outside their own institutions? . . . We clearly need a complete restructuring of the losing war against cancer. Prevention must get the highest priority. Industrial carcinogens must be phased out or banned. Innovative non-toxic therapies must get independent evaluation."
— **Dr. Samuel Epstein** (*USA Today*), **1992**

". . . No disseminated neoplasm incurable in 1975 is curable today."
— **Albert S. Braverman MD** (*The Lancet*), **1991**

The unkindest cuts

In 1991, the *Honolulu Star-Bulletin* reported the case of the 46-year-old woman who "didn't want to wait for ovarian cancer to kill her." [1]

Her grandmother, aunt and cousin had died of ovarian cancer in their 40s, hence giving the woman — according to the "best" medical minds — a "fifty percent chance of getting the disease," noted the newspaper.

So, "I got up the courage to ask my doctor if he could remove my ovaries, uterus and fallopian tubes as a preventative measure." Apparently, he obliged. She now believed her chances of getting ovarian cancer had dropped to "zilch." The newspaper reported the woman had spent the foregoing nine months getting grass-roots support in seven states for similar research efforts.

In January 1992, the *Wall Street Journal* reported [2] that about 20 percent of 800 mastectomies (breast removals) per year at the famed Memorial Sloan-Kettering Hospital, New York, were "prophylactic" — that is, they had been carried out to *prevent* breast cancer under the oncological theory that if cancer "runs in families" and if the location of a tumor mass at a single site represents cancer as defined by that site, organ or tissue, then it made sense to remove the site, organ or tissue.

By that time, reported the *WSJ*, the "prophylactic" mastectomy was also being carried out at other well-known cancer research hospitals.

That same prophetic month, the British medical journal *Lancet* reported [3] that in a worldwide analysis of breast cancer it was found that removal of a woman's healthy ovaries following breast surgery (a total mastectomy or simple lumpectomy — removal of the lump only) improved the 10-year survival rates of cancer-stricken women under 50 by 11 percent.

Still and all, *USA Today* quoted [4] Memorial Sloan-Kettering's Larry Norton as saying that such a double-whammy surgical approach was not without "major disadvantages" — including osteoporosis, increased cholesterol, and higher risks of heart attack and stroke.

(Some observed how interesting it was that such medical opinions on what women should do with their bodies were being rendered primarily by men).

While an incredulous public found it difficult to believe that there could be such a thing as selective, authorized self-mutilation to prevent cancer even in the absence of any signs and symptoms of the disease (Faulkner Breast Center surgeon Susan Love in Boston was quoted as saying, "I think the idea of removing a body part preventively is really crazy") it unfortunately was a natural result of the linear thought processes of standard or allopathic medicine's cancer subdivision — oncology (whose name, from the Greek *onkos*, really means "the study of bumps.")

The falsest premises

Since American oncology still believes, indeed insists on, the notion that there are hundreds of "forms" or "kinds" of cancer (definable by tumor and tissue type), then there is a kind of primeval logic in the notion that a cancerous tumor in a mammary gland is "breast cancer," that a cancerous tumor in the lower digestive tract is "colon cancer," that a cancerous tumor mass in the cerebrum is "brain cancer" . . . etc. The concept that there is a single, underlying, subclinical *malignant process* (the unitarian theory) is still held by only a handful, though growing, number of researchers. If unitarianists are right, of course, then tumors are not the disease process itself — they are only symptoms, albeit in many cases life-threatening ones, and therefore the basic thrust of oncology, which years ago some of us baptized "cut, burn and poison" (surgery, radiation and chemotherapy), is not only conceptually wrong — it is lethally, fatally wrong. If unitarianists are anywhere near the mark, removing a tumor in the breast is no more a "cure" of cancer than, more than a hundred years ago, was poisoning an ulcerating skin lesion with gold or arsenic a "cure" of syphilis, even though such surgery may in fact "buy time."

An endless carnage

However, unitarianists do not have to be either right or wrong in the American debate over cancer:

Cancer is the fastest-growing, most life-threatening disaster of all the disasters of the plague of chronic, systemic, metabolic disorders sweeping not only the United States and North America but indeed of the Western "civilized" world. It does not take a doctorate in logic, philosophy or statistics to figure out that the basic premises on which American oncology has mounted its disastrously failing campaign against "the big C" not only are wrong, but are *very* wrong.

For, any way one measures the statistics, and from any angle, there is more cancer, both in terms of incidence and fatalities, and more people are dying from it at ever earlier ages than ever before in the history of our planet. Given the conservative 1993/1994 projections of a minimum of 700,000 new American fatalities annually from the malignant process, following the earlier half-million which had been reported for several years, then even the analogy we used for several years had become passé:

Going into the decade of the 1990s, it was appropriate to assess a new cancer death every minute (60 seconds) in the USA, with *two* new diagnoses roughly in the same period, meaning that in any 24-hour period there would be upwards of 1,500 cancer deaths or 3,000 diagnoses of the disease. This added up to the approximately 550,000 annual deaths and more than 1 million new diagnoses being reported or estimated by "the experts."

Even then, the analogy our own Committee for Freedom of Choice in Medicine Inc., had used through the foregoing decade — daily cancer deaths were the approximate equivalent of what would be occurring if two jumbo jets collided every day, killing all aboard on both airplanes — was somewhat conservative. If such a thing were happening, the American people would demand a full-scale investigation. That was then.

By 1993, the officious if not official American Cancer Society (ACS), which has heavily dominated what Americans know, think and believe about cancer and which has done such yeoman work in broadly disseminating the very likely false premises on which US oncology is built and nurtured, projected almost 1,900,000 cancer cases for the year — a catastrophically high figure, even though 700,000 were thought to be what the oncological establishment calls "curable," that is, non-melanoma skin cancer, non-spreading lesions in the cervix, and a few others. The remaining 1.2 million were of the "metastatic" (that is, spread-capable) "forms" of the disease.[5]

But even those figures may have been conservative, because the rapid growth in non-melanoma skin cancer in the United States was so seemingly uncontrollable that dermatologists were reporting much higher projections by 1994, with a rapid spread of the common basal cell skin carcinomas appearing in ever younger people.[6]

Such projections suggested roughly 1,900 cancer fatalities and 5,200 cancer diagnoses per day as of 1994 — one death from cancer every 45 seconds!

There were various ways to describe what all this meant:

Cancer was now striking 1 out of every 3 Americans, at least statistically, up from 1 out of 4, which had been the level for many years, but was expected to be killing 1 out of 5, or down from 1 out of 4. This meant, in oncological parlance, a slight improvement in "cure" rates. It was still occurring in two out of three families. Other ways to assess the figures were that as many Americans were dying monthly from cancer as died during the entire Vietnam War, and that the disease was the biggest killer of the middle-aged, the second biggest killer of the elderly, and the major "natural" killer of children through age 14.

There was no stretch of semantics by which American medicine could truly deflect the central reality — failure — either by arguing that there was more cancer because people were living longer (which indeed explained a small amount of new cases) or even, more appropriately, that improvements in diagnostic techniques (the major bright star in cancer "progress" in the USA) were detecting more cancer than could have been detected earlier (which also was true for a small part of the rise).

Giving the devil his oncological due, it is also not specifically the single guilt of organized medicine or organized oncology that cancer incidence ballooned in the USA, other than — as we will see — those areas in which cancer *treatments* actually helped cause "secondary cancer" years later. The reasons for the mass explosion of cancer incidence and fatalities are societal and collective in nature and far transcend even the medical miasma.

Year by year, the incidence of cancer, quite aside from the fatalities therefrom, has risen inexorably in terms of cases per 100,000 and this has been true since reliable cancer statistics began being tracked earlier in this century, or at about the time the American Cancer Society (ACS) was established as a fairly unimportant fund-raising group for what was at the time a fairly unimportant medical problem. Neither the rise in population nor the fact more Americans are living (that is, surviving) longer can account for this increase.

Indeed, in 1994, Assistant Secretary for Health Devra Lee Davis and statistician/epidemiological colleagues reported that increases in cancer in white people between 1973 and 1987 could not be explained either on the basis of age or smoking patterns.

"In light of these results and similar studies in Sweden, changes in carcinogenic hazards in addition to smoking are likely to have occurred and need to be studied further," Davis *et al.* concluded.[7]

They were not long in being criticized by other elements of the cancer research establishment for the "models" used, but there still was no "positive spin" on the fact ever more Americans were developing and dying from cancer than ever before.

In 1991, the American Hospital Assn. predicted[8] that by 2000 cancer would bypass the constellation of pathologies called "heart disease" as the leading cause of death in the USA (as it had already done in Japan), so that oncology will replace cardiology as the number-one medical specialty and cancer incidence may be 1 out of 2.

The Association publication *Meditrends* was even being conservative: it estimated that 1.6 million Americans would be diagnosed with cancer throughout each year of the 1990s, and that cancer would soon be gobbling up to 20 percent of the nation's healthcare costs. That would now conservatively mean that cancer currently constitutes approximately $200 billion a year of the nation's healthcare cost crisis. This would take into account the 1992 estimate (Dr. Samuel Epstein) of $110 billion in direct costs, and add on billions more in lost productivity and indirect costs. The 1992 estimate was that cancer (industrially described) was about 2 percent of the entire gross national product (GNP). It had, said a group of experts questioning progress against the disease, increased in incidence a frightening 44 percent since 1950, with breast cancer having increased 60 percent during that time, and cancers of the testis, prostate and kidney up by 100 percent.[9]

In fall 1994, a 15-member panel made up of representatives of the cancer industry — asked by Congress to explain why cancer was still on the rise after the expenditure of $23 billion since 1971 — called for a sweeping overhaul of the entire anti-cancer effort (shades of 1971) including, of course, additional monetary outlays. The panel did seem convinced about the necessity of encouraging "translational research" — that is, actually putting some worthwhile scientific leads into practice more quickly — and emphasizing preventive aspects more.[10]

A ministry of misinformation

While cancer incidence and fatality levels have risen year by year with no real end in sight, the constellation of elements we style "Cancer Inc." has constantly and with gnat-like tenacity force-fed and spoonfed the American public an endless battery of statements, statistics and projections. These have attempted to put what Washington politicians would describe as the best possible "spin" on an otherwise disastrous situation.

This has been done through the ministry of propaganda and anti-"alternatives" misinformation which the ACS so often simply has been — despite the charitable instincts of its many volunteers, the objectives of its original founders, the undoubtedly good intentions of its well-paid executives and lesser officials and also the good intentions of the great majority of researchers, doctors and analysts within the American oncological paradigm or belief system. It also has been carried forth through the federally funded National Cancer Institute (NCI), conduit of tax-supported research into cancer yet second in societal impact to the private ACS. From both we have heard an endless symphony of optimism.

Cancer has been variously described as "among the most curable of diseases" (true if we mean five years without symptoms constituting "cures," and most of these related to nonmelanoma skin lesions or small local "primary" tumors which have not yet spread and have been surgically or otherwise removed). It has also been called a disease condition susceptible to a fifty-percent cure rate, and the disease for which the "light at the end of the tunnel," the "turnaround" or "breakthrough" have been predicted annually, sometimes monthly.

Though more Americans than ever are dropping like flies from cancer, Cancer Inc. — the ACS, the NCI, the industries which turn out toxic chemotherapeutic drugs, major research and treatment centers, the medical discipline of radiology, oncological surgery, the multi-billion-dollar cancer detection and diagnosing business, the animal research industry, special cancer insurance plans, and on and on — has kept assuring the citizenry that the nation's commitment to high technology (gene splicing, monoclonal antibodies, recombinant DNA, etc.) — will lead to the super-tech knockout of the disease. And perhaps it or they will.

But in the meantime, such high-handed rhetoric and bombast are redolent not of any solid achievement in cancer but more of the Vietnam War — with the troops to be home by Christmas, lights constantly appearing at the ends of tunnels, a turnaround in body counts, and all that went with it, before the negative realities set in.

In fact, the oncological revolution is occurring as much from within as without — credentialed "experts" from within the entrails of allopathic medicine can no longer remain silent or passively acquiesce to the propaganda bilge. They are speaking out and breaking ranks, as we shall see.

Some modest gains

Yet, the hype and hoopla of it aside, there *have been* tiny advances against cancer, though hardly matching the billions of dollars committed in 1971 to the "Conquest of Cancer" program of President Nixon, let alone the many more billions spent in private research. Diagnostics and monitoring have improved, though they mostly confirm just how much more cancer there is, and how little it basically responds to therapeutic oncological orthodoxy. The touted gains in five-year survival rates are noticeable in childhood leukemia and Hodgkin's disease, yet these "forms" of cancer hardly comprise more than 2 to 3 percent of total cancer.

Some "forms" of cancer, such as stomach malignancy, seem to have dropped all by themselves (or, some would say, due to the unexpected anti-cancer effects of certain food preservatives in the otherwise highly carcinogenic Western diet), and some "forms" remain highly "curable" if, again, by "cure" one means five years free of symptoms. Such is the case, for example, with most non-melanoma skin cancer, testicular cancer in teenage males, and even early primary breast cancer.

It is the *metastatic*, or easily spread-capable, "forms" of cancer, the killer cancers, which are devastating the Western population, where so little progress has been seen despite however semantics are twisted or rhetoric deployed.

Malignant truth-twisting

As we see throughout the Allopathic Industrial Complex (AIC), the deft manipulation of semantics — tortured language to hide a simple truth — is employed time and time again either consciously (deceit) or, more often, unconsciously (paradigm capture/cognitive dissonance) to obscure realities.

Ah, semantics, semantics — how its twists and turns can be used to obfuscate.

In cancer, we are presented with the only case of a disease in which "cure" means five years free of symptoms. The fact a patient drops dead on the first day of the sixth year leads to the dumbfounding reality that, by this kind of logic, a person can be listed as both "cured" of, yet dead of, cancer at the same time! It is also true that the five-year gold standard has been altered somewhat — in certain "forms" of the disease (particularly among the elderly, whose overall life expectancy is much less anyway) it has been argued that even two or three years without symptoms might be "cures," thus inflating "cure rates."

And, for decades, Cancer Inc. has played fast and loose with arithmetic, giving support to the notion of "rubber" numbers:

By including non-melanoma skin cancers and localized primary tumors whose surgical removal might indeed correlate to five years or more without a recurrence of cancer-related symptoms, and perhaps forgetting that such "forms" of cancer have been "curable" since the days of Hippocrates, Cancer Inc. can, virtually at will, inflate its "cure rate" to lead the American Cancer Society and others to talk about the possibility or even likelihood of "curing" at least "half" of all cancer.

(In the laetrile wars of the 1970s, court testimony by my friend and long-time cancer statistician and physiologist, the late Dr. Hardin B. Jones of the University of California-Berkeley, was introduced which showed that, incredibly enough, if cancer patients were placed into two categories — the treated and the untreated — the latter lived longer and felt better![11])

But such realities have seemingly had little impact on the cancer establishment.

Ponder, for example, the outright gobbledegook issued to explain the perpetual rise in, and failure in the therapeutic control of, adenocarcinoma of the lower gastrointestinal tract — that is, "colorectal cancer," one of the major killers in the United States:

A "consensus conference" of the National Institutes of Health (NIH), the sprawling federal bureaucracy which oversees the NCI, informed one and all in 1990 that "despite the high resectability [*that is, surgical removal*] rate and a general improvement in therapy, nearly half of all patients with colorectal cancer will die of metastatic tumor."[12]

The "general improvement" referred to seemed to be a slight increase in efficacy from toxic chemotherapy, burning radiation and the new component in oncology, immunotherapy, together with improved longevity rates of those who survived initial surgery of a "Stage I" tumor and lived out their normal lifespans. The quality-of-life level of such patients was apparently not measured.

Yet in an intriguing use of linear logic the experts summarized that "patients with Stage III colon cancer or Stage II/III rectal cancer are at a high risk for recurrence and warrant adjuvant therapy."

But, we are informed in the second breath, "optimal adjuvant therapy for Stage II and III colon cancer has not yet been devised" (!) so that "continued clinical trials in this disease are essential to discover more active adjuvant therapies."

In an introduction to the analysis, the experts frankly opined that

> ... over the past three decades, many clinical studies have failed to demonstrate benefits from adjuvant therapy. Claims of efficacy have been viewed with skepticism [although] recently, new data from several studies have demonstrated delays in tumor recurrence and increases in survival for specific groups of patients.[13]

Translating all the extensive verbiage, one is left with a simple overview: orthodox oncology is mostly failing most of the time in metastatic (spread) colorectal cancer. Simply expressing this crude fact in plain English seems to be extremely problematical for the experts.

Lies, damned lies, and statistics

In the past few years, Cancer Inc. has made much of the probably correct statistic (though, as Benjamin Disraeli observed, falsehoods come in three forms — "lies, damned lies, and statistics") that slightly more than 50 percent of cancer victims are surviving their disease more than five years, the odd number by which oncology defines "cure."

The 1991 figure indicating this first important crossover event (50.9% five-year survivals vs. 49.1% years prior) was said to be an indication — however irrelevant — of some kind of payoff for the vast investment in private and public funds to rein in cancer.[14]

Yet, as probing experts have long argued, the increase in five-year survival rates may be viewed as a "statistical artifact" — not as a proof of any real improvement in therapeutics.

This is because improved diagnostics simply move the survival clock backward — a tumor or pre-cancerous condition discovered *earlier* will lengthen the time between diagnosis and death *despite* whatever therapies are employed. Earlier detection hence artificially inflates five-year survival rates which thus artificially sustains Cancer Inc.'s dubious claims to impressive progress against cancer.

In September 1993 the President's Cancer Panel, a top-drawer, blue-ribbon group of individuals supposedly set up as a kind of presidential palace guard to report on "progress" against cancer, convened once again. The mood was — as *Scientific American* reporter Tim Beardsley put it — one of "euphoria" since so many new research breakthroughs and experimental therapies were being talked about (as they had been each year prior).

Then entered the room John C. Bailar III, professor of epidemiology and biostatistics at Canada's McGill University.

Bailar, who seemed constantly unfazed by both cancer euphoria and propaganda, had created a major stir in 1986 by publishing a report on the "Conquest of Cancer" program and finding an utter lack of progress in the pull-out-the-stops effort unleashed in 1971 the American way: hurl enough money at the problem and it will be solved.

This time, he was back for another assessment of the American cancer program. Beardsley recorded it:

> *"In the end, any claim of major success against cancer must be reconciled with this figure,"*

[Bailar] *said, pointing to a simple graph that showed a stark continuing increase in US death rates from cancer between 1950 and 1990. "I do not think such reconciliation is possible and again conclude, as I did seven years ago, that our decades of war against cancer have been a qualified failure. Thank you."*[15]

His numbers had been provided by the NCI itself and they had been adjusted to account for the changing size and age composition of the population, so they could not be blamed on Americans' dying less from other diseases. The statistical extrapolation was chilling: US cancer death rates went up 7 percent between 1975 and 1990 despite all efforts at control and therapy, all statistical and semantical legerdemain, and all the $25 billion expended on the "war on cancer" so far. Dr. Bailar was simply as candid and logically direct in 1993 as he had been in 1986: the "war on cancer" was — is — a "qualified failure."

He and other experts have argued whether nationwide campaigns to detect possible precancerous conditions earlier (mammography for breast, Pap smear for cervical, PSA for prostate) can be said to have precipitated or, paradoxically, *caused* a decline in the reported numbers of such "forms" of cancer.

If one is oncologically oriented — that is, considering cancer to be hundreds of different kinds of tumors — then by 1993 (NCI figures monitored between 1973 and 1990) it could be said that cancer death rates were impressively down for testicular cancer, Hodgkin's disease, cervical and uterine cancer; that they were drastically up in lung cancer (so drastic, in fact, as to offset the combination statistical progress in all other "forms" of cancer), melanoma and other skin cancers, non-Hodgkin's lymphoma, and brain cancer; rates were moderately up for liver, prostate, esophageal, kidney and brain cancer; holding their own in breast and leukemia; and were moderately down in colorectal, mouth and pharynx, thyroid and stomach cancer.[16]

It should be pointed out that these figures antedated estimates of an allegedly mass increase in prostate cancer (primarily because of the PSA test) and sudden surges in breast cancer (the mammography controversy reaching white-hot proportions in 1993/1994), two examples in which it could not truly be determined whether there was vastly more cancer of these "kinds" or simply that they were being detected earlier and in greater numbers.

Shaking up The Club

By any measure, the oncological division of allopathic medicine is that which most reflects the scientific bankruptcy of the allopathic paradigm or mind-set. While the "heart disease" calamity has improved, at least in terms of falling death rates (*X*), and still constitutes, for a time, the number-one killer in the United States and the Western world, it is cancer which is growing either geometrically or exponentially and hence dimming the optimism for standard medicine against chronic disease in general. We will see (*XIII*) that this is even truer, on a so far lesser numerical scale, for the calamity of AIDS.

Yet, ironically, it is precisely because of the failure of oncology, more than any other element, that the entire apparatus of the AIC has been profoundly shaken. It is because of the failure of orthodox oncology that so-called "alternative" medicine, sparked primarily by the laetrile revolution of the 1970s (*XII*), became a major challenge to organized medicine itself and began to work its way into the mind-set of orthodoxy, so much so that by 1993, incredibly enough, there actually was an Office of Alternative Medicine (OAM) established within the federal NIH — something utterly unthinkable a decade prior.

It is because of oncology's manifest failure in the West's most rapidly advancing killer chronic condition that physicians, researchers and observers from within the ranks of the AIC itself have strongly questioned key elements of the American health paradigm, have actually argued that prevention of disease should take priority over treatment, and have observed that promotion of health should be the central target of medicine. In questioning the existing establishment apparatus, such doctors, researchers and observers have unavoidably begun to vindicate, validate and justify decades of practices and observations made by outside-the-pale practitioners and others dismissed by so many for so long as eccentrics at best, quacks at worst.

It is thanks to the cancer disaster and the laetrile revolution it spawned that more interest in dietary aspects of health and disease are now being seriously looked at both from within and without orthodoxy in just a few years' time than ever before in the history of American medicine.

In parallel fashion, the elephantine awkwardness of Cancer Inc. in attempting, often viciously, to suppress "alternative" cancer treatments, and to lie, cheat and obfuscate on the utility of dozens of worthwhile (if often non-allopathic) modalities and techniques against cancer, has helped generate a political freedom-of-choice backlash which is entirely salutary to the health of the republic.

Even so, Cancer Inc. still remains committed to its central premises, probably all of them false, mostly false, or misleading. It is committed because the greed factor is so enmeshed therewith — far more money is made off treating cancer than preventing it, far more people have profited from "looking for the answer" than from finding it, and a cancer patient with metastatic disease (the majority of cancer) may conservatively be said to represent a $100,000 profit — minimally — for organized medicine. Long-term cancer bills into the high six-figure and even low seven-figure range are by no means rare, and in state after state the "oncological surgeon" is often the best paid (sometimes the most egregiously paid) of the "healthcare delivery team." He is trained to cut, wants to cut — so he cuts.

The big business of Cancer Inc.

By any aspect, cancer is big business — and probably bigger by now than the total cardiovascular industry, with no signs of letting up.

Part of its 20 percent take of the trillion-dollar "healthcare delivery cost crisis" still resides in the use and promotion of toxic drugs (chemotherapy) despite an avalanche of credible research questioning just how useful such chemicals are.

Former Sloan-Kettering public affairs officer Ralph Moss PhD, a hero of the laetrile era and since that time an author of two major books exposing the economic side of Cancer Inc., has written and testified that as recently as 1991 cancer drugs brought in $3 billion in profits in the USA annually and that such compounds had a 22 percent growth in "profitability" in a year's time.[17]

We discuss here and elsewhere (*VIII*) the sudden advent of PSA (prostate-specific antigen) screening for prostate cancer, the linchpin of an estimated $28-billion-a-year new industry in this "form" of cancer alone, with no clear evidence that earlier detection (if in fact that is what the PSA provides) leads to a meaningful decline in death rates.

In 1990, a private market research analysis primarily brought to light by Moss in his newsletter[18] gave some indication of just how big the big business of cancer is:

The profit in cancer treatments and devices was estimated in 1989 at $1.03 billion in 1989 with a projection of $1.74 billion in 1993.

Many of the facts and figures were from market researchers Frost & Sullivan and published in an incredibly expensive 641-page report called *Market for Cancer Therapy Products*.

After noting how cancer products and devices had topped $1 billion for the first time in 1989, Frost & Sullivan added that chemotherapy at the time currently had three-quarters of the market share, with radiation second at 17.1 percent. In descending order were hyperthermia techniques, "immunoproteins" and various experimental items. Chemotherapy's share of the cancer pie was projected to drop to 52.3 percent by 1993 and radiation's to 12.3 percent.

These figures suggested astute observation or inside information or both and took into account the rapid rise of immunotherapy through high technology, just beginning to be highly noticeable in the cancer armamentarium:

The market for such synthetic immune boosters as alpha-, beta-, and gamma-interferon, as well as interleukin-2 and tumor necrosis factor (TNF), was expected to jump from a 5.8 percent share of the 1989 market (or $60 million) to a 24.6 percent share (or $428 million) by 1993. "Monoclonal antibody conjugates" were expected to be marketable by 1991 and to command a 9.1 percent market share (or $158 million).

Moss observed:

> ... [T]he market report, not intended for public consumption, is refreshingly candid about radiation and chemotherapy's drawbacks, such as "lack of specificity, with adverse side effects caused by damage to normal cells and tissue." Radiation equipment is "extremely expensive, and sales at present are suffering from cost containment pressure," the study says.[19]

It should be recalled that various interleukins and interferons were rushed onto the market in the late 1980s and early 1990s with great fanfare amid hopes that each would constitute the breakthrough, the big payoff in biomedical high technology which would win the "war on cancer." As of this writing, all had failed to do so.

In terms of breast cancer, a summer 1993 US Office of Technology Assessment (OTA) *Washington Post* survey found[20] that annual manual breast cancer screening for all women between 55 and 65 meant a $15,500 "net cost" per woman for every one-year extension of life, and that if mammograms (specialized X-rays of the breast) were added to the same age group, the "incremental cost" per year of life extension per woman was $84,000 — and this, based on 1988 data.

It should be pointed out that mammograms are at the root of a decades-old controversy pitting various parts of Cancer Inc. against each other. Early suggestions were that mammograms might cause as many cancers as they detected, and that their track record in detecting early cancers was not all that confidence-building to start with.

By 1993, the NCI, long dominated by the ACS, had split with the latter on the need for annual mammograms in women between age 40 and 50.[21] The American Cancer Society had for years made the pushing of mammograms one of its major public relations campaigns, on a par with its attack on the tobacco industry.

(A central ACS/NCI excuse for runaway increases in lung cancer, particularly among women, has been laid at the door of the American tobacco industry, with the implied argument that if all cigarettes could be banned lung cancer rates would plummet and this would greatly enhance cancer survival statistics. Usually not discussed is the nettling reality that in some other countries, higher rates of cigarette smoking — as in Japan — do not correlate with higher rates of lung cancer. This is not a defense of cigarette smoking, so replete with pathological perils, but it is a suggestion that Cancer Inc. has often used the tobacco industry as a convenient scapegoat to excuse its own failures.)

And more test traps

The same *Post/OTA* survey also found that Pap smears for cervical cancer conducted every three years for women aged 20 to 75 cost about $13,300 for every year of life saved and that if done annually resulted in an "incremental cost" of $1 million per each additional "life-year" saved.[22]

In 1993, a medical journal report of a six-year observation of 1,017 post-surgical colorectal cancer patients found[23] that monitoring through the CEA (carcinoembryonic antigen) test not only had identified only 39 percent of recurrences (that is, a failure rate of 61 percent) while finding "elevated CEA levels" in 16 percent of cases in whom *no* recurrence was found — but that the financial costs were significant.

In an editorial note in the *Journal of the American Medical Assn. (JAMA)*, Robert H. Fletcher MD observed that the financial costs of CEA monitoring are "considerable — almost $500,000 per possible cure . . . and perhaps much higher."[24]

There remains, thus, a huge business in cancer screening programs let alone the costs of "managing" cancer once the unlucky victim enters the "medical loop," from which he will be fortunate to escape without coming out feet first, particularly if he has "metastatic disease" (spread cancer).

For it is in the "spread cancer" cases where so little meaningful progress has been made, and which has led to an all-out attack on standard cancer therapies even by allopathic experts themselves, many of whom have no truck with "alternatives" and would not be caught —er—dead using or recommending apricot seed extract (laetrile) or Vitamin C.

The roots of illogic

Currently, the "big three" — some call it the Terrible Triad — of American (and therefore, Western) oncological treatments remain "cut, burn, poison" — surgery, radiation, chemotherapy. These three are based on the ancient observation that the tumor *is* the disease. In fact, the spread of surface tumors over the body in a shape approximating that of the crab led to the Latin definition of the disease — *cancrum*, or crab. It was an understandable mistake to believe that if the "crab" could be cut off or burned away by fire (the actual conceptual basis of surgery and radiation in the twentieth century), and if the patient seemed to survive either treatment for a credible amount of time, that this was the way to "cure" the disease.

This physical observation was enhanced by the 17th-century guiding notions of allopathy (the Cartesian-Newtonian postulates) as they related to what would later become "the scientific method" and to the overall paradigm of allopathy itself — cancer, whether conceived of as a single wayward cell or a tumor or a swollen spleen or any number of aberrations in elements of serum — is an externally produced disease "caused" by a thing or things; therefore the answer is to kill or block those things. If the disease is mistaken for its most notorious symptom, the tumor, as it usually is, the "cure" means getting rid of the tumor. After microbiology and high-resolution microscopy entered the field in the twentieth century, a parallel goal became somehow getting rid of every last cancer cell in the body — a feat more likely to be accomplished with a Smith and Wesson (through total extinction of the host) than through the ministrations of cut-burn-and-poison.

Treatments worse than the disease

Perhaps the factors which most militate against the "big three" cancer treatments are their ancillary effects — they range from being painfully disfiguring to producing nausea, hair loss, skin lesions, liver and other internal damage, and at one point or another depress immune functions, sometimes profoundly so. It has long been a common observation that while toxic chemicals might indeed attack or slow down the advance of cancer cells, the corollary damage done to host defense is such that simple infections which might otherwise have been held in check or stopped outright are now killing the patient, despite the condition of his tumor or tumors.

As an information officer for a south-of-the-border hospital specializing in cancer, I was visually exposed to hundreds of cases in which it was horribly clear that the damage done to the patient (internal organs literally cooked with radiation, for example; botched surgeries which had done irreparable harm to the body) in the name of "treatment" had been worse than the disease process itself. I heard to the point of exhaustion horror stories of patients sickened and terrified even by the prospect of one more round of "chemo" or one more assault by X-rays, and I could assess by the 1990s that I had heard literally hundreds of patients state that they preferred death or no more treatment to being further subjected to medical orthodoxy.

As a California pathologist friend told me (and I have heard similar estimates elsewhere): "Half the bodies I autopsy are of cancer patients. And half of these were killed by chemotherapy." When I inquired, "Will you go public with that?" the response was, "Of course not. I'm in the AMA."

Death due to the *treatment* of cancer is not routinely

mentioned on a death certificate, even though death due to "complications of" cancer may be.

Until the 1990s, hardly any meaningful method had been devised — or could be, due to the lack of randomized, crossover, placebo-controlled, double-blinded studies demanded in the interest of "the scientific method" — to attempt to measure the *subjective* effects on the patient of cancer therapy. *Objective* evaluations could indeed measure shrinking tumor masses, more normalizing white-cell counts, better ranges of platelets and hemoglobin, more normalizing spleens. But since there was no way to truly measure how the patient was faring subjectively, the question of greatest importance to the multiply assaulted cancer patient remained that held to be the least "scientific" of all — *how do you feel?*

The rapid growth of so-called nutritional/metabolic approaches to cancer was due as much to the fact that, as a group, cancer patients simply *felt better* under such therapies as it was to claimed miracle successes of such treatments or even the ever-more-noticeable failures of orthodoxy.

"Quality of life" became a very real, very palpable element for consideration among cancer patients. I am personally aware of hundreds of cases in which, even though the advanced cancer patients eventually expired due to some complication of their disease, they felt their involvement with "alternative" therapies of a nutritional nature, so intrinsically benign, had literally made all the difference in the world. For the first time they had less or no pain, had recovered much of their appetite, had more energy; some had been able to go back to school or work for extended periods of time. But these were "non-quantifiable" elements to Cancer Inc., "subjective responses" somehow hypnotized into the unwitting cancer patient by "quacks" who were applying "unproven" or "dubious" or "unscientific" modalities.

From microbes to viruses to genes

As cancer incidence exploded in the USA and the Western world, allopathy's obsession with "causes" shifted from the more generic "microbes" to the "new kids on the block" — viruses — and it was preached for a long time, and in some cases still is, that viruses "cause" cancer. Part of this allopathic assumption lies in the confusion between correlation and causation — because certain viruses *do* seem to correlate with certain "kinds" of cancer, it is a linear allopathic leap of faith to conclude that this correlation implies a causation. (A Texas medic puckishly put this line of thinking to me this way, as it related to the obsessive notion that a single virus "causes" all of AIDS: broken twigs in the barnyard absolutely correlate 100 percent with a tornado, but only virologists might argue that the broken twigs actually *caused* the tornado. But such is the allopathic thought process.)

By the late 1980s and early 1990s, while viruses were still uppermost on the list of suspects in cancer causation, advances in genetic research began to accord genes — these tiniest of all little sacks of replicatory information and even tinier than viruses (though at the submicroscopic level, actual mass recedes in importance) — an increasing role in "causing" cancer, either on their own or through mutation or absence of the same. Hence the rise of *oncogenes* (literally, bump-genes).

Under current genetic theory, an unknown number of genetic events is implicated in causing a normal cell to turn into a cancer cell. Involved are various genes which may seemingly induce or suppress the chain of events leading to the conversion of a cell to its primitive cancerous state. Some initiating event or events will somehow alter a gene in the chromosome within the nucleus of a normal cell as step one in the process.

From here on, ideas get somewhat murky: some of these "altered" or "mutated" genes are the real culprits; in some cases, the *absence* of certain genes is considered to be key.

By mid-1994, as highly funded genetic research blossomed across the biomedical horizon with the same rapidity that had marked viral research earlier, two different research teams claimed to find that a loss of a "suppressor" gene variously called p16 and MTS1 was "detected" in 60 percent of breast cancer cases, 82 percent of one "type" of brain cancer, and might play a role in many other "forms" and "types" of the disease. Thus, they seemed to be replacing in importance the recently discovered p53 gene which had been thought by some to be the genetic *sine qua non* of cancer induction.[25]

Experts were not of one mind in claiming that the absence of these "suppressor" genes directly caused cancer (though some believe they do) but they, and other newly found genes, seemed to be proof of why at least hereditary cancers — cancers that "run in families" — might occur.

Just as decades earlier biomedical high technology pursued the viral cause, the ever-more-expanded biomedical high technology now pursues the genetic cause — and that is where the lion's share of cancer research is directed, at least as of the middle of this decade.

But, as usual, the devil is in the details, exceptions — and defectors from the research establishment.

First, one of the "fathers" of retrovirology and "discoverer" of oncogenes, Berkeley molecular biologist Peter H. Duesberg PhD — perhaps better known as a heretic against the theory of AIDS causation by a "new" retrovirus (*XIII*) — has stated plainly:

> *There is still no proof that activated proto-oncogenes are sufficient or even necessary to cause cancer.*[26]

It is Duesberg who, more than any other, has forced the AIC to ponder the chasm between correlations and causes — be it of viruses in AIDS or oncogenes in cancer.

In 1994, Gerald B. Dermer PhD, long-time cancer researcher (cell biologist turned cancer pathologist), ripped into the high-technology American cancer research establishment on many fronts in a book:

> *. . . There is absolutely no evidence from observations of human tumors to indicate that the mutation of any proto-oncogene is essential for any cancer . . . The evolution of the viral theory of*

cancer into the oncogene theory of cancer is a classic example of how the cancer establishment manages to preserve its image even in the face of evidence that refutes its doctrines and favorite models. [27]

Dr. Dermer was not saying there is no role for genes in cancer (particularly in the seemingly "inherited" childhood cancers) — but he argued strongly that the research establishment was pinning its hopes for the conquest of cancer on a series of catastrophic scientific miscues — one of the most notorious being reliance on "immortal cell lines" synthetically developed in petri dishes. He found such reliance essentially devoid of honest-to-God science, but nonetheless a fad (along with the earlier obsession with viruses and various forms of high-tech immunotherapy) helping to keep nourishing a $100 billion governmental-academic-medical-industrial complex which has developed around cancer research and treatment and whose "heart" is the National Cancer Institute (NCI).

Reliance on petri dish-produced "unnatural cells as a model for the human disease has been directly responsible for our ongoing defeat," he wrote. "These cultures . . . give incorrect and clinically useless information about cancer."

As a victim of the system itself, he noted that

Research proposals that do not conform to the status quo are deemed invalid and left unfunded. Papers that openly criticize the reigning model rarely see the light of day on journal pages. By controlling the purse strings, the cancer establishment also controls the direction of all cancer research, crowding out innovation and real advancement in favor of the status quo. In essence, the system rewards mediocrity instead of excellence. [28]

The biomedical high-technology pursuit of genes as underlying disease itself was in full flower by the middle of the decade, and several had been found to be possible "causes" of several diseases.

With ethics now entering the picture (if refined new tests can detect aberrant genes which are expected to *cause* a disease, should the carrier be treated even in the absence of symptoms and/or should couples sharing the trait be denied marriage or procreation because they will surely "pass it on"?) some sober minds must be heard.

One of them belongs to University of Michigan geneticist Dr. Charles Sing, who told *Newsweek*:

"What is a good gene and what is a bad gene depend on how you treat it. Genes don't wake up until they are exposed to some environmental factor ... We're overselling. We're not going to be able to deliver [on promises to predict and prevent disease.] *We're being dishonest."*[29]

As one gene after another appears in research labs as the "cause" of something, the same unanswered question about so many viruses continues to be raised a decibel or two: is correlation causation? Inquiring medical integrationists want to know.

In 1994, the National Institutes of Health's National Advisory Council for Human Genome Research — overseer of an ambitious project aimed at "mapping" each and every gene in the body — warned against going overboard about genetic testing.

In a statement, the council noted that "it is premature to offer testing of either high-risk families or the general population as part of general medical practice until a series of crucial questions has been addressed."[30]

This was a sobering recommendation to stop and look before leaping and bring some sanity to the obsession:

Without doubt, genes have a role to play in disease induction — but are they central causes or machinery through which true causes are mediated?

Our own research group proposed "the primordial thesis of cancer" as a unitarian concept of malignancy — that is, cancer can be described more than anything as the reversion of a normal, aerobic (oxygen-using) cell to the most primitive, genetically "remembered" life form on the planet, an *anaerobic* (non-oxygen-using, acid-oriented) cell. This process assuredly involves a series of repressing and de-repressing genetic events. A true *cause* of cancer would be that which sets this chain of events into play; a true *cure* of it would be that which prevents such a chain of events.[31]

In this particular view, the "environmental factor" — or factors — which might directly or indirectly influence a cell to begin its genetic reversion are the culprits. And there are many of them — carcinogenic chemicals, radiation, for example — but, as we shall see, the central element is almost certainly nutrition (excesses and deficiencies).

As we also shall see, even cancer orthodoxy itself is now according vastly more importance to lifestyle and diet as "causes" of cancer, the most salutary developments to come out of the oncological disaster.

But in the meantime, American oncology, by its nature, training and persuasion, remains committed to the Terrible Triad in attempting to "cure" the disorder. In the last decade or so, the advent of immunology/immunotherapy has provided oncology with a fourth leg. Up to now it has largely meant highly expensive and potentially toxic manufactured proteins aimed at manipulating human immunity since most of organized allopathy, blinders on, does not like to admit the flood-proportion biochemical research data and massive empiricism attributing immune-boosting and immune-modulating properties, let alone anti-carcinogenic effects, to an ever-growing range of naturally-occurring nutrients.

Indeed, nothing seems to be more viscerally terrifying to Cancer Inc. than the concept that cancer can be treated by unpatentable, natural nutrients — unless it is the more sweeping concept that cancer can largely be *prevented* by the same, thus bringing to an end a $200 billion element in the nation's "healthcare delivery cost crisis."

A litany of failure and disaster
But what of the "standard" or "accepted" or "scientifically

proven" therapies?

— In 1989 and 1990, information gathered or published by the medical establishment itself was so negative to chemotherapy (including synthetic hormones) and radiation that in some quarters there was raised the question of just how much longer chemotherapy would still be around. This was not only because of the lack of very much efficacy from such toxic compounds but the ever-more-obvious fact they helped *increase* the likelihood of cancer.

A *New England Journal of Medicine* study, for example, found[32] that the administration of chemotherapy for Hodgkin's disease and ovarian cancer enhanced the chances of leukemia developing later. The same learned journal had reported a year earlier that the use of X-rays during infancy significantly increased women's chances of developing breast cancer when they reached their 30s.

— The US General Accounting Office (GAO) found in 1989 that despite an increase in the US of chemotherapy since 1975 there had been no detectable increase in survival rates in breast cancer and that "the benefits of chemotherapy are small and therefore difficult to detect."[33]

— Leading surgeons, sharply challenging the NCI, argued[34] in 1989 that women with breast cancer should not necessarily undergo chemotherapy, with one stating that for many cancer patients "high costs and side effects probably outweigh the benefits" of the toxic drugs.

(It should be pointed out that, despite the appearance of a united front of surgeons, chemotherapists and radiologists against the "cancer quacks," many of whom believe cancer can largely be prevented let alone managed by nutritional factors, the three schools in private often detest each other with the vigor of Yale vs. Harvard. Surgeons, who were first on the scene as virtually the sole managers of cancer — even engaging in a ghastly technique called the "hemicorporectomy" [cutting the body in half to halt advancing tumors] in the 19th century — felt threatened first by the radium industry early in this century [with its insistence on burning out, rather than cutting off, tumors] and, decades later, by the chemotherapists, who believed cancer could be poisoned away.)

— A Swedish/NCI study concluded[35] that long-term treatment with estrogen (female hormones or their artificial analogues) seemed to be associated with an increased risk of breast cancer.

— By 1990, the "war on cancer" had a new skipper, Dr. Samuel Broder, and at a cancer treatment conference in Tucson he was blunt about the campaign: since declaration of the "war" in 1971, overall cancer incidence had risen by 14 percent and the death rate had gone up by more than 5 percent, he said.

"There are several [cancer] diseases [in which] by any measure there has been inadequate or no progress — areas where we have gotten nowhere," he forthrightly stated.[36]

A Bristol Myers Co. cancer researcher was equally on-target: "The process of drug discovery and drug development over the past 20 years has had very little effect on the evolution of drug treatments. The progress has been very slow, and our strategies may need re-evaluation," he said.[37]

By 1991, the utility of chemotherapy was attacked head-on in *The Lancet* by Albert S. Braverman MD, division of hematology-oncology, Division of Medicine, Health Sciences Center of the University of New York at Brooklyn, who wrote:

> *. . . The time has come to cut back on the clinical investigation of new chemotherapeutic regimens for cancer and to cast a critical eye on the way chemotherapeutic treatment is now administered . . . No disseminated neoplasm [cancer] incurable in 1975 is curable today . . . Many medical oncologists recommend chemotherapy for virtually any tumor, with a hopefulness undiscouraged by almost invariable failure . . . The oncology community should respond to the data of the past decade by scaling back the whole chemotherapeutic enterprise. Chemotherapy should be prescribed only when there is a reasonable prospect either of cure or benefit in quantity and quality of life.*[38]

Earlier that year, an *Annals of Internal Medicine* had reported[39] on Italian studies showing that three chemotherapeutic drugs given in breast cancer might lead to esophageal cancer later, and American research on leukemia therapy published in the *New England Journal of Medicine* showed that treatments with the chemotherapy agent doxorubicin could result in "clinically important heart disease in later years" through "progressive increase in left ventricular afterload."[40]

The same year, data gathered by the National Academy of Sciences (NAS) and the ACS found[41] a surge in breast cancer — now it was said to affect 1 out of 9 instead of 1 out of 10 women, while rates of lung cancer, melanoma, multiple myeloma, brain and central nervous system cancers were up across the Western world, with no downturns in sight and no appreciable impact made by therapy.

The same year, Heidelberg cancer biostatistician Ulrich Abel unleashed through the widely distributed German magazine *Der Spiegel* another roundhouse attack on chemotherapy.

Abstracted from his 1990 data, Abel insisted:

> ... *[T]here is no evidence for the majority of cancers that treatment with these* [chemotherapeutic] *drugs exerts any positive influence on survival or quality of life in patients with advanced disease . . . The almost dogmatic belief in the efficacy of* [chemotherapy] *is usually based on false conclusions and inappropriate data . . . Ten years of activity as a statistician in clinical oncology . . . and a . . . sobering and unprejudiced analysis of the literature have rarely revealed any therapeutic success by the regimens in question. . .*[42]

He also hit oncology in its tenderest of concepts:

Contrary to standard oncological thought, he added, "reduction of tumor mass does not prolong expected survival."

(Here was an appropriately credentialed attack on a concept at least off-handedly suggested by oncologists to their patients — that somehow there is a correlation between what happens to the tumor [did it go "up" or "down"?] and their life expectancy. The major proponent of laetrile long called this, correctly, "the false criterion of tumefaction.")

1991 was also the year when the NCI released the startling news that "secondary" cancer was on the rise, primarily because of the success of "cures" for "primary" cancer — again, a twist of semantics that left honest minds groping to make sense of it all:

An NCI survey showed[43] that 1 out of 8 cancer-stricken, orthodoxy-treated children would develop "secondary" cancer within 25 years, and that for Hodgkin's patients the risk of developing a "secondary" cancer in 15 years was greater than 1 in 6. It hence argued that chemotherapy and radiation, "treatments of choice," increased the risks of cancer later.

This was not a surprise to many researchers, since virtually every toxic chemotherapy drug on the market had been shown, or suggested, as a cause of cancer in animal tests (assays of dubious validity, to be sure) and, even in humans, were suspected of inducing cancer unless carefully monitored.

In 1993, the NCI had new data on a five-year followup of 1,100 cancer survivors:[44]

While more children were surviving the disease, many faced learning disabilities, memory loss and even stunted growth and possibly heart failure because of the aggressive chemotherapy and radiation which had ostensibly "cured" their malignancies.

Radiation came in for some of the worst criticism since, as Dr. Paula Lemper, director of the Late Effects Clinic at Children's Hospital, Orange CA, put it: "we used to radiate everyone" as a precautionary measure but "now we radiate the heads of only 20 to 25 percent of child cancer patients."[45]

The most damaged survivors are still those who had radiation to the brain.

The NCI data also parenthetically raised the issue: *is* there "secondary" cancer, or simply a continuation of the underlying malignant process which has either been slowed — or exacerbated — by aggressive treatment of childhood tumors? Even so, the fact that children who might have died faster in an earlier era were surviving long enough to develop "secondary" cancer later was, in its own strange way, a net plus for cancer orthodoxy.

Belling the cat

By 1992, unquestionably the cancer establishment's primary failure-baiter was Dr. Samuel Epstein, professor at the University of Illinois School of Public Health and author of a major book *(The Politics of Cancer)*, which belled the cat, at least partially.

In a Feb. 4, 1992, press conference in Washington, Dr. Epstein and 65 other American cancer experts in an open statement denounced the US cancer establishment, claiming that it had "misled and confused the public and congress" by continually claiming significant progress against the disease.[46]

Epstein told the media that "the public has been hoodwinked" and that "Congress was sold a bill of goods by the cancer establishment. 'Give us the money,' they said, 'and we'll cure cancer.' Congress was bulldozed into funding massive amounts for supposed 'cancer cures.'"

Earlier, in *USA Today*, Dr. Epstein was even more explicit:

> This *"cancer establishment" pushes highly toxic and expensive drugs, patented by major pharmaceutical firms which also have close links to cancer centers. Is it any wonder they refuse to investigate innovative approaches developed outside their own institutions? . . .
>
> We clearly need a complete restructuring of the losing war against cancer. Prevention must get the highest priority . . . Until then, Congress must refuse to fund NCI and the public should boycott the bloated American Cancer Society.*[47]

Dr. Epstein's long-time battle has been to convince the public that it is cancer-causing industrial and agricultural chemicals (carcinogens) far more than smoking and dietary fat which are linked to rapidly rising cancer rates in the West.

(Which of course pits two branches of the cancer research community against each other: those who generally downplay the role of industrial, synthetic chemicals in the environment and those who, like Epstein, believe they may be paramount.

(The widespread chemicalization of not only the food supply but practically everything else in the environment strongly correlates to the plague of man-made or man-altered "modern" disease conditions which have in common profound dysregulation of the immune system(s) — see *XIII*. Whether chemicalization leads to cancer is a less important question than is the reality that such chemicals, to which we are continually, consistently, and *cumulatively* exposed, *do* correlate with chronic disease conditions across the board. The record is clear: industry absolutely does not want to have such connections looked at too closely, and therefore is happier with the conclusion that dietary problems and too many cigarettes are more to be blamed.

(When researchers many of whose grants directly or indirectly come from one or more wings of vested interests — be they the food industry, the drug industry, the chemical industry, the power industry — pontificate on any of these connections to, say, cancer, it is always appropriate to wonder how objective the data really are. The interplay between vested interests does *not*, however, necessarily mean that research with which such interests are somehow involved is bereft of meaningful contributions to our knowledge about cancer.)

In the *Washington Post*, Epstein added:

> *While explaining away soaring cancer rates, the establishment, abetted by cheerleading science journalists, grossly exaggerates treatment successes. Periodic announcements of dramatic advances are based on initial reduction in tumor size rather than on prolonged survival. For most cancers, survival has not changed for decades. Contrary claims are based on rubber numbers.*

> *Furthermore, the establishment is financially interlocked with giant pharmaceutical companies (grossing $1 billion annually in cancer drug sales), with inherent conflicts of interest...*[47]

The General Accounting Office (GAO) was back in the news in 1992 with a cold assessment that "there have been no gains in preventing breast cancer over the past two decades, and its relentless rise, primarily among American women, cannot be explained on the basis of earlier diagnostics."[48]

Word games and cognitive dissonance

None of the above should suggest that American cancer orthodoxy always fails: there *are* cases of long-term survival through the cut-burn-poison approach to advanced cancer, just as there increasingly are cases of long-term survival *without* such approaches — the institutional difference is that the former successes are called "statistics" and the latter are dismissed as "anecdotes."

This has been a standard technique for downplaying seeming cancer victories by an ever-growing list of "unproven" or "unscientific" modalities, and it has always run this way:

If a patient with advanced cancer (meaning spread from one site to another) seems to be doing very well on an "unorthodox" program, and is approaching, or bypassing, the five-year survival rate ("cure"), then one of three things must be true —

• He was either misdiagnosed (lack of a "histopathologically confirmed" tumor) by his standard or orthodox physician, let alone by the "quack" now claiming victory or

• He was somehow belatedly responding to earlier "orthodox" therapy even though the failure on same is what probably led him to the "unorthodox" practitioner in the first place; or

• Should he be a "virgin case" — that is, cancer confirmed by an "accepted" cancer research facility but *no* orthodox therapy having been done — it must be a clear case of "spontaneous remission." This is a religious term which would normally have no place in "science" except for orthodoxy's urgent need to sweep away every last crumb of doubt.

As we argue throughout, the "spontaneous remission" argument is generally not deceitful or of malicious intent but rather a reflection of what psychologically may be called *negative cognitive dissonance* — inability or unwillingness of the observer to process unwanted or startling new information. The new information in this case would be, for example, that laetrile, proteolytic enzymes, various vitamins and diet seemed to have clinically eradicated an obvious case of cancer. The mental mechanism is: since what seems to have occurred cannot possibly have occurred (because "quack" therapies do not work), then what did occur really did not occur — the answer must lie elsewhere.

(I am reminded of a case south of the border in which an American gentleman from an Eastern city seemed to be doing spectacularly well on an all-natural program with an advanced "form" of cancer [mesothelioma] which medical orthodoxy has never "cured." He came to the Mexican hospital with a confirmed diagnosis by a well-known cancer expert. His prognosis, by orthodoxy, was a few weeks to live at most. Upon his return home, his original doctor was so startled to see him in such seemingly good condition that he pondered the most self-deprecating reality of all for a physician — perhaps he had made a diagnostic mistake. Searching through medical tomes to find some pathology which seemed to match the symptomatology of advanced mesothelioma, he hit upon a rare tropical disease, and announced that this might very well have been what the man had had. The fact the gentleman had never been in the tropics was only an irritant to this workout in a form of cognitive dissonance.)

When any of the above arguments do not work, then it is easy for orthodoxy to point to some orthodox component of a total integrative program (for example, a synthetic hormone suppressor administered along with vitamins, minerals, enzymes, fatty acids, laetrile and diet in prostatic cancer) and explain the good success thanks exclusively to the hormone suppressor. Conversely, should the patient *not* be doing well on the same program, hormone suppressor and all, failure can then be attributed to the "useless" metabolic therapy.

This form of brain-scrubbing is of course more successful when those who control the information and research channels in the cancer industry have the greater access — as they do — to the media.

As we explore in the discussion on heart disease (*X*), among cardiology's various failings have not only been inappropriate or even dangerous therapies which frequently either fail or otherwise harm the patient — the diagnostics alone leave a great deal to be desired.

So it is for cancer.

Keeping abreast of a scandal

The decades-old controversy over mammograms for breast cancer reached critical mass in 1993, when, as mentioned, the NCI, splitting with the ACS, declined to advise women in their 40s to have mammograms every year, as recommended by the Society. At an earlier time, there were suggestions that women even younger have annual or biannual trips to the mammogram specialist — the only "sure" way to find the tiniest of mammary malignancies before they became problematical. The ACS had made promotion of the same (at between $50 and $150 per imaging) a major public relations effort for decades.

In 1992, a Canadian study of 90,000 women at 15 hospitals conducted by the University of Toronto failed to find that women between 40 and 49 received any benefit from the technique.[49] By 1993, analyses of new data from around the world supported the Canadian findings.

The *Lancet* editorialized:

There are no reliable data to suggest that screening [mammograms] *reduces mortality in the youngest or* oldest [author's emphasis] *age groups, so this leaves us with a 30 percent or so reduction in breast cancer specific mortality for the middle group.*

Even a 30 percent reduction in the relative risk of relapse or death following local treatment of breast cancer, important though this may be in public health terms for so common a disease, still means that most patients with clinically overt breast cancer still will die of their metastases if followed for long enough...

So, if we acknowledge the failures of primary therapy and secondary intervention, our frustrated attempts at primary intervention, and the true increasing incidence of the disease, we should not be surprised by the static overall mortality from carcinoma of the breast.[50]

In 1994, the Canadians were back in cancer news again with research indicating that the mammogram procedure itself — the painful squeezing of the breast into a kind of vise whereby it can be properly "scanned" — is so traumatic to the mammary tissues that it can induce the spread of cancer on its own.[51]

(As we shall shortly see, the mammogram element in breast cancer is but the tiniest tip of a massive iceberg involving radiation scandals galore, and the controversy is far from over.)

More worthless tests

At about the same time, Mayo Clinic researchers were reporting that the widely used screening test for colon cancer, the Hemoccult test (which checks for cancer in the stool) was practically worthless: a three-year study of 13,000 patients showed it missed more than 70 percent of colorectal cancers that were later diagnosed through X-rays or colonoscopic examination. Blood in the stool equated with cancer less than 10 percent of the time.[52] Two months later, a 13-year University of Minnesota survey of 46,000 people reached contrary conclusions and said the test had reduced colon cancer deaths by 33 percent.[53]

And the earlier-mentioned 1993 Moertel study on CEA monitoring of post-surgical colorectal cancer not only found this long-used assay to be mostly irrelevant, as well as expensive, but in an editorial which accompanied the study's release, Robert H. Fletcher MD noted:

> *But it is not just a matter of money. There is also the inconvenience and discomfort of repeated blood tests, worry over what the result may be, extra surgery, and knowing about recurrence of cancer earlier than one would ordinarily, even though many of these patients cannot be cured. I am skeptical that the benefits outweigh the costs, all things considered.*[54]

The great PSA caper

The taker of the cake in terms of relevance of screening, however, was the launching with fanfare (*VIII*) of the PSA (prostate-specific antigen) test to detect prostate cancer in men.

Since the age levels of men thought to be incubating possible or probable prostate cancer keeps ranging downward — to around age 50 — the use of a test which could detect the tiniest "marker protein" for the disease should ideally alert middle-aged men to what might be upcoming. (It naturally also increases the market for PSA tests). It was already generally known, at least in North America, Australia, New Zealand and much of northern and western Europe, that if a man lived long enough, he would surely develop prostate cancer. This was not true, of course, for males in many other societies, many of whom lived as long or longer than Western males.

But the development of yet another new test with a new number to be worried about posed the most serious of dilemmas:

Since there had been no meaningful improvements in prostate cancer therapies, and they ranged from the more mutilating orchiectomies, castration and complete prostatectomies to the less destructive but unpredictable and far from risk-free TURP (trans-urethral resection of the prostate), as well as radiation and application of female hormones, and often would be followed by impotence, incontinence or both, the question remained:

Why would a middle-aged to elderly man really want to know if he had the problem when its "management" was so devastating and results so uncertain, and when it was also not at all clear that simply "having" prostate CA would necessarily be much of a problem, particularly if the growth were confined to the prostate?

By 1992, the Sacramento *Bee* could synthesize the prostate cancer mishmash thus:

> *Physicians treating prostate cancer face an unusual medical problem: 40 percent of [American men] have prostate cancer but only 10 percent are diagnosed. And while 3 percent of American men will die of prostate cancer, most of those who have the disease never know it and are not affected by it.* [55]

Some studies had already shown that, particularly due to the advanced age of men with diagnosed prostatic cancer, survival outcomes were not much influenced, if at all, by therapy. And some research showed no treatment at all to be just as good.

In a key study, Swedish researchers following a group of 200 men whose prostate cancer remained localized in the prostate gland, which was initially left untreated, found[56] that (a) only 8.5 percent had died of prostate cancer after 10 years while (b) almost half died of some other cause during the time of the study, and (c) of a subset of men who 10 years earlier had met current standards for radical prostate surgery but did not receive it, the survival rate was an impressive *88 percent*.

H. Ballantine Carter, author of a Johns Hopkins study, opined:

> *The bottom line is, we don't know which patients are going to get into trouble from the disease. It's very, very difficult to tell a patient he may do just as well without any treatment, but we can't assure him of that.* [57]

And, added Dr. John Wasson, who participated in two studies whose results were published in 1993: "We have, in essence, an epidemic of treatment and no scientific proof that it's valid."[58]

Seemingly throwing up their hands over all of this, some researchers were ready, by 1994, to suggest "watchful waiting" (also known as "expectant observation") in men with diagnosed prostate cancer.

In yet another report, this one a survey of six separate studies of early-stage prostate CA in 828 men, University of Chicago surgeon Gerald Chodak claimed[59] that the analysis "shows that watchful waiting is a reasonable option."

In late 1994 the FDA licensed Eli Lilly's Hybritech unit to make PSA prostate cancer screening tests available. The federal agency thus approved the test kits for the actual detection of cancer (they had been accepted as monitors of the disease and as detectors of the BPH condition before.) Approval followed on the heels of the FDA's agreeing that PSAs could be used for detection — but only in combination with the vintage digital examination. Despite the fanfare, the FDA's Susan Alpert noted that both tests had a "combination predictive value" of about 50 percent — meaning they could miss prostate cancer half the time![60]

No sooner had the FDA approvals been announced than a University of Toronto study claimed that "screening for prostate cancer cannot be justified as a rational health policy" and that mass PSA screening would cost anywhere from $113,000 to $729,000 in doctor, hospital and other bills simply to gain one year of life-expectancy from early treatment, while lowering the quality of life for many men.[61]

But, since the PSA had already been estimated (*VIII*) as the linchpin of a new $28 billion per year industry, the new figures seemed unlikely to deter Cancer Inc.

And now, drugs as preventives!

True to allopathic linear logic, the oncological establishment through the NCI by 1993 had launched two programs involving synthetic drugs (neither free of possible side effects) in order to *prevent* breast cancer and prostate cancer in otherwise healthy people.

Tamoxifen, considered useful in breast cancer, was being tested for five years on 16,000 randomly selected healthy women thought to be at some kind of higher risk for the disease, to see if the synthetic hormone would prevent the disease. Should the tests check out, women would be advised to stay on tamoxifen (at $3.60 per day) *for the rest of their lives.* The Women's Health Network found the effort "a perversion of women's health."[62,63]

And the NCI began a 10-year, $60 million assessment of finasteride (Proscar), which had already shown some utility against the most common (and non-malignant) form of male prostate problems, BPH (benign prostatic hypertrophy), to see if it could prevent prostate cancer.[64]

Both notions are allopathic thinking writ large.

It is essential to bear in mind that even as orthodox oncology was running up the white flag in breast cancer and was baffled over what to do about prostate and to some extent colon cancer, and while the use of potentially toxic synthetic drugs as preventives was being catapulted into taxpayer-subsidized research, information was pouring in linking fatty diets to cancer in general and to various vitamins as well as (of all things) aspirin to prevention of various "forms" of the disease. A race between biological wisdom and drug company profits had thus broken out, with the cancer-stricken public caught in between.

Tamoxifen ran into trouble almost from the start — as plans for its preventive use moved ahead in the USA and Canada and as similar trials were about to begin in the United Kingdom, Australia and Italy, a thorough review of the extant literature by Adriane Fugh-Berman and Samuel Epstein found links between the drug, a synthetic steroid, and endometrial cancer, retinopathy, clot-forming events, liver problems and menopausal symptoms.[65,66]

Claiming widespread use of the compound constituted not so much disease prevention as disease substitution, they argued:

Tamoxifen is too dangerous to use in healthy women. The Breast Cancer Prevention Trial, by accepting the concept of disease substitution in place of disease prevention, sets a dangerous precedent in public health research. The priorities of the cancer establishment need fundamental reform . . . [67]

British researchers also found cause for concern.[68]

Perhaps even more ominously, it became clear in 1994 (as Cox News Service reported[69]) that in 1992 the Food and Drug Administration (FDA) had dismissed warnings from one of its own safety officers that women taking part in the tamoxifen trial were being misled about the risks of taking daily doses of the stuff.

In fact, Cox reported, by Oct. 28, 1992, the very day that safety officer Paul Goebel wrote a memorandum claiming that a consent form female volunteers were required to sign downplayed the risks and overstated potential benefits of the drug, four uterine cancer victims from an earlier tamoxifen trial had already died of the disease.

The carcinogen-of-the-month club

In the meantime, in terms of "causes" of cancer, what we began to call "the carcinogen of the month club" continued to terrify the American (and in general the Western) population with every new disclosure that this chemical or that was linked to cancer development, usually based on animal studies.

To some extent, the hunt for carcinogenic chemicals had reached *reductio ad absurdum* proportions by the 1980s, for data derived from using proportionally gross amounts of potentially harmful chemicals on animals was being extrapolated to the infinitesimally small amounts of the same that humans might be receiving.

This did not, of course, undercut the possible dangers of continual, *accumulated* buildup of chemicals and synthetic hormones dumped into the nation's food chain (see *XIV*) nor mitigate the real possibility of overexposure to all manner of industrial chemicals, pesticides, herbicides and insecticides.

The span of opinion ranged from that of Dr. Epstein, who spent a lot of time alerting the public to the understated dangers about and links between cancer and industrial chemicals, and chemical company-backed researchers and apologists who liked to pooh-pooh such attacks and were happier to blame cancer almost exclusively on tobacco. Added to both was scattered research over several years suggesting correlations between certain "forms" of cancer and exposure to electric power lines, extremely low electromagnetic frequencies (ELFs) and to everything from television sets and electric curlers to cellular telephones, in addition to the increasingly obvious connection between cancer and prior exposure to nuclear radiation.

The radiation holocaust — 'security' and coverup

By the mid-1990s the nuclear radiation exposure matter was assuming research dimensions which implied a much vaster problem and was becoming far too great to be considered other than as a series of nationwide scandals.

The scandals had a whiff of political agenda since they bore on women's issues — particularly breast cancer (though, in fact, a small and even more aggressive "form" of breast cancer occurs in men) — and, as a subdivision, on higher breast cancer rates in "minority" women. But the scandals implicated the perils of radiation and cancer *in general*, a point often missed in the political hoopla.

As we noted in *II*, the dangers of radiation via X-rays and through the touted mammography program were noted years ago, although not too much attention was paid to them at the time. But subsequent research went on, and it produced worrisome questions: *is* there a "safe" dose of radiation? How long does it take for the accumulated effects of radiation to show up? How much radiation can one absorb in what amount of time before serious problems occur?

John W. Gofman MD PhD, professor emeritus of molecular and cell biology, University of California-Berkeley and former associate director of California's Livermore National

Laboratory, has relentlessly kept up his crusade to warn of the downside of "medical exposure to ionizing radiation" — one, he noted, that "is barely ever mentioned as a prime explanation for the current high rate of breast cancer."[70]

By the mid-1990s, the ever-quotable Dr. Epstein was on hand to warn of "mammoscam" — his assessment of "national breast cancer awareness day" for women — and to argue forcefully that there simply had not been demonstrated, as late as 1994, any benefit from mammography in premenopausal women even as the radiation industry and hawkers of radiological products were plumbing the "pre-menopausal market."[71]

Even more ominously, data released in 1993 by Ernest J. Sternglass, professor emeritus of radiology, University of Pittsburgh, and Jay M. Gould, of the Radiation and Public Health Project, New York, found "highly significant rises" in breast cancer over time among women who lived near nuclear reactors. Breast cancer mortality rates in 268 counties within 50 miles of reactors were studied.[72]

At a San Diego meeting, Dr. Sternglass asserted:

For the period between 1950 and 1989, the age-adjusted breast cancer mortality rate rose 10 percent near the reactors and only 4 percent for the average in the US. Of the 51 sites involved that began operation before 1982, the five oldest operated by the Department of Energy such as Hanford and Oak Ridge known to have had the largest releases registered an even greater increase of breast cancer mortality of 41 percent, from 20.7 deaths per 100,000 women in the five-year period 1950-54 to 29.2 in 1985-89.[73]

The scientists pointed out that in the case of Oak Ridge TN, one of the oldest sites of atomic bomb development

... for the downwind counties within 40 miles, the breast cancer mortality increased by 39 percent, in striking contrast to a 4 percent decline for women living in four nearby upwind counties. The same

pattern exists for all cancers combined (emphasis mine).[74]

The Sternglass-Gould research — admittedly "in response to the call by the National Breast Cancer Coalitiion for an increase in investigator-initiated research to find the cause for the recent sharp rise in breast cancer" — used official data from the Nuclear Regulatory Commission (NRC) and the National Cancer Institute (NCI) to reach its sobering conclusions and cannot be said to have juggled figures to prove a point.

The work bore a great deal on "very low concentrations of radioactivity in milk, meat and drinking water" and the nuclear fission products strontium-90 and iodine-131. Such "tiny emissions are almost as dangerous as the Hiroshima explosion and nobody wanted to believe it," said Dr. Sternglass.[75]

Abstracting from copious data before them, Drs. Sternglass and Gould summarized that nuclear fission products in diet and drinking water constituted "the previously neglected factor in the rise of breast and other types of cancer that has accelerated since the operation of large nuclear reactors began" and that

Tragically, the desire to build and test ever larger numbers of nuclear weapons and therefore to suppress all research and epidemiological studies of very low dose effects of nuclear fallout . . . because of fear that serious health effects of nuclear fallout would lead to a demand for an end to nuclear weapons testing . . . led to the premature construction of nuclear plants near large population areas before the seriousness of free-radical damage to the cells of the immune system produced by strontium-90 and other bone-seeking fission products was recognized . . .

Failure to face these mistakes of the cold war will not only cause further increases in human suffering, but it will also prevent us from slowing the enormous rise in health-care costs brought about by the combination of costly medical technology and

the rising incidence of cancer and other chronic diseases now known to be caused by the action of free radicals that are produced by the fission products, often acting synergistically with other toxic agents and hormones that we are continuing to release into our milk, our drinking water and our diet.[76]

(One of the synthetic hormones added to milk, gonadotropin-releasing hormone [GRH], may, according to Dr. Epstein, induce osteoporosis, and its advocacy among California scientists to counteract the "incessant ovulation" that some argue is a "cause" of increased breast cancer, "promotes the interests of Imperial Chemical [a United Kingdom-based pharmaceutical giant.]"[77])

The charges made by various investigators looking into the hidden-radiation peril are that as early as 1943, or even before the first atomic bomb was exploded, American scientists knew that there were extreme dangers involving nuclear fallout — and that the US government secretly experimented in hundreds (and probably thousands) of tests on humans to attempt to determine what the dangers were.

In a "preliminary report" released Oct. 21, 1994, the 14-member "Advisory Committee on Human Radiation Experiments," a group of investigators reviewing the history of government-sponsored atomic experiments, found that

Cold War secrecy and bureaucratic sprawl created a patchwork of policies that unwittingly exposed many humans to potentially dangerous radiation [and that] government officials extensively debated the need for human experimentation and the policies that should govern it. But because that debate was often secret, many contractors and university researchers apparently were unaware of the legal and ethical concerns surrounding the experiments they were paid to conduct.[78]

Johns Hopkins University medical ethicist Ruth Faden, a

panel member, claimed that the group had documented 400 government-sponsored radiation experiments that exposed humans to radiation between 1947 and 1977 but that by the time the huge data-gathering effort was to be completed the number of experiments probably would turn out to be "in the thousands."

Such research explains in part the unusually high rates not only of cancer in general but also elements of immune dysregulation (*XIII*) in such areas as New Mexico, home of Los Alamos and many other experimental nuclear outlets — a state where, I was staggered to learn in fall 1994, more than a tenth of the entire adult population is on the federal payroll, particularly that of the Department of Energy (DOE).

It is in vintage nuclear-experiment New Mexico where, quite aside from above-normal levels of breast and other "forms" of cancer, so many victims of alleged "e.i." (environmental illness) cluster that it may become increasingly difficult to find a truly healthy resident of the state. It is also true that clusters of "e.i." patients moved there from other polluted areas of the USA seeking open spaces and better air. To a great extent, they have not found them.

Intriguingly, the onrush of information as to radiation (obvious, low-dose or occult) and its connection to cancer and to immunological disarray in general points to the increasing validity of oxidology (*XIV*) as a vital medical subspecialty — both in explaining the nature of many chronic disorders and their resolution.

There is also increased information to suggest that various toxic chemicals, as well as synthetic hormones, particularly estrogens — and of various substances the human immune system(s) may "scan" *as* estrogens — may interact with radiation. Given the frequent disturbance of a woman's hormone pool by steroids and "the pill," quite aside from enforced life-long dependence on estrogens and/or progesterone following hysterectomies or other medical events, and the interplay of substances the body may detect *as* estrogens let alone alterations already underway due to accumulated low-dose or other radiation, there can be little wonder that breast cancer rates are so stratospheric that the actual incidence may soon be closer to 1 out of 8 rather than the (as of 1994) officially recognized 1 out of 9 in the USA.

In the meantime, the chemical industry itself is not too entranced with research which may indicate a malignancy-"organizing" role for the multiple substances of industry and agriculture — yet testing them for possible carcinogenicity has itself become a major industry in the hunt for "causes" of cancer.

Suffer the little animals

The animal research industry, itself a multi-billion-dollar undertaking involving the breeding and cross-breeding of animals, typically mice, rats and rabbits, and also of chimpanzees and monkeys, was usually the conduit through which information on alleged carcinogenic dangers developed.

In the oncological industry, in alignment with allopathic thinking and the dictates of the Food and Drug Administration (FDA), there arose an imperative to test both suspected cancer-blocking drugs as well as suspected cancer-causing agents on animals — which, when one thinks of it for more than five seconds, is frankly irrational.

The extremes of oncological inanity occur as tumors taken from another species are transplanted into animals already bred to have no significant immune response. Then potential anti-cancer drugs are used on such animals (that is, against their transplanted tumors) to see "what will happen." If there seems to be tumor reduction, this evidence is then transferred to the human species — an allopathically sound, FDA-approved chain of linear thought. A major reason for testing cancer drugs on animals, of course, is that, given their inherent toxicity, it somehow would be immoral to try out a suspected toxic drug on humans willy-nilly — so why not force it on animals, however far removed by species they might be from *Homo sapiens*, to establish an "LD50" (code for "dose at which 50 percent of a given lot of test animals will die of lethal effects")?

A similar cascade of linear thought has occurred in testing compounds thought to be cancer-causing (carcinogenic): use amounts of the substance at biologically unreasonable levels in animals to test their possible carcinogenicity. If found to be carcinogenic, announce this fact to the world.

There certainly are *some* reasons to follow both lines of reasoning — but they pale alongside the central consideration: the only appropriate test model for a human being as it relates to that which might "cause" or "cure" cancer or anything else is man himself. This simple truth dislodges much of the underpinning of the heavily funded "vivisectionist" industry (experiments on sentient animals for either drug or cosmetic development, sometimes reaching levels of horrific cruelty).

But in the medical/pharmaceutical world of cancer — since virtually *every* alleged cancer-blocking drug *is* toxic or potentially toxic, even at a relatively modest level — there is no escaping a certain amount of animal tests before a compound may be "cleared" for human use.

(The same system, parenthetically, makes it frankly either impossible or unreasonable to test non-toxic, natural, nutritional factors on animals. How measure the anti-cancer or antioxidant effects of exogenous Vitamin C, for example, on test animals, most of which already produce their *own* Vitamin C? How *really* test for "toxicity" in naturally-occurring laetrile in a test rat, let alone determine what the "useful dose" of apricot-seed extract is on a human while injecting it into a hybrid animal in which a tumor has been transplanted?)

In *Science* in 1990, research scientists not known for being unfriendly to industry dismissed as "bankrupt" the idea that cramming test animals with carcinogenic compounds and issuing the results, thus "scaring the country sick," is a rational thing to do.

University of California biochemist Bruce Ames, who has long argued there are as many or more "natural" carcinogens in plants and the pristine environment than produced by the chemical industry, said in new research that there was a growing body of biological evidence to suggest that often it was not the chemical makeup of a substance, but the high dose of it, which produced cancer in laboratory animals.[79]

And in 1991, the federal Environmental Protection Agency (EPA) came up with research showing that male rats have a special protein (alpha-2U-globulin, not found in humans) that makes them particularly *prone* to cancer — a disclosure which, it was thought, might very well invalidate literally millions of tests of chemicals, herbicides, pesticides, preservatives and additives which have been banned because of their cancer-causing potential in rats.

In its own peculiar language, the EPA stated that cancer found in laboratory rats is a "species-specific effect inapplicable to human risk assessment."[80]

The ACS: propaganda central

The great amount of what Americans know or think about cancer is heavily influenced by the American Cancer Society (ACS), whose name suggests a degree of officialness which it does not have. Hardly any literate American is unaware of ACS smokeouts, celebrity yacht cruises, elegant fund-raising events of all kinds, and the noisy campaigns against cigarette smoking and in favor of mammograms. Most news media are well aware of the annual "science writers' conferences" at which the ACS wines, dines and "informs" science writers and assorted journalists so they can be kept "updated" on the latest breakthroughs in cancer research and application.

The vision of selfless volunteers going door to door soliciting coins for the endless war on cancer constantly comes to mind. And, truth to tell, the marching troops of the ACS are indeed well-meaning volunteers — just as the marching troops of the originally anti-polio March of Dimes, American Heart Assn. (AHA) and American Lung Assn. (ALA), plus lesser charities, are well-meaning volunteers.

But time, vested interests, the establishment of bureaucratic monoliths and, naturally, the management of money, take their toll on *any* organization, be it charitable or not (see *III*).

In 1990, charities critic and economics professor James T. Bennett reported that the ACS held land valued at $14 million, $42 million worth of buildings and leasehold improvements, and $6 million in buildings under construction."[81]

In 1992, the ACS — whose influence over the smaller, federally funded NCI has long been described as the classic example of the tail wagging the dog — was kept scrambling to explain away a piercing article by University of Tennessee-Chattanooga economics professor Thomas J. DiLorenzo.

In the *Wall Street Journal*, DiLorenzo charged that "ACS affiliates have diverted substantial sums away from providing cancer service in order to accumulate large holdings of cash, securities, land and buildings."[82]

He claimed that "the typical affiliate spends more than 52 percent of its budget on salaries, pensions, fringe benefits and overhead" and that "chief executive officers earn six-figure salaries in a number of states."

He added:

> ... *For every $1 spent on direct service, approximately $6.40 is spent on compensation and overhead ... The financial statements ... reveal that Cancer Society affiliates are wealthy organizations, despite their fund-raising appeals, which stress an urgent and critical need for donations to provide cancer services.*
>
> *As of 1990 the California affiliate ... had accumulated $36 million in cash, certificates of deposit and securities; Florida had set aside $20 million; Texas, Ohio and Colorado held about $10 million each. The average affiliate in this sample of 10 held $10.8 million in cash reserves.*[83]

He reported that, in terms of land and buildings, the Texas ACS affiliate had $11.3 million in such assets, the California and Florida affiliates more than $3 million in property.

The current ACS president, responding in the *WSJ*, called

ACS financial statements a "snapshot in time" which reflected both program expenses of a current year and funds accumulated for the following year's programs and made much of the fact the Society was the "first non-profit health organization to use an independent auditor and issue a combined national financial annual report."[84]

The Society, he said, "does not spend money it does not have," although how this could be used to "categorically refute each of the allegations by Thomas J. DiLorenzo" was not clear.

In 1994, DiLorenzo and Dr. Bennett noted that for every $1 spent by the ACS for research, Americans paid $15 — and that the National Cancer Institute was spending more on cancer research each year than the ACS had in the past half century. They added that at the end of 1993 the ACS had a net worth of $520.3 million — and owned more than $61 million in real estate.[85]

The ACS had earlier been looked at with a critical eye by investigative reporter Peter Barry Chowka, who wrote in 1978 that in fiscal 1976 the Society had spent $114 million while its assets totalled $181 million and that between 1970 and 1973 ACS' net profit doubled.

Moreover, he noted:

With so many millions of dollars invested and deposited in checking and savings accounts, ACS is a prime banking customer. At least eighteen members of the ACS Board of Directors and House of Delegates are executive officers or directors of banks. As of August 31, 1976, 42 percent of ACS' cash and investments, totalling $75 million, were maintained in banks with which these eighteen men were affiliated.[86]

In summer 1977, as part of its ongoing review of the national "Conquest of Cancer" effort, the House Committee on Governmental Operations, while investigating the NCI, found that the federal agency and the ACS in effect had interlocking directorates — though neither side had taken particular pains to hide this fact, and it was not a crime.

As this writer noted in 1983:

> *The most obvious example of the comfortable relationship between the NCI as a spender of taxpayer monies in the cancer war and the major lobby for conducting that war in the first place was the hiring of former NCI Director Frank Rauscher as an ACS senior vice president — at a doubling of his annual salary.*[87]

The spectacular fund-raising successes of the American Cancer Society (ACS) and its strong influence over how research funds are ultimately used is due to the fact it has long been dominated by experts in advertising, public relations and business.

Indeed, the PR volleys which the ACS annually fires off in a most professional way can largely be attributed to the virtual takeover of an otherwise lackluster charity (founded in 1913) by Albert Lasker, "father of modern advertising," and his socially well connected wife, Mary, and Elmer Bobst, "father of the modern drug industry."[88]

Some rays of hope

In defense of the ACS, it can be said that the Society, for all its excesses, took cancer — once a whispered-about malady rarely mentioned in polite society — out of the closet. As cancer rates climbed, it was infinitely better to draw attention to it than to try to obscure the reality. And the ACS campaign against cigarette smoking — over-done in that ACS has been too quick to blame cancer in general on tobacco, hence providing the oncological industry with a partial excuse for failure (people just won't stop smoking) — has been salutary to the extent that there are a lot of health problems connected with lighting up and nicotine addiction appears to be the toughest of all to overcome.

It is also true that, despite the fact that the Society has been a heavy hitter against "alternative" cancer therapies and a major voice of disinformation against such "unapproved" approaches as laetrile, it has nonetheless been more open to integrating new information than certain other elements of Cancer Inc.

After arguing for years that anybody who connected cancer with diet was deluded at best, a charlatan at worst (the Cancer Inc. general "line" for decades), the ACS, yielding to a torrent of epidemiological, biochemical and empirical research to the contrary, gradually switched its position.

While in the 1950s it had actually lobbied Congress to hold hearings to investigate what it considered to be false claims that there was a connection between nutrition and cancer, by 1989 the Society had zig-zagged by about 180 degrees and could baldfacedly state:

> *There is strong evidence that perhaps people can be protected from cancer by what they eat or drink, or by other substances or lifestyles that serve as defense mechanisms . . . This is a new and important area which needs further research so that recommendations can be developed on how people should change their lifestyles to reduce their chances of getting cancer.* [89]

By the 1990s, the Society was running ads and television spots *in defense* of the concept that a more vegetarian, more fruit-oriented, lower refined carbohydrate, lower animal fat and protein, higher natural fiber diet might be associated with the prevention of cancer!

For long-time ACS watchers and observers of Cancer Inc., this campaign represented a quantum leap away from earlier established doctrine that it was just plain insane to make any connection between cancer and diet. It also, of course, strongly validated what numerous physicians and researchers long derided as "cancer quacks" had been saying for decades.

By this writing, the ACS was not quite ready to take the next leap (bearing in mind the aphorism that "that which prevents, also cures") to actually *suggest* elements in the cancer-prevention diet might also be used to *treat* it, despite growing evidence to that effect from biochemistry — a discipline always a decade or more ahead of medical application. But it *was* "studying" the idea. Hope springs eternal . . .

The fact that major executives of the ACS, AHA or ALA have large salaries, or that such operations as the ACS have bulging bank accounts and heavy investments in real estate and buildings implies neither criminal nor immoral behavior — it simply points to one of the ambivalent elements in the American healthcare mess:

There is a lot of money to be made in "charity" fund-raising, and organizations aimed at solving a problem, no matter how noble the cause or effort, will, when exposed to hard cash, tend to self-perpetuate.

By mid-decade, Cancer Inc.'s continuing attacks on "alternative therapies" — the vast majority of them involving nutritional approaches to cancer — was beginning to ring hollow, despite the enthusiasm and barbarity with which the FDA and other federal state and local agencies continued to raid nutritional-therapy clinics, arrest offending doctors and terrify patients.

It was simply clear that a wide range of nutrients, including some veteran standbys (Vitamins A,C,E, beta-carotene, selenium, certain B vitamins) and some "non-nutritive food factors" in the plant kingdom (phenols, indoles, isothiocyanates) by themselves and/or within whole foods, where they were joined by other ingredients, and even some spices and condiments,[90] were associated with the prevention of cancer.

Research around the world said so and, most importantly, research at home said so.

By 1992, on the heels of an assessment by the NCI of strong links between cancer prevention and dietary factors in an impressive 156 studies, a national survey to examine eating habits was launched by the Cancer Society (*XIV*).[91]

And, in 1994, nutritional aspects in cancer constituted a major theme at the annual convention of the American Assn. for the Advancement of Science (AAAS).

There, the aforementioned Dr. Ames was on hand to note that of 172 studies in the orthodox scientific (that is, "Club") literature examining the role of fruits and vegetables in cancer prevention, 129 had shown a "significant protective effect." He and others noted that while the general overview is that one can cut one's risk in half "for every major cancer" by eating far more fruits and vegetables, virtually no research money was going in to bolster such stupendous conclusions.[92]

Diet and malignancy
How diet might affect cancer causatively let alone therapeutically falls into several areas:
— Ways in which refined carbohydrates or other aspects of a chemically altered food supply may directly influence cellular integrity so that a cell, in allegiance to the implied primary directive of life itself — adapt or die — may adapt by reverting to its primitive (that is, cancer-like) stage.
— Ways in which toxic chemicals used to treat or process food may, by accumulation, lead to a possible cancer-organizing cascade, including factors which the body may scan as hormone-like and hence respond to by altering its own "pool" of such messenger substances, leading to "hormone-dependent" expressions of cancer, particularly breast and ovarian in women.
— Ways in which overly fatty diets may help provide reservoirs for toxic synthetic chemicals which in turn can initiate the cancer process.
— Ways in which specific dietary and nutritive deficiencies deplete the body's store of natural scavengers of toxic oxygen ("free radicals"), allowing the latter to proliferate and damage every system in the body (cancer itself utilizing the "free radical cascade" as a way to spread) and possibly to induce the malignant process itself via genetic damage.
— Ways in which various nutrients may enhance host defense and aspects of immunity indirectly against the malignant process.
— Ways in which excesses (for example, of animal protein)

may interfere with a natural defense system (proteolytic enzymes) against cancer, enhancing the malignant process.

(As we shall see [*XII*], the "laetrile theory" has much going for it since a class of compounds described as *nitrilosides* or "Vitamin B17" seems strongly linked to the prevention of clinical cancer and, in the form of laetrile, to be useful in its management — the heart of one of this century's major medical controversies).

Each of these areas presents a world of biochemical possibilities which in their totality add up to the importance of diet in the induction and/or suppression of the malignant process, with some relevance at every step of the process.

The dietary element — by this reckoning — would be involved regardless of all other aspects — presumed hereditary predispositions (genetics), possible "organizing" events such as radiation, inadequate wound healing, and even mental stress, the effects of a universe of manmade synthetic chemicals affecting both the internal and external ecology of human beings, and alterations in the hormone pool, part of which may be directly related either to dietary or chemical factors.

For 'control' rather than 'cure'

For decades, practitioners who usually call themselves "metabolic therapists," whether their view of cancer is unitarian or not, have been more likely to seek the "control" of cancer than the "cure" — for, as we have seen, "cure" is at its best a supremely deceptive and tricky word which, to many people, means the entire eradication of a disease and the likelihood it will never occur again.

Many of the views of metabolic doctors have focused on the reality that cancer is itself not an interloper, not a foreign invader (the probable reason why an immune response is *not* mounted against it, at least in the early phase) — and hence not "curable" in the classical sense of the word.

Such physicians — and metabolically oriented writers, including the present author — have stated that the maximum goal in cancer management, therefore, should be *control* — and that the most common analogy is diabetes. The latter is a chronic, systemic condition which is not basically "curable" but which can be controlled for the whole of an individual's genetically predisposed span of life by diet alone or diet plus insulin. A diabetic may thus live a life that is within 90 percent of "normal". Most metabolic physicians argue that the same is true for cancer.

Cancer should be controllable and manageable for the whole of a person's life. This is the strong suggestion from long-term survivors of even very advanced malignancies who have been on nutritionally-oriented, essentially natural, metabolic treatment regimens.

Such doctors and researchers, for so long denounced as quacks, could only express some satisfaction when the Western cancer establishment began, in 1993 and 1994, actually to start speaking in the same terms.

In a 1994 *Journal of the American Medical Assn. (JAMA)*, a "commentary" by Alan B. Jastrow, St. Vincent's Hospital and Medical Center, New York, was called "Rethinking Cancer." In it, Dr. Jastrow further expanded on arguments made by a Canadian research group in 1993 — namely, that the goal of cancer therapy might better be "controlling" rather than "curing" malignancy.[93]

In a spring 1994 *Time*, Dr. Lance Liotta, described as "the [NCI's] leading metastasis expert," stated something oncologically unthinkable just a few years before:

"After all, we don't cure diseases like diabetes and hypertension. We control them. Why can't we look at cancer that way?"[94]

This was conceptual progress by any definition.

Later the same year, a Canadian investigator, assessing the calamity of breast cancer in women, seemed to be undergoing virtual holistic catharsis in a "viewpoint" editorial in *The Lancet*. Dr. James E. Devitt observed:

In focusing on the breast lesion, the tree, have

we failed to see the forest, the whole patient with her plethora of growth-restraining factors, both systemic and local, and of the growth potential directed by the chromosomes in each cell? If the breast lesion is not the cause of the disease but merely the local expression of a combination of changes in both local and systemic growth-restraining factors, and if such a combination was more or less specific for producing breast-tissue-like growths, they would be more easily induced and occur earlier in breast tissues. . .[95]

But research is one thing. Politics and economics is another.

While dramatic new ideas of cancer were developing, Cancer Inc. was not about to let natural therapies go unchallenged.

More tigers in the jungle

The new tigers in the jungle that Cancer Inc. was seeking to exterminate by mid-decade — believing (incorrectly) that it had gotten rid of laetrile — were 714X (essentially a camphor-based product promoted in Canada and finding numerous adherents elsewhere); the late Canadian nurse Rene Caisse's Essiac herbal tea, which had been around for decades and was now being produced by several companies while gathering many supporters; shark cartilage, since both Cuban research and national publicity, as well as an insightful book by William Lane, indicated the notion behind it (blocking the process whereby tumors can create their own circulatory systems) was of value; and, in the USA, the outside-the-Club therapies propounded and used by Emanuel Revici MD in New York and Stanislaw Burzynski MD PhD in Texas.

To say nothing of a special vegetarian soup, metallurgy-derived "chondriana," the "Greek serum" of the late Hariton Alivizatos, and even a special herb combination designed to help wipe out flukes (flatworms), said by one theorist to be a "universal cause" of cancer. True, patients threatened by death from cancer often caromed from one off-the-wall "cure" to another and many an opportunist paraded this or that "magic bullet" against a multifactorial disease state which by its very nature could *have* no such resolution. However silly some of the ideas and however much opportunists crowded the field, the real guilty party remained made-in-America Cancer Inc. through its abject failure to stem the pandemic.

Other older tigers kept growling too: there still was the never-convincingly-described CanCell, which had its own share of living and breathing true believers and which the FDA kept trying to stamp out. There was still the late Dr. Lawrence Burton's IAT (immunoaugmentative therapy) in the Bahamas, other immunity-bolstering techniques as well as ozone machines and "Rife instruments," speaking to lines of research which at least had highly interesting pedigrees (*XV*), and so many herbal concoctions of both domestic and foreign origin that suppressing them all was turning out to be a "compliance" impossibility.

And there still was laetrile — which, more than any other single factor, had so shaken Cancer Inc. that it would never fully recover.

References

1. *The Choice*, XVII:2, 1991.
2. Cited in *The Choice*, XVIII:1, 1992.
3. Cited in *The Choice*, XVIII:1, 1992.
4. Cited in *The Choice*, XVIII:1, 1992.
5. American Cancer Society, January 1993.
6. Weinstock, MA, *J. Am. Aca. Derm.*, May 1994.
7. Davis, DL, *et al.*, *J. Am. Med. Assn.*, Feb. 9, 1994.
8. *Meditrends 1991-1992*, American Hospital Assn., May 1991.
9. *The Choice*, XVIII:1, 1992.
10. Cimons, Marlene, *Los Angeles Times*, Sept. 30, 1994.
11. Culbert, ML, *What The Medical Establishment Won't Tell You That Could Save Your Life*. Norfolk VA: Donning, 1983.
12. *J. Am. Med. Assn.*, cited in *The Choice*, XVI:4, 1990.
13. *Ibid.*
14. National Cancer Institute national cancer survey, August 1991.
15. Beardsley, Tim, "A war not won." *Scientific American*, January 1994.
16. National Cancer Institute chart, in Beardlsey, *op. cit.*
17. Testimony before "Cancer treatment: new directions for the 1990s" seminar, convened by Staten Island Borough President Guy V. Molinari, New York, September 1993.
18. *Cancer Chronicles*, cited in *The Choice*, XVI:2,3, 1990.
19. *Ibid.*
20. *The Choice*, XIX: 3,4, 1993.

21. *Ibid.*
22. *Ibid.*
23. Moertel, Charles, in *J. Am. Med. Assn.*, Aug. 25, 1993.
24. Fletcher, RH, in *J. Am. Med. Assn.*, Aug. 25, 1993.
25. *The Choice,* XX:1, 1994.
26. Dermer, GB, *The Immortal Cell.* Garden City Park NY: Avery, 1994.
27. *Ibid.*
28. *Ibid.*
29. "When DNA isn't destiny." *Newsweek,* Dec. 6, 1993.
30. Lehrman, Sally, *San Francisco Examiner*, March 6, 1994.
31. Bradford, RW, and Allen, HW, *The Primordial Thesis of Cancer.* Chula Vista CA: Bradford Research Institute, 1990.
32. *New Eng. J. Med.,* Jan. 4, 1990.
33. *The Choice,* XVI:1, 1990.
34. *Ibid.*
35. *Ibid.*
36. *The Choice,* XVI: 2,3, 1990.
37. *Ibid.*
38. *Lancet,* April 13, 1991.
39. Sartori, Sergio, *et al., Ann. Int. Med.,* February 1991.
40. Lipschultz, SE, *et al., New Eng. J. Med.,* March 21, 1991.
41. *The Choice,* XVII:1, 1991.
42. Cited in *The Choice,* XVII: 1, 1991.
43. *The Choice,* XVII: 3,4, 1991.
44. *The Choice,* XIX:2, 1993.
45. *Ibid.*
46. *The Choice,* XVIII: 1, 1992.
47. *USA Today,* Dec. 23, 1991.
48. General Accounting Office (GAO), January 1992.
49. Canadian National Breast Cancer Screening Study, Nov. 13, 1992, cited in *The Choice,* XVIII: 3, 1992.
50. "Breast cancer: have we lost our way?" *Lancet,* Feb. 6, 1993.
51. *The Choice,* XX: 1, 1994.
52. *The Choice,* XIX: 1, 1993.
53. *The Choice,* XIX: 2, 1993.
54. Moertel, *loc. cit.*
55. The *Sacramento Bee,* Nov. 8, 1992.
56. *J. Am. Med. Assn.,* cited in *The Choice,* XVIII: 2, 1992.
57. *Ibid.*
58. *J. Am. Med. Assn.,* May 26, 1993.
59. Chodak, Gerald, *New Eng. J. Med.,* Jan. 27, 1994.
60. *The Choice,* XX: 2-3, 1994.
61. Winslow, Ron, "Prostate-cancer test may be more costly than beneficial." *Wall Street Journal,* Sept. 14, 1994.
62. *The Choice,* XVIII: 2, 1992.
63. *The Choice,* XX: 1, 1994.
64. *The Choice,* XIX: 3,4, 1993.
65. Fugh-Berman, Adriane, and Samuel Epstein, "Tamoxifen: disease prevention or disease substitution?" *Lancet,* Nov. 7, 1992.
66. Fugh-Berman, Adriane, and Samuel Epstein, "Tamoxifen for breast cancer prevention: a cautionary review." *Reviews on Endocrine-Related Cancer 43,* 1993.
67. *Ibid.*
68. Kedar, RP, *et al.,* "Effects of tamoxifen on uterus and ovaries of postmenopausal women in a randomized breast cancer prevention trial." *Lancet,* May 28, 1994.
69. Cox News Service, Aug. 18, 1994.
70. Gofman, JW, "A prime cause of breast cancer: what did we know, and when did we know it?" Presentation, the American Academy for the Advancement of Science (AAAS), San Francisco CA, Feb. 22, 1994.
71. Epstein, Samuel, presentation, Women's Health & the Environment: Action for Cancer Prevention, Albuquerque NM, Oct. 15, 1994.
72. Sternglass, EJ, and JM Gould, "Summary of study on the relation between breast cancer and nuclear fission products in the diet and drinking water." *Int. J. Health Serv.,* Oct. 1993.
73. Sternglass, EJ, "Breast cancer linked to nuclear releases." Presentation, American Assn. of Naturopathic Physicians, San Diego, CA, Sept. 8, 1994.
74. *Ibid.*
75. *The Choice,* XX: 2-3, 1994.
76. *Ibid.*
77. Epstein, presentation, *loc.cit.*
78. Healy, Melissa, "Cold war secrecy tied to radiation peril." *Los Angeles Times,* Oct. 22, 1994.
79. *Science,* Aug. 31, 1990.
80. *The Choice,* XVII: 3,4 1991.
81. Bennett, JT, *Health Research Charities: Image and Realities.* Cited in *Pittsburgh Courier* and *The Choice,* XVI: 4, 1990.

82. *Wall Street Journal*, March 13, 1992.
83. *Ibid.*
84. *Wall Street Journal*, April 6, 1992.
85. "Uncharitable charities." *USA Today*, July 19, 1994.
86. Chowka, PB, "The cancer charity ripoff." *East-West Journal*, July 1978.
87. Culbert, *op. cit.*
88. *Ibid.*
89. *Cancer Facts and Figures 1989*, American Cancer Society, 1989.
90. Bradford, RW, and Allen, HW, "The significance of diet in cancer prevention." Chula Vista CA: Bradford Research Institutes. Abstracted in *The Choice*. XIX: 3-4, 1993, and XX: 1, 1994.
91. *The Choice*, XVIII: 3, 1992.
92. *The Choice*, XIX: 1, 1994.
93. Jastrow, AR, "Commentary," *J. Am. Med. Assn.* Feb. 26, 1994.
94. Nash, Madeleine, "Stopping cancer in its tracks." *Time*, April 25, 1994.
95. Devitt, JE, "Breast cancer: have we missed the forest because of the tree?" *Lancet*, Sept. 10, 1994.

XII
APRICOT POWER:
Laetrile as the Marine Corps of the 'alternative' revolution

> *"At no time in American history has there been a more effective challenge to medical expertise and authority than that mounted by the contemporary laetrile movement. Despite opposition from the FDA, the American Medical Association, the American Cancer Society, and virtually all of the American medical community, support for this purported cancer cure* [sic] *continues to grow..."*
> — **Sociologists G.E. Markle and J.C. Peterson, to the American Association for the Advancement of Science (AAAS), 1979**

> *"Laetrile completely eclipsed any other unorthodox therapy ever used for any disease in our time."*
> — **Charles G. Moertel MD, The Mayo Clinic, 1982**

> *"Although... Laetrile utilization in this country is proceeding... in spite of FDA prohibitions, it is even more so because of unwarranted FDA procedures, and lack of FDA scientific and medical justification for its stand, extending to probable unconstitutionality... I have hundreds of letters sent to me enclosing FDA information sheets and pronouncements, in which the senders of these letters point to the extensive falsification, duplicity, deviousness, red herrings and literal lies... promulgated by the FDA with respect to Laetrile, as well as similarly on the part of certain high officials... of the American Medical Association, the American Cancer Society, the US Department of Health, Education and Welfare, and state agencies..."*
> — **Dean Burk PhD, National Cancer Institute, to Rep. Louis Frey Jr., 1972**

> *"You may wonder, Congressman Roe, why anyone should go to such pains and mendacity to avoid conceding what happened to the NCI-directed experiment* [involving laetrile on a tumor system.] *Such an admission is crucially relevant. Once any of the FDA-NCI-AMA-ACS hierarchy so much as concedes that Laetrile anti-tumor efficacy was indeed even once observed in NCI experimentation, a permanent crack in the bureaucratic armor has taken place that can widen indefinitely..."*
> — **Dean Burk PhD, National Cancer Institute, to Rep. Robert A. Roe, 1973**

An apricot kernel shakes things up

There was a strangely dominant theme in the 1979 convention of the prestigious American Association for the Advancement of Science (AAAS):

Laetrile.

Not if, how, why or why not laetrile, the most recent "unproven" remedy found "anecdotally" useful against cancer while opposed by the totality of the forces we call Cancer Inc. actually "worked."

But why so many people could be led to believe that it did — when medical orthodoxy and oncological expertise insisted it did not.

No less than five papers on "the laetrile phenomenon" were presented at the AAAS convention that year — and they came not from physicians, biochemists or oncologists but from Western Michigan University sociologists. The latter abstracted:

> *At no time in American history has there been a more effective challenge to medical expertise and authority than that mounted by the contemporary laetrile movement. Despite opposition from the FDA, the American Medical Association, the American Cancer Society, and virtually all of the American medical community, support for this purported cancer cure [sic] continues to grow...*
>
> *The first paper takes a case-study approach and focuses on the recent laetrile controversy at the Memorial Sloan-Kettering Cancer Center illustrating the richness and complexity of the dispute. The next paper provides an historical context to the recent success of the movement. The third paper examines the conceptualization of the laetrile problem and attempts to explain a variety of legal issues, including the right of privacy; the rights of physicians, informed consent, and government control, are considered. The final paper examines the social context of the controversy and attempts to*

answer the following question: Why has the laetrile movement been so successful in the late 1970s?[1]

Even Mayo Clinic cancer researcher Charles Moertel (dead of cancer himself in 1994), who led the team in the federal "amygdalin (laetrile) clinical trial" in 1980-81 which was used to wreck the laetrile movement, observed that "Laetrile completely eclipsed any other unorthodox therapy ever used for any disease in our time."[2]

The issue: freedom of choice

The sociological savants could have saved themselves an enormous amount of research hours had they simply switched their paradigm meter over to "common sense":

Laetrile was fast becoming a dominant issue because, for the first time in the long and tortured history of suppressed cancer "alternatives" in the United States, it had, unlike its predecessors, "gone political."

A personal note here: I began my involvement as a science writer and health-rights activist on the laetrile issue, which I entered as a trained — and skeptical — journalist. As the primary writer/journalist of what became the Committee for Freedom of Choice in Cancer Therapy Inc. (later, Committee for Freedom of Choice in Medicine, Inc.) I decided very early that the issue was neither scientific nor medical but political. And that issue was — is — simple:

What right does the state have, or should it have, to intervene in medical decisions between a patient and his doctor, particularly if that patient is dying of a "terminal" disease for which there is no known, or guaranteed, cure?

The marching slogan of the CFCCT became, as agreed by the rough-hewn self-taught visionary who founded the organization, Robert W. Bradford, several collaborators and myself, a simple one:

Freedom of choice, with informed consent, for physician and patient.

It was *this* issue, the freedom of choice concept, which so captivated the public and which led to many regional public opinion polls and, more impressively, such national samplings by those of the Harris (1977) and Roper (1978) organizations in which clear majorities of Americans believed at the very least in the *right* to have laetrile.

It was this basic, horse-sense approach, so consonant with the public at large, which lofted laetrile into the most impressive anti-establishmentarian phenomenon of a medical nature in this century and which set off what many would later call "the metabolic revolution" — the forcing, from the grass roots, of the Allopathic Industrial Complex (AIC) to begin to look at dietary elements in the prevention and management not only of cancer but of chronic disease in general.

What opponents styled "the political success of a scientific failure" — for the AIC would bestir itself to attempt to thwart the upstart laetrile movement with prostituted "science" of a high order — was the catalyst for increasing interest at all levels in nutrients against disease.

Laetrile captures 24 states

By the time of the 1979 AAAS convention, and usually led by the Committee for Freedom of Choice, pro-laetrile forces had "captured" one statehouse after another and were causing state legislatures to write into law various statutes either to protect doctors from punishment should they prescribe laetrile, or to protect patient access to the substance, or simply to make it an available option in cancer treatment and prevention.

Between 1976 and 1981, in a series of frequently stunning political events which shook the AIC and the nation at large, some 24 states covering more than half the population of the United States approved legislation which in one way or another either "decriminalized" or "legalized" laetrile. In others, such as New York, pro-laetrile laws passed the legislature only to be vetoed by state governors, actions which, as in the Empire State, were sometimes impossible to overturn.

Actually, those of us in "the laetrile movement" more or

less stealthfully planned it that way — we decided *against* federal legislation (for what the federal government enacts on Wednesday it can repeal on Thursday, while also strengthening that very level of government) and decided on "legal guerrilla warfare" at the state-by-state level, beginning with Alaska in 1975/1976.

Uniting Left and Right

The movement was also a populist revolution and strongly ideological, because much of the early leadership of the Committee was drawn from the ultraconservative John Birch Society (JBS), many of whose members took the freedom of choice issue to heart and, already experienced in lobbying and politicking, provided an unofficial support mechanism for the Committee.

Yet, much to the chagrin of some of the major media and various apologists of the AIC, neither the laetrile movement in general nor the Committee in particular were "Birch fronts" — support for individual freedom of choice in medical matters spanned all shades of the political landscape, all religions, races and socioeconomic levels.

As a journalist, I was drawn from the early days to the broad spectrum of the controversy, and was uniquely positioned to become informed:

It was the arrest of my *own* physician and friend, the late John A. Richardson MD, of Albany CA, on State of California charges involving laetrile, which was the actual catalyst for the formation of the original Committee for Freedom of Choice in Cancer Therapy Inc. "Dr. John" was a long-time Birch Society member. Yet at his initial hearings and trials within the Berkeley-Albany municipal jurisdiction — perhaps the most *left*-leaning in the country at the time — it was common to see youthful student radicals and hippies with McGovern-for-President buttons showing up *in support of* an outspoken Birch Society physician. Hence, from its ancestral origin in 1972, the Committee confounded the AIC just as the laetrile movement confused the scientific intelligentsia of the AAAS who so desperately wanted to know just how or why the American public could be "for" laetrile when the massed forces of institutional expertise so opposed it.

Laetrile, of course, had been kicking around long before the Richardson arrest and the advent of the Committee.

An ancient background

The history of the laetrile concept and the use and application of the substance were covered by myself in two books[3,4] as well as by Kittler[5] and Griffin.[6]

Permit me to synthesize:

In modern times, the word "laetrile" (apparently concocted by the major modern-day proponents, the late Ernst T. Krebs Sr. MD and his biochemist son, Ernst T. Krebs Jr., from the biochemical terminology "*lae*vo-mandeloni*trile*") has usually referred to the chemical amygdalin, first isolated and studied in the 19th century. The term "laetriles" has also been used to cover what the State of California calls "substantially similar compounds," particularly prunasin, linamarin, dhurrin, and several others.

These, plus sambunigrin, lotaustralin and more exotic compounds, have variously been described as "cyanogenetic glucosides," "cyanophoric glycosides" and, particularly as championed by Krebs Jr., "nitrilosides." They are impressively abundant in nature, as in all the black and brown bitter fruit seeds in North America, and are in many other seeds as well, and are found in many varieties of beans, peas, berries, tubers and grasses.

Whatever their names, the compounds have in common one or more sugars attached to benzene or acetone "rings" and carry a "cyanide radical" — that is, they are cyanide-bearing sugar compounds. They are so widespread in nature that the Krebses, the earlier McNaughton Foundation (first in Canada, then in California, as a research apparatus for the development of laetrile) and the late Dean Burk PhD, the peppery biochemist who for years headed the cytochemistry division of the National Cancer Institute (NCI), decided that altogether they constituted one or a complex of B vitamins — which they agreed should be the 17th in order of definition: Vitamin B17.

They argued that ubiquity in nature of such compounds was a proof, but not the only proof, of their vitamin nature. Their essential non-toxicity and solubility in water are other characteristics, Dean Burk always argued,[7] that added to their B-vitamin status. But the crux of the vitamin argument was whether or not their absence or depletion led to a pathological condition. For the laetrilists, their absence or depletion did indeed lead to a pathological condition: cancer. Not only that, but laetrile and its breakdown products are involved in a host of other metabolic processes.

Beyond that, amygdalin was known in medical history as both a poison, as implemented by the Egyptians, and as an elixir, as utilized by the Romans, and had been first successfully used on its own against cancer by the Russians even though amygdalin-laden black and brown bitter fruit seeds were described as anti-tumor agents in the herbal pharmacopeia of ancient China.[8]

Proofs from epidemiology

The notion of nitrilosidic prevention of cancer had enough adequate study in the current century to stand on its own and not simply as the excuse for developing a product.

Whether assembled by the Krebses, the McNaughton Foundation, or various independent researchers, the epidemiological aspects of "Vitamin B17" — correlations with much lower rates of cancer to no appreciable cancer at all in studied population — are impressive:

Essentially cancer-free or minimally cancer-afflicted populations have been studied, including, in South America, the Ecuadorian Vilcabamba Indians in particular (though numerous peoples of the Andean highlands and the Amazon Basin have been known to be either without cancer or to be minimally afflicted with it), the apricot kernel-popping Hunzakuts of

Pakistan (observed by several investigators over decades), various tribes and peoples of Southeast Asia (including at least one group in the southern Philippines which, I found on-site, had no word for the disease itself but, when explained what it was, called it "the Christian disease" — of meat-eaters), the Abkhasians of the former Soviet Union, Arctic Circle Eskimos prior to their "civilizing" by the Dutch Reformed Church and other entities; various American Indian tribes in the Southwest and in Mexico.

Krebs Jr. and the McNaughton Foundation gathered data on the essential absence or modest presence of cancer in other groups and in wild animals of many species (contrasting them with domesticated animals in the civilized West, among which cancer is highly present and growing.) They and others have pointed out that Western eating habits and the food processing industry have essentially eliminated nitrilosides from the common dietary — historically, the change from consuming nitriloside-rich millet for higher consumption of wheat in the making of bread and the Western habit of depriving North Temperate peoples high sources of nitrilosides (as in fruit seeds) by spitting out or throwing away the same are milestones in the history of dietary nitriloside depletion. At the same time, the continuing high presence of "B17" compounds in grazing grasses (sudan, arrow, etc.) on which range animals feed may clarify why these animals are cancer-free while their human handlers are often cancer-stricken.

The existing data can be construed several ways: laetrile compounds consumed in the natural diets of "primitive" peoples (as certain tribes in Southeast Asia for which B17-rich cassava is a staple food — "the poor man's bread") are part of a total eating regime which is best encompassed by the term "the poor people's diet." It consists not only of natural laetriles, but dozens of other natural-state nutrients in a diet largely built around non-chemically-treated fresh vegetables, unrefined grains, fresh fruits and berries, and a much lower prevalence of animal meats and proteins, the virtual non-existence of refined carbohydrates and few or no stimulants.

This *entire* dietary lifestyle in general terms highly correlates to the absence not only of cancer but of the chronic, metabolic diseases of the "civilized" Western world in general.

The foods bearing "B17" compounds also usually contain a treasure trove of many other useful nutrients — including the apricot kernel itself, the usual source in the Americas for the extraction and manufacture of laetrile. It becomes clearer with time that various of the factors in these foods, perhaps captained by the nitrilosides, are specific against malignancy, and are even more effective in combination.

The earlier developers of laetrile were as beholden to the pharmacologically-inclined allopathic thought process as anyone else in attempting to find "the" anti-cancer element. Perhaps not one, but many, were found — and an entire complex of compounds, some clearly within the nitriloside category and others simply similar to it, may work synergistically either to prevent the establishment of an incipient subclinical malignant process or, at the very least, to thwart or slow down one already in place.

Prevention, of course, is one thing — a nutrient construed as a "drug" is quite another.

For Cancer Inc. laetrile — almost always defined as the better-known chemical amygdalin, occurring in virtually all black and brown bitter fruit seeds in North America — is everything a cancer treatment should not be:

It is a natural nutrient, not a patented drug (though American and British patents have defined various refined and/or synthesized amygdalins which have never been marketed and may not even be producible), it is allegedly effective both in cancer prevention and therapy, it is not toxic at least in the doses long recommended and utilized, and it is usually provided as a central part of a "metabolic" program involving dietary change, protein-digesting enzymes, and other natural components.

Cancer as a nutritional deficiency

The rationale of laetrile against cancer also strikes at the very root of oncological wisdom:

It suggests that cancer is, more than anything else, a dietary deficiency disease (the deficiency being "Vitamin B17"), that cancer is unitarian in nature (there are not 300 or more "kinds" of cancer), that cancer is not "tumor disease" *per se* and that thus what happens or does not happen to tumors is not a fair determinant of the efficacy of an anti-cancer program, that cancer is easily preventable, that cancer treatments should be natural.

It is, hence, too simple, too "unscientific" and — worst of all — far too inexpensive for the AIC, let alone the orthodox oncological establishment, which now lays claim to an incredible $200 billion per year of the nation's trillion-dollar "healthcare delivery" bill (*III*).

Adding insult to injury, Ernst T. Krebs Jr., the biochemist, has also been a major proponent of another fruit seed derivative, which he and others baptized "pangamic acid" or Vitamin B15, which has a shorter, but equally controversial, history in against-the-grain unorthodoxy, and of the "trophoblastic thesis of cancer."

John Beard and the trophoblasts

The latter, as an updated version of an idea put forward at the turn of the century by Scots embryologist John Beard, states that cancer is nothing more or less than misplaced trophoblast, a birth cycle-related tissue essential to the fetal development of mammalian life. Under "Beardian" thinking, whatever naturally inhibits the natural trophoblast tissue in the birth cycle should also inhibit cancer. Since pancreatic enzymes are apparently involved in the inhibition of trophoblast, they should be useful against human cancer — hence the German/American and modern-day twin theories espoused by the Krebses and, for a long time, by the modern laetrilists: proteolytic enzymes and the body's host defense system constitute the "endogenous" first line of defense against cancer; the nitrilosidic food compounds, "Vitamin B17," serving as a second team or backup, constitute the "exogenous" second line of defense.

The AIC detested Vitamin B15 (probable active factor: N,N dimethylglycine), which received rave notices in Europe and the ex-Soviet Union, where much research on it was conducted and where it has been widely used. And, of course, Cancer Inc. seemed terrorized by the trophoblastic, vitamin-nature and/or any other unitarian explanation of cancer. Simple economics alone ultimately explains the institutional aversion, particularly to the vitamin theory of cancer.

There is increasing evidence to support a unitarian — if not necessarily trophoblastic — understanding of cancer (including the discovery of the "immortalizing enzyme" telomerase in most "cancer types") and abundant evidence that either laetrile or laetrile-like compounds, and other natural nutrients, are protective against cancer and hence useful in its management.

It is not the province of this study to explicate the multiple controversies of laetrile, which we have done elsewhere. What we demonstrate here is that laetrile became a major challenge not only to the scientific claims of oncology in general but, far more importantly, to the authority of the Allopathic Industrial Complex (AIC) or The Club, wounding the AIC in its tenderest of tissues — the economic one — and hence had to be destroyed scientifically, conceptually, legally, administratively, and every other way.

The Laetrile War, then, is a template for the AIC vs. its challengers — be they homeopathy, as in the last century, or chiropractic, as in the present.

Cancer Inc.'s war on 'unprovens'

Historical background is essential:

The primary "red flag" in "alternative" medicine in the United States during most of this century has been *cancer*. While "unproven" or "dubious" methods have been developed against other chronic diseases, nothing has seemed to excite such a frenzy of institutional, ideological and legal responses as the open advocacy of a "cancer cure" developed outside the parameters of the AIC.

Hence, the history of what the medical establishment derides as everything from "quackery" to "unproven remedies" in cancer is tangled, extensive and disgusting. Medical and research careers have been ruined and innocent people prosecuted and persecuted in an allegedly free society for involvement with, or the purveying of, "unapproved" "cancer cures."

There seems almost a visceral reaction from within the AIC to strike out at the same, probably because cancer (even before AIDS) was the most noticeable failure of American (and Western) "scientific medicine" and was growing exponentially through Western society. There seemed to be an unstated fear that any attack on the basic tenets of oncology (cancer as tumors — hence the destruction of tumors equating to the "curing" of the disease) somehow meant an attack on the doctrines of allopathic medicine itself. Worse, since the greater amount of the "unproven" remedies usually involves natural substances or ultimately simple and inexpensive techniques, the enormous profitability of Cancer Inc., under construction for many decades, has sensed in the non-toxic "unprovens" the greatest of threats.

In an excellent recounting of the cancer industry, Ralph Moss PhD — who was fired from his public affairs position at Memorial Sloan-Kettering Cancer Center in New York over the laetrile affair — summarized the American Cancer Society's list of "unproven remedies" (commonly called the "quack list").[9]

(The concept of "unproven" therapies suggests that there are "proven" ones — that is, chemotherapy, radiation, surgery and a few high-tech immunology boosters. With between 1,500-1,900 Americans dying per day from cancer by 1993/1994, with more than 5,000 being diagnosed with the disease at the same time and with historic highs in both the fatalities from and incidence of cancer, the notion of a "proven" cancer remedy provokes as much funereal humor in the unbiased observer as does the hoary Cancer Society concept of "unproven" methods.)

Moss found that of 63 ACS-listed "unproven techniques," by the 1990s an incredible 44.4 percent had undergone no investigation by the ACS or any other agency, public or private, before having been condemned as "unproven" — which is to say, "quack."

Moreover, among some 70 advocates of "unorthodox therapies" — often described by Cancer Inc. as "snake-oil salesmen" (a phrase which needs some updating inasmuch as some Asian research has demonstrated actual anti-cancer efficacy *from* "snake oil") — Moss noted that over 77 percent were or are medical doctors or doctors of philosophy in various scientific disciplines.

And, further, as he has noted with some humor, when at the National Cancer Institute (NCI) — the federally funded government research unit largely brought into being by the private ACS and long dominated by it — a researcher seeks a new lead into cancer management he is apt to reach first for the "unprovens" list.[10]

Cancer was grist for the mill of genuine quackery in centuries gone by — when cancer rates were tiny compared to those of today — simply because it was then, as today, mostly incurable. As I discovered while researching my first book on the laetrile affair, there even was, in the 19th century, an American Indian anti-cancer remedy with the suspiciously familiar name *Leotrill*.[11]

To be sure, the mysterious nature of cancer and its seeming incurability made it a target for con men and opportunists, so we are not here making the case that all suppressed would-be cancer "cures" were indeed legitimate research efforts: *of course* there truly was charlatanry involved in some of them. Yet, given the dismal record of the "scientifically proven" cancer remedies it has often been appropriate to draw a fine line between "unapproved quackery" and "approved quackery."

We note elsewhere (*V*) the triumph of the allopathic paradigm in medicine, backed by solid financial considerations, toward the end of the 19th century. In terms of cancer, allopathy's victory meant the institutionalization of the notion that cancer is tumors, and that there are hundreds of different kinds of tumors, each requiring its own "cure," and that the latter surely would be found in surgery, and then radiation, and then toxic chemicals. That is, mechanical assaults on the tumor mass were understood to be "scientific" approaches to a disease whose Greek-derived specialty name (oncology) means "the study of bumps."

The notion that homeopathics, fever therapy, special serums, let alone plant and other natural nutrients, might "shrink tumors" met with shrill opposition.

The beginnings: Coley, Warburg, Gerson
In the US, from the advent of Coley's toxins, one of the first "unprovens" — and later removed from that category in modern times for further research since it belatedly became obvious that the theory and practice of the same had some genuine value — "unproven" remedies against cancer grew parallel to the geometric rise in cancer incidence and deaths.

Both cancer rates and "unproven remedies" boomed in the immediate post-World War II years.

Dietary theories concerning cancer and how to manage it are not new: Otto Warburg in Germany described a dietary connection to malignancy decades ago. Straddling Germany and the United States, the late Max Gerson MD probably did more than any single physician/researcher to bring dietary and nutritional elements to light in the management of the disease, and was among the major challengers to the allopathic paradigm.

Despite widespread evidence of efficacy against cancer through Gerson methods of detoxification and dietary manipulation, the German physician in the 1940s underwent an all-out attack by the then-fledgling Cancer Inc.: neutralization, isolation, and professional elimination. So "Gersonism" was one of the first of the widely used "unprovens" to abandon the United States and reappear in Mexico as well as in other countries around the world.

An "unproven" method called the Lincoln bacteriophage therapy helped the cancer-stricken son of Senator Charles Tobey recover in the 1950s, leading the legislator to attempt a full-scale investigation into the American cancer industry — one definable as that even as early as 1953. Just years prior, in 1946, American

Medical Assn.-influenced legislators had blocked a proposal by Senator Claude Pepper for a $100 million research effort into *all aspects* of cancer therapy.

As chairman of the Senate Interstate and Foreign Commerce Committee it was Tobey who hired attorney Benedict F. Fitzgerald Jr. of the Justice Department as special counsel. Senator Tobey died of a heart attack before his cancer-probe project could get underway, and his successor, Senator John Bricker, proved to be far more favorable to the AMA. Even so, Special Counsel Fitzgerald's investigation of cancer treatments in the United States resulted in the first general "official" overview of what was going on, and it was the first time the word "conspiracy" was used to describe the activities of Cancer Inc. in an official forum.

By the time Fitzgerald's report was published in the *Congressional Record* in 1953, several "alternative" cancer therapies had had or were in the process of having an appreciable impact on United States medicine aside from the Gerson controversy. The major ones:

— Dr William F. Koch's Glyoxylide, one of the first examples of an "alternative" therapy hounded into near-extinction internationally and which we now recognize as an early precursor of oxidative treatments.

— Krebiozen, an animal blood serum-derived therapy pioneered in the United States by physiologist Dr. Andrew C. Ivy, vice president of the University of Illinois, after having been introduced to it by Yugoslav physician Stephan Durovic.

— The Hoxsey herbals, perhaps — second only to laetrile — the best-known, long-running controversy pitting Cancer Inc. vs. a natural method.

The campaign against Glyoxylide

Dr. Koch's treatment had such support earlier in this century that by 1921-22 the AMA was, of course, lobbying against it. No one at that time had any inkling of either "free radicals" or oxidative treatments. Koch's work had continued through the 1930s and 1940s with major research and use of this modality occurring in Canada, whose Ontario Cancer Commission in 1939 and 1940 provided objective forums in which to indicate Glyoxylide efficacy.

Dr. Koch worked in Mexico and Brazil in 1940 and 1941, using the substance also for treating mental conditons. He was arrested in Florida in 1942 on a charge of false labelling, with a district attorney noting that his (for the time) high bail of $10,000 was set at that level in order to keep him from returning to Brazil to finish research work.

Despite thousands of case histories in support of Glyoxylide — "anecdotes," as Cancer Inc. calls such testimonials — Dr. Koch was subjected to Food and Drug Administration (FDA)-triggered trials in 1942 and 1946 which led to a permanent injunction against the treatment in 1950. Nobody could understand his ahead-of-his-time approach, out of which the kindred product Rodaquin (later available in Mexico) was developed. Harassment, legal fees and the lack of any political savvy on the part of Glyoxylide's supporters spelled the essential demise of what had been a promising avenue of research.[12]

Taking on Harry Hoxsey

Between the 1920s and 1940s thousands of Americans were successfully treated with many "forms" of cancer with the herbal preparations originally developed in the 19th century by John Hoxsey and promoted in the United States by his descendant, Harry Hoxsey.

Because of early support by several physicians of the Hoxsey method, and also because the flamboyant Harry Hoxsey refused to turn over the herbal formulations to another doctor, American medical officials began a lengthy persecution of the maverick in Illinois, Pennsylvania and Texas, all of which at one time or another had Hoxsey clinics to which thousands of Americans turned for at least partial remedies of their cancer cases.[13]

While the Krebiozen controversy was just beginning and as

Fitzgerald was investigating cancer in general, laetrile was also being quietly looked at by various physicians in several countries. Dr. Krebs Sr. had pioneered it in the 1920s when it was developed as an unexpected byproduct in efforts of the San Francisco innovator to make Prohibition Era whiskey taste better. Compounds, of which amygdalin may have only been one, and later compounds which turned out to be refined amygdalin, were seriously studied in several countries, as the laetrile research-sponsoring McNaughton Foundation pointed out. But by the 1950s laetrile was not the "news" that the Koch compounds, Krebiozen and the Hoxsey herbals were.

Dr. Ivy and Krebiozen

Dr. Ivy, one of America's most prestigious scientists and scholars, found Krebiozen to be useful in terminal cancer patients and went on to promote its use as a major anticancer medicine, one which reportedly was sought by two major drug companies whose takeover offers he spurned. Despite some 20,000 cases attesting to Krebiozen usefulness, including 530 described by Fitzgerald, the US government, equipped with an amended Food, Drug and Cosmetic Act, took Dr. Ivy to court in 1964.[14]

Even though he was cleared of all the counts against him in an expensive, 289-day showcase trial, the negative publicity from Cancer Inc. virtually ended Krebiozen in the USA.

By the time Fitzgerald issued his *Congressional Record* assessment of cancer research in 1953, there had been considerable hoopla generated by the Hoxsey, Krebiozen, and Glyoxylide controversies. They were larger challenges to Cancer Inc., which also had to fend off many other unwanted approaches, compounds and techniques.

The pattern was ever similar: a lone researcher or doctor would stumble upon an apparently useful anticancer compound, test it, then attempt to gain federal licensing and recognition. Suddenly the representative of a drug company would appear bearing sufficient gold and would attempt to induce the inventor to turn over the formula or share in the profits. Failure to do so would often mean actual harassment of the inventors and compounds.

Occasionally, unpleasant truths slipped out. In the 1980s I was intermittently researching and writing a still-unpublished account of the incredible story of the development of anti-cancer compounds derived from the head-shrinking process of the Jivaro Indians of South America, as researched over many years by "white medicine man" Wilburn Ferguson.

In the not-commercially-available recounting of his professional life among the Jivaro (or Shuara)[15] and in many interviews with me, he described how an officer of a major drug company in the USA had actually told him that to legalize the Jivaro compounds would put cancer drug development out of business. This was why, Ferguson felt, that despite years of effort and a bureaucratic runaround, he had received little federal support to follow up on highly promising cancer research which at one point had been supported by the Ecuadorian government.

Fitzgerald lets a cat out of the bag
This is the kind of backdrop against which Benedict F. Fitzgerald's report should be read, and the laetrile controversy understood.

The attorney summarized in the August 28, 1953, *Congressional Record* that:

There is reason to believe that the AMA has been hasty, capricious, arbitrary and outright dishonest [in its statements against various "unapproved" therapies] *and could involve the AMA and others in a conspiracy of alarming proportions . . .*

Behind and over all this [apparently successful response to Krebiozen in hundreds of cases] *is the weirdest conglomeration of corrupt motives, intrigues, selfishness, jealousy, obstruction and conspiracy that I have ever seen . . .*

Should we sit idly by and count the number of physicians, surgeons and cancerologists who are not only divided but who, because of fear or favor, are forced to line up with the so-called accepted view of the American Medical Association, or should this Committee make a full-scale investigation of the organized effort to hinder, suppress and restrict the free flow of drugs which allegedly have proven successful in cases where clinical reports, case history, pathological reports and X-ray photographic proof, together with the alleged cured patients, are available?

Accordingly, we should determine whether existing agencies, both public and private, are engaged in and have pursued a policy of harassment, ridicule, slander and libelous attacks on others sincerely engaged in stamping out this curse of mankind . . . My investigation to date should convince this Committee that a conspiracy does exist to stop the free flow and use of drugs in interstate commerce which allegedly (have) solid therapeutic value. Public and private funds have been thrown around like confetti at a country fair to close up and destroy clinics, hospitals, and scientific research laboratories which do not conform to the viewpoint of medical associations. How long will the American people take this?[16]

The answer was: at least several more decades.

Between the Fitzgerald report and the laetrile outbreak of the 1970s, the Food, and Drug and Cosmetic Act was amended (see *IX*), a move which, among many things, made it extremely difficult for a natural substance to be federally licensed as a "new drug" — unless a proponent group had many millions of unrecoverable dollars to spend on the effort.

Even so, the McNaughton Foundation made an effort to secure FDA licensing for laetrile, only to be sandbagged at the last moment.[17]

Enter Dr. Dean Burk

The entry into the laetrile field of National Cancer Institute

(NCI) cytochemistry chief Dean Burk, PhD, a biochemist, added a variety of clout to laetrile that its predecessors and contemporary challengers to the medical orthodoxy never had:

"The Dean" was uniquely credentialed and positioned to defend laetrile from within the very bowels of the American research establishment, and he did so repeatedly and incisively.

While scattered laetrile research in the United States and other countries had been strongly favorable for what was in essence a derivative of apricot kernels, the compound was receiving a major boost with the opening of an anti-cancer clinic in Tijuana, Mexico, and official interest by the Mexican government.

On May 30, 1972, Dr. Burk wrote to Congressman Louis Frey Jr. that

Although . . . Laetrile utilization in this country is proceeding . . . in spite of FDA prohibitions, it is even more so because of unwarranted FDA procedures, and lack of FDA scientific and medical justification for its stand, extending to probable unconstitutionality, concerning which many thousands of cancer-afflicted persons and their relatives and physicians are rapidly becoming aware.

. . . I have hundreds of letters sent to me enclosing FDA information sheets and pronouncements, in which the senders of these letters point to the extensive falsification, duplicity, deviousness, red herrings and literal lies . . . promulgated by the FDA with respect to Laetrile, as well as similarly on the part of certain high officials . . . of the American Medical Association, the American Cancer Society, the US Department of Health, Education and Welfare, and state agencies . . . It is becoming evident that the current generation of cancer sufferers is coming to regard the intransigence and palpable lies of the FDA and the above-indicated

related organizations with a marked measure of contempt on the basis of prima facie evidence provided by these organizations themselves as to their integrity and credibility and that something of a Boston Tea Party mode of action is being undertaken by an increasing number of cancer sufferers in this country, who intend to be hoodwinked no longer; in short, an active backlash is developing even at the grass-roots level...[18]

My friend and mentor was quite prescient — for just a few days later, in June 1972, an event occurred in Northern California which would change the American medical landscape forever.

A newspaper editor gets hooked

As a checkup patient of Dr. John A. Richardson and as editor of the *Berkeley Daily Gazette*, I was suddenly thrust into an awkward position when a friend in the Alameda County district attorney's office called to inform me, just as he had other media, that a "cancer-quack bust" was in the works for tomorrow.

When I inquired just who the cancer quack to be "busted" was, and he told me, "that Dr. Richardson out in Albany, the one using the laetrile," I gulped. I had a moral quandary: I was given privileged information in my role as a journalist, yet the information directly bore on my own physician, who was also a friend.

I agonized over what to do and decided that it was not my role to interfere with the "bust." It took place — police swarmed into the Albany clinic to arrest Dr. Richardson on various counts involving violation of specific California codes aimed at laetrile. True enough, Dr. Richardson had ballooned into prominence (together with the pioneering Ernesto Contreras Sr MD in Tijuana) as a major laetrile-using doctor with a rapidly growing caseload of essentially satisfied patients.

It was the arrest of Dr. Richardson, a John Bircher, which ignited the firestorm of national agitation not so much over laetrile as over the issue of freedom of medical choice, a concept not only near and dear to Birchism but to Americans of many political persuasions. When fellow medics in the San Francisco Bay area, Stanford University scientist Robert Bradford, Birch writer G. Edward Griffin, and various patients and businessmen rallied to the legal-defense cause of Dr. Richardson the first Committee for Freedom of Choice in Cancer Therapy Inc. was set up.

Dr. Richardson ultimately went through three trials involving laetrile, losing one and tieing two, litigations which sparked the explosive growth of the original committee into a nationwide movement. Eventually, there would be committees for freedom of choice in all 50 states with an activist membership variously estimated at anywhere from 20,000 to 50,000.

On July 3, 1973, more than a year after the Richardson raid and as the committee was congealing as a national movement, Dr. Burk wrote to Congressman Robert A. Roe that laetrile had been successful in NCI-directed studies of the compound against Lewis mouse lung cancer even while the federal agency, Dr. Burk's employer, was consistently denying overall efficacy from the substance. Wrote Dr. Burk:

You may wonder, Congressman Roe, why anyone should go to such pains and mendacity to avoid conceding what happened to the NCI-directed experiment. Such an admission and concession is crucially relevant. Once any of the FDA-NCI-AMA-ACS hierarchy so much as concedes that Laetrile anti-tumor efficacy was indeed even once observed in NCI experimentation, a permanent crack in the bureaucratic armor has taken place that can widen indefinitely by further appropriate experimentation.[19]

By this time, more and more "anecdotal case histories" of Americans responding to the "laetrile program" of oral and intravenous laetrile, proteolytic enzymes and special diet were coming forward and gaining media attention. Initially as a skeptic, I also was interviewing several dozen laetrile users, most of them Richardson and Contreras patients, for my first book, being consistently amazed by what I found, heard and saw.

When I asked state authorities for the official version of what was wrong with laetrile, I was referred to an aging 1953 report on some 44 dying, terminal cancer patients who had received tiny doses of experimental laetrile in the early 1950s. Since the patients died this was taken as a sure sign of a lack of efficacy. Yet I was bewildered to read that improvements in overall well-being and cessation of pain had occurred in many of these terminal patients. Even as a non-MD journalist, it seemed clear to me that this obviously harmless substance should be further studied if only for its apparent ability to reduce pain and enhance subjective feelings of improvement.

The laetrile juggernaut

From 1973, the laetrile juggernaut began to roll with an intensity which had never been experienced by any other anti-establishmentarian medical movement in America:

It was learned that collaborative trials between the Mexican government and the prestigious Memorial Sloan-Kettering Cancer Center (MSKCC) in New York were in the offing and that more physicians were coming forward admitting they were finding merit in laetrile in their cancer patients. The "guru" of the movement, indefatigable San Francisco biochemist Ernst T. Krebs Jr., was joining Committee national chairman Robert Bradford and laetrile-using doctors on speakers' platforms around the country.

The rapid proliferation of Committees for Freedom of Choice became a phenomenon in its own right, and it was matched by politicking — the very thing in which proponents of earlier cancer unorthodoxy in the United States had not engaged.

In 1975, three events galvanized the movement:

First, US District Court Judge Luther Bohanon, Oklahoma City, ruled that the FDA had no right to keep US patients from being able to secure their own supplies of foreign laetrile and that "the FDA has abdicated its duty to make a clear determination as to whether Laetrile should or should not be placed in commerce since the drug has been in use for many years." The legal move entered by attorney Clyde Watts on behalf of terminal cancer patients as a class instantly allowed Kansan Glen L. Rutherford (described as "cured" of bowel cancer by Dr. Contreras' laetrile program) "legal" access to Mexican laetrile. The legal fight would go on for years, twice reaching the Supreme Court, allowing American cancer patients an affidavit system through which foreign laetrile could be procured.

Then, an underground research group at Sloan-Kettering revealed a "coverup" of seven series of animal tests of laetrile which had shown efficacy even as the New York research center was denying that its testing program had shown any benefits. (In my 1974 book, a Sloan-Kettering vice president had confirmed to me that there had in fact been beneficial results, so much so that further trials were planned.[20]) I was one of the newspapermen to whom the data were anonymously "leaked." I immediately confirmed (by speaking with Sloan-Kettering's veteran biochemical researcher, Dr. Kanematsu Sugiura) that the results were valid and were his.

That the nation's foremost cancer research facility would fudge on positive test results with an essentially non-toxic cancer compound provided a major piece of evidence that Cancer Inc. was alive and well. Not long afterward, the "underground" at Sloan-Kettering would emerge as disgruntled staff members openly opposed what they saw as a front-office effort to suppress positive test results with "Vitamin B17." It worked out that Ralph Moss PhD, assistant public affairs director at MSKCC, was a key element in the "underground." In a bold move, Dr. Moss — sent by MSKCC to a press conference in part sponsored by the Committee for Freedom of Choice in Cancer Therapy — took advantage of the conference to announce his disagreement with MSKCC's laetrile coverup. He was promptly fired.

The MSKCC disclosures also galvanized me personally and radicalized me on the subject: no longer was this simply a journalistic exercise — life-and-death issues revolved around the fight over freedom of choice let alone the possible efficacy of laetrile. 1975 was the year of my moving from "straight" journalism into the advocacy camp of the Committee.

The 'great laetrile smuggling trial'

The third major event occurred in Christmas Week, 1975, when federal officials conducted a nationwide crackdown of the incipient laetrile movement: Robert W. Bradford was among 16 individuals ultimately arrested and/or indicted on charges of smuggling Mexican laetrile into the United States. The police deployment was considerable: at least 20 federal agents in a dozen vehicles were involved in a surveillance operation stretching from the Mexican border to the San Francisco Bay Area in the effort to nab Bradford. In Minnesota, an entrapment scheme involving US-ordered, US government-dispatched, US government-seized and US government-followed laetrile was used to raid two private residences and set up the arrests of presumed laetrile distributors there.

The "international laetrile smuggling ring" trial was to become the lengthiest federal conspiracy case ever tried in a San Diego federal court. While the principals were ultimately found guilty, no prison time was meted out, and the court record was replete with the scandalous efforts of US federal authorities to induce, entrap and set up presumed laetrile distributors as if they were heroin importers or vicious criminals. Court testimony brought out that the federal side paid Mexican "mules" (professional smugglers) to bring clandestine laetrile (apricot seed extract) into the United States in order to aid in the entrapment of members of the "ring."

In the seeming acting out of a Greek drama, each new element of the controversy simply set the stage for an even greater element later.

A revolt starts in Alaska

In 1976, the next major element dramatically occurred in

Alaska:

The state legislature passed a law protecting physician/patient freedom of choice in cancer therapy, with laetrile clearly the target. The American Cancer Society, the American Medical Assn. and the FDA, all of which opposed the bill, did not fully realize that the Alaska action, spurred by Committee chapters, was only a shot fired across the bow. Cancer Inc. and American medical orthodoxy failed to assess the symbolic importance of the Anchorage legislation and for that reason unexpectedly ceded so much terrain to the laetrile movement that the Allopathic Industrial Complex (AIC) would ultimately have to go to the greatest — and dirtiest — lengths in its history to suppress what became the stiffest-ever challenge to its power and authority.

For, between 1976 and 1981, bills either "decriminalizing" laetrile (that is, barring the state from punishing a physician for administering, or a patient from having, laetrile) or outright "legalizing" it (accepting it as a useful medication, allowing its distribution and, occasionally, its manufacture) were approved in 24 states, which encompassed more than half the population of the United States. Pro-laetrile bills also passed twice in New York, only to be vetoed by the governor with the vetoes not overturned. In some states, laetrile legislation was simply appended to existing medical statutes; in others, whole new statutes were written and passed. Following the rapid-fire approval of laetrile-connected legislation in Indiana, Florida and Texas, Cancer Inc. and the AIC began to note that they had a considerable problem on their hands.

The Committee-spearheaded efforts at taking one statehouse after another, activities also backed by other health-freedoms groups, captured media attention and popular interest. The Committee stuck to a single sweeping principle — that the issue was not so much freedom for laetrile as it was freedom of informed consent in cancer therapy in general for physician and patient. In virtually every professional opinion-sampling poll taken, be it national, state or local — and including Roper, Harris and Gallup — the concept of freedom of choice won by margins ranging from 2 to 1 to 12 to 1. The revolt drew scorn and shock from the AIC, fresh rounds of police action by the FDA (which even circulated Post Office "wanted"-style posters called "Laetrile Warnings" across the country), and such reflections of academic concerns as the laetrile-dominated AAAS meeting of 1979.

Since I was an eyewitness to, and frequent participant in, these state-by-state campaigns, I am fully aware — as the opposition slowly came to recognize — that we had a considerable populist tiger by the tail: an upsurge of grassroots rejection of the institutional, scientific and academic forces of the American establishment not so much over the issue of laetrile efficacy or lack of same but over the burning, central issue of freedom of choice. One observer after another joined the conceptual battle and usually remained clear on the separation of the issues of freedom of choice in medicine vs. the efficacy of laetrile: by what stroke of logic or presumed vested interest does the state have the right to intervene in life-and-death decisions between a physician and a patient, particularly when the patient is said to be "terminal," as with cancer? The AIC and the establishment in general never could offer a sound, coherent answer to that question. It still cannot. Hence, the tactics of the opposition changed.

From the scientific side, famed Mayo Clinic researcher Charles Moertel MD opined publicly that even though there was no proof of laetrile efficacy, at least in "accepted" circles, neither was there sweeping evidence *against* the compound. He and other front-rank researchers suggested there might be sufficient "biochemical background noise" to suggest the "valid sign of efficacy," the "shred of evidence" which Cancer Inc. kept arguing did not exist for laetrile — increasingly recognized as amygdalin and often described as "Vitamin B17." There were too many doctors stepping forward with case histories, some published in book form, too many dissident scientists claiming there was some merit in the notion of anti-cancer efficacy from glycosidic compounds, and far, far too many "anecdotes" from patients treated in Mexico or even within the USA to be able to make the claim the apricot kernel extract was totally without value. With a US district court protecting citizen access at least to foreign laetrile, with one state after another either legalizing or decriminalizing the use of laetrile products in total disregard of the official positions of the FDA, AMA and American Cancer Society, with doctors and patients in ever greater numbers saying good things about the substance, and with cancer death rates ever worsening even after the Nixon Administration declaration of a "war on cancer," it became obvious that Cancer Inc. had to take another position.

The Establishment counterattack

In the earlier years of the controversy, the general establishment "line" on laetrile had been that it was worthless yet essentially harmless and that its only real danger lay in diverting cancer patients from "useful" treatments — a dodge argument inasmuch as the great majority of laetrile treatment seekers were advanced cases whose likelihood of being "cured" by "useful" therapies was quite low.

But given the political successes of the laetrile movement, the worthless-but-harmless argument needed to be amended. The new position was that it was not only useless but harm*ful* — the harm primarily attributable, to nobody's surprise, to the fact that an excess amount of the oral product could indeed produce a low-grade cyanide toxicity. Even though virtually no laetrile-using physician prescribed oral doses above the presumed therapeutically useful maximum oral amount (1.5 grams daily), and intravenous laetrile was regarded as so essentially non-toxic at even huge levels (one Mexican hospital once slow-dripped a breathtaking 97,000 milligrams — 97 grams — into one patient over 24 hours), the cyanide component of laetrile became the cornerstone argument.

We have recounted[21] how Cancer Inc. scoured world literature ("anecdotes" by any measure) to find scattered accounts of seeming "laetrile poisoning." These included the intoxication of garbage-plundering Turkish waifs years before who may have eaten too many fruit seeds, and the intoxication of a "hippie" couple in California who became ill after drinking a slurry of ground-up apricot kernels kept in a glass of water left standing in an open window the night before. Even the case of a woman who, averse to injections, broke open several vials of injectable laetrile and drank the contents before becoming fatally ill, made the news. While accounts of several hundred babies per year dying of aspirin intoxication was clearly not news, the mere suggestion that laetrile overdoses *might* be dangerous *became* news.

Major research centers turned to celebrated animal tests to attempt to alert the people to the "dangers" of laetrile.

In 1978 studies in Ohio, toxicity from oral amygdalin was said to have occurred in test animals when up to 1.3 grams *per kilogram of body weight* was provided for monkeys and up to 6.4 grams *per kilogram of body weight* for dogs. These enormous levels, extrapolated to humans, meant that from *five to 300 times* the normal oral dose of amygdalin for a 150-pound man were provided to the test animals. No doubt about it: toxicity occurred.[22]

Results of the incredible "laetrile toxicity study" at the University of California-Davis in 1978 were provided to the press and public at large as evidence that the consumption of certain vegetables together with oral laetrile could kill, and that even the "laetrile diet" recommended to laetrile patients was dangerous.

But the test was actually a sophisticated effort to produce cyanide intoxication in animals: dogs were starved, drugged (to suppress vomiting), and then administered by inserted gastric tube a mash of sweet almonds mixed in a plastic blood bag with amygdalin at a temperature sufficient to allow an enzyme within the almonds to "hydrolyze" the amygdalin, causing cyanide release. This tactic did indeed intoxicate several dogs — but it had nothing to do with the ways in which either dogs or man eat or how they consume "B17" compounds.[23]

By the time of the laetrile trials, American orthodoxy had taken a belated interest in potentially toxic chemicals in the plant kingdom, very much including the nitrilosides, and no effort was spared to serve up frightening new evidence that overdosing on such compounds could indeed be life-threatening. Scattered research also suggested that inappropriate uses of such compounds might be *mutagenic* — that is, change-causing and hence predisposing to cancer — as if such information constituted important new discoveries.

Most of these findings, of course, were already well-known to chemists and biochemists who were fully aware that too much of anything, including air and water, and/or the misuse of virtually any compound, herb or medication could lead to serious problems, even death. Yet the AIC was forced, by sheer weight of laetrile's political successes, to overkill the issues of danger from cyanide-bearing compounds and to track down, and extrapolate from, every isolated datum that could be found which might produce a negative for laetrile. No such campaign of any such dimension had ever been mounted before in American medical history.

The medical establishment continued to write off laetrile case histories pointing to seeming successes the time-honored way — such cases were either misdiagnoses, belated responses to earlier orthodoxy therapy or, when all else failed, "spontaneous remissions," the line of defense used consistently throughout this century against the "unprovens". (*XI*)

It also made certain that notable failures of laetrile-centered therapy got plenty of press attention, particularly if the failures came from the growing caseloads of Drs. Contreras and Richardson. Such negatives were indeed reported in gruesome detail — yet it was only an occasional journalist who dared contrast failures on laetrile therapy with failures on vincristine, 5-FU, adriamycin, radiation and surgery, since somehow a failure on an orthodox modality was somehow less a failure than one on unorthodox therapy.

The establishment also chose most of the time to overlook

the fact that modern-day laetrilists absolutely denied that amygdalin was a "cure" of cancer (even if the original proponents of laetrile seemed to have believed it was), and that the maximum claim being made for its use by the great majority of doctors and researchers was that laetrile, as part of a total "metabolic program," might lead to the lifelong "control" of the disease.

But for every "establishment" setback of laetrile research there were countermoves by "unorthodoxy" — even when well-credentialed. Cancer Inc. seemed particularly enraged when Loyola University (Chicago) biochemist Harold Manner PhD and a team of graduate students released data in a "non-standard" publication on tumor shrinkage in laboratory rats with a combination of amygdalin, proteolytic enzymes and vitamins.[24] Tests conducted at Salisbury State College in Maryland suggesting cancer prevention by *ad libitum* consumption of apricot kernels by test rats not only were not followed up on but got the key researcher in hot water.[25]

Harold Manner would fall under heavier attack after he started inducing foreign cancer clinics to utilize his "Manner cocktail" (not very divergent from the laetrile "metabolic therapy" already in place) against human cancer, in which he claimed striking success against breast cancer in particular.

Independent-minded researchers frequently tried to bring reason out of the war. University of California-Berkeley chemist James Cason PhD, who found merit in the "B17" theory, wrote in a scientific publication in 1978:

> *If I believe that eating 100 mg of nitriloside and 2 g of vitamin C per day will prevent me from becoming a cancer victim, and I live according to my stated convictions, and* I am wrong, *I suffer no penalty for my poor judgment, because I am doing nothing other than eating food that is commonly regarded as nutritionally beneficial.*
>
> *If one who believes that all this stuff about cancer resulting from nutritional deficiencies is nonsense, lives by his convictions, and* he is wrong,

that individual stands a very good chance of paying an awesome penalty for his faulty judgment.[26]

This was just the kind of argument, as advanced by a properly credentialed American scientist writing in a properly credentialed scientific journal, that Cancer Inc. did not wish to hear — but could do little about.

Attempted KO: the 'laetrile clinical trial'

The laetrile controversy, simmering both politically and scientifically, had a final denouement in the scientific arena with the federal 1980-81 "laetrile clinical trial," an outgrowth of Senate subcommittee hearings in 1977 (another landmark event for an "unapproved" remedy). With the trial, the Committee for Freedom of Choice took a calculated risk: providing the government with the tools to test a compound already found anecdotally useful for thousands of patients could either vindicate or destroy it.

Even so, as I reasoned, the mere fact that such a trial had to be done in the first place was an unprecedented event by itself, and it seemed unlikely that such a study would be uniformly negative.

The laetrile movement wandered into the trial quicksand poorly prepared: there were arguments about the proper manufacturing procedures for intravenous laetrile, there remained differences of opinion even over the definition of the word "laetrile," and too often laetrile proponents had explained theories as to how amygdalin "worked" as facts rather than as educated speculations.

And, too, as in any orthodoxy-denied activity (prostitution, alcohol consumption at an earlier time), there were commercial pimps and criminal elements ready to take advantage of a legally unserviceable market: there were indeed phony laetriles, cases of fifty-dollar vials of bootleg laetrile, and some manufacturers of both vials and tablets were not always honest in reporting true weights and contents of tablets and vials.

The presence in the contraband market of numerous

laetriles of uncertain origin both compounded the fight for acceptance and provided the AIC with propaganda targets.

Yet such presence bespoke a greater reality: there was a growing popular clamor for access to laetrile, whose legal availability — and therefore the nature and purity of which — could not be guaranteed *because of* state-sanctioned interference with the availability. Such a situation was a most well-fertilized breeding ground for con men, opportunists, and criminals. Yet these were exploiters rather than causers of the situation, the true creator of which was the Allopathic Industrial Complex (AIC).

The "laetrile clinical trial" was conducted on 178 patients at four major research centers after a "retrospective analysis" conducted by the National Cancer Institute (NCI) turned up evidence of laetrile efficacy (as understood by orthodoxy) in nine of 93 case records submitted, somewhat timorously, by US physicians.

American Biologics, a California company which in no small part was an outgrowth of the Committee for Freedom of Choice in Cancer Therapy Inc., had offered to provide for free a Mexican-manufactured supply of laetrile — certainly a risky maneuver if in fact the company, as a major proponent of amygdalin, knew the material to be worthless. The government refused the offer, only later admitting the material to be used was a reproduction of Mexican laetrile seized during a confiscation and that the injectable form was not pure amygdalin but in fact a "racemic" form of it. Our group attempted unsuccessfully to block the trial in court when evidence surfaced that the material originally planned for use would not release cyanide. It is not clear exactly which material was ultimately used, or if the same material was consistently used.

The "laetrile clinical trial" was wholly unprecedented in American medical history and — as our group noted in a point-by-point rebuttal of its findings[27] — wound up being in essence a US government-sponsored test of an uncertain laetrile product whose application was in the hands of doctors and scientists known to be or assumed to be hostile to laetrile, whose patients were anonymous, and the test results of which, being coded, could not be individually released or cross-checked. Worse, the patients accepted for entry into the program were variously described as "terminal" or beyond the hope of cure by conventional means, yet not at the "final stage."

The government also saw fit to release data on the test before the trial results were published — itself an unprecedented move — before a special audience as a kind of slide presentation. But a Committee observer at the event was able to photograph the relevant slide which showed that a significant amount of test patients had remained "stable" while on the injectable part of a program whose oral protocol, we had every reason to believe, was not very strongly adhered to (and parts of which, as in suggested Vitamin A levels) seemed not to have been followed at all.

By the time the results were published, in the *New England Journal of Medicine*,[28] an abstract of them summarized that the clinical trial had shown laetrile to be ineffective as a cancer treatment — yet the fine print did not truly substantiate the analysis. For, depending on how the numbers were read, either a small majority or a large plurality of patients had remained "stable" while on the injectable part of the program, and only advanced into further disease after the 21 days of injections ceased. It later surfaced "anecdotally" that at least one patient was urged not to continue on the program (claiming he had "done too well".[29]) As a corollary, a preliminary test found amygdalin not to be toxic, at least in the ranges suggested for therapeutic use.

In all, the results, far from putting laetrile to rest, raised far more questions than they answered. Yet the press was provided with an abstract-based account which had the desired effect: "LAETRILE FAILS" and similar headlines greeted the release of the findings. The *New England Journal of Medicine* subsequently allowed brief dissents by cancer researchers Edwin Bross, acclaimed scientist Linus Pauling, and myself, but the damage was done, and it was extensive.

Laetrile's real victories

Despite the fact that for the first time ever the AIC and Cancer Inc. had had to play unusually rough to quench an unwanted competitor, and despite the fact that for a time the Mayo Clinic-centered "laetrile clinical trial" had a chilling effect on use of the substance itself, it had all been a matter of too little, too late:

Just as plans for the trial were getting underway, Rutgers University, in diabetes-oriented research, came up with a finding it seemed almost too flustered to report — that amygdalin is a useful natural "scavenger" of the deadliest of the "free radicals," hydroxyl radical.[30] This finding substantiated laetrile's role as an antioxidant (scavenger of free radicals), an activity being seen of increasing importance in the way cancer spreads (metastasizes). Then, just as the test furor was hottest, the National Academy of Sciences (NAS) published an incredible, federally funded study appropriately called *Diet, Nutrition and Cancer*.[31]

In it, essentially American research (most of it from the University of Minnesota) found a wide spectrum of plant kingdom factors apparently useful in the prevention of cancer, including Vitamin C. Among the more prominent, widely dispersed plant compounds was a class of what researchers called "non-nutritive food factors" and among these a key family was referred to as "benzyl-aromatic-isothiocyanates" — or, as we reported it, BAITs, for short. However much anti-laetrilists wished to gloss over the fact, BAITs refer to compounds which at the very least are structurally similar to "Vitamin B17" even though their mode of action against cancer has not been well elucidated. It seemed a kind of hollow scientific victory for our side in the propaganda war, and of course went essentially unnoticed by the media and certainly by the major organs of the AIC: laetrile might be a "dirty" but a benzyl-aromatic-isothiocyanate was a "clean."

While the NCI laetrile trial was widely reported to have "put laetrile to rest," use of products said to be laetrile, in natural or manufactured form, continued apace — and still do. It was up to such entities as our Bradford Research Institutes (BRI) to place the use of the cyanide-bearing sugar compounds (natural laetriles) into their proper position within a total metabolic program and to publish by far the most definitive study on how amygdalin might or might not work against cancer, which we did in 1981 in a research paper which helped to demystify "Vitamin B17" but remained essentially unknown.[32]

Research in the 1980s, primarily in Japan,[33] indicated that benzaldehyde — usually a considerable portion of "B17" compounds — had anti-cancer properties on its own. The institutional observation that BAITs, "benzaldehyde inclusion compounds" — and other natural factors which tended to metabolize in the body to laetrile-like substances — has only tended to strengthen the overall concept of a dietary-deficiency theory of cancer.

That oral "B17" compounds convert to *thiocyanate*, a chemical useful in almost two dozen natural body functions, including regulation of blood pressure, also bolstered the notion of a natural "surveillant, antineoplastic" mechanism against cancer. It may be that the "real" Vitamin B17 is in fact thiocyanate, and that the cyanogenetic glucosides or nitrilosides are "pro-vitamins." Whatever the research outcome, the case for laetriles and laetrile-like compounds as useful against the malignant process — and useful in numerous *other* processes — has been enhanced over time.

Scientifically, laetrile's victories have thus been confined to a kind of pyrrhicness: the substance itself remains a kind of Cinderella compound, yet the plant families in which it and similar substances are often found (as in the *Brassica, Rosaceae, Prunasae*) are those families in which modern-day research has isolated indoles, flavones, phenols and many other compounds in addition to BAITs as useful anticarcinogenic agents.

Too, what for years laetrile doctors called the "laetrile diet" is, broadly speaking, the diet now promoted by, of all things, the American Cancer Society and Cancer Inc. in general: less animal fat, less animal protein, fewer stimulants, more natural fruits and vegetables in as natural, raw or sprouting a stage as possible, and more fiber and unrefined grains. And aspects of the metabolic program of which laetrile is usually a part — as beta-carotene and Vitamin C — have come under close scrutiny for increasing evidence they are useful against cancer.

It is as if laetrile gave a party it was not allowed to attend — or, as one long-time "laetrilist" put it, "modern, establishment-accepted nutritional therapy against cancer and without laetrile is rather like Christianity without the Virgin Birth."

Even so, long-term "laetrile/cancer survivors" — people with advanced malignant states who used laetrile as a central part of a total metabolic program — abound. Some have written books about their experience with the apricot-kernel derivative, including long-term survivor Helen Curran of Laguna Hills CA, whose inspiring book carries the same name as this chapter.

And there was Kansas' Glen Rutherford — the man for whom the original US Supreme Court case involving freedom of access to laetrile in the 1970s — is named.

In 1994, Rutherford was a self-described "seventy-seven years young," and 23 years away from the prognosis of fatal colorectal cancer that had sent him to Mexico in the first place. Along with his oral laetrile, Rutherford daily consumed upwards of 80 supplements a day and was a stickler on the "cancer diet." Not only had colorectal cancer not returned in more than two decades — neither had he had the flu, he was pleased to report.[35]

But perhaps laetrile's major victory was, as our group analyzed, at the political level.

The fight for freedom of choice for laetrile ballooned into a much broader fight for freedom of choice in medicine itself. The attempt by Cancer Inc. to suppress the growing "anecdotal" efficacy of Vitamin C against cancer followed on the heels of the Laetrile Revolution, and paralleling both was a substantial increase in the use by physicians of natural nutrients in both the prevention and management of chronic diseases, including cancer. Laetrile had let a major cat out of the bag, and it would never go back in.

The apricot kernel extract had become the Marine Corps of the integrative medical revolution — first on the beach, first to be bloodied, first to open the door to what would come after.

References

1. Markle, GE, and Petersen, JC, five papers, American Assn. for the Advancement of Science, January 1979.
2. Moertel, CG, et al., "A clinical trial of amygdalin (laetrile) in the treatment of human cancer." *New Eng. J. Med.*, Jan. 28, 1982.
3. Culbert, ML, *Vitamin B17: Forbidden Weapon Against Cancer*. New Rochelle NY: Arlington House, 1974.
4. Culbert, ML, *Freedom from Cancer*. New York: Pocketbooks (Simon & Schuster), 1977.
5. Kittler, GD, *Laetrile — Control for Cancer*. New York: Paperback Library, 1963.
6. Griffin, GE, *World Without Cancer*. Westlake Village CA: American Media, 1974.
7. Burk, Dean, *A Brief on Foods and Vitamins*. Sausalito CA: McNaughton Foundation, 1975.
8. Halstead, Bruce, *Amygdalin (Laetrile) Therapy)*. Los Altos CA: Choice Publications, 1978.
9. Moss, RW, *The Cancer Industry*. New York: Paragon House, 1991.
10. Testimony, Cancer treatments seminar, sponsored by Staten Island Borough President Guy Molinari, New York, September 1993.
11. Culbert, ML, *Vitamin B17, op. cit.*
12. Culbert, ML, *What the Medical Establishment Won't Tell You that Could Save Your Life*. Norfolk VA: Donning, 1983.
13. *Ibid.*
14. *A Complaint Against Medical Tyranny as Practiced in the United States of America: American Medical Genocide*. San Francisco CA: Committee for Freedom of Choice in Medicine, Inc., June 1984.
15. Ferguson, Wilburn, *Tsanza*, unpublished memoirs, 1982. Also, Ferguson, Wilburn, *The Jivaro and His Drugs*. Quito, Ecuador: Editorial Casa de la Cultura Ecuatoriana, 1957. And extensive private communications.
16. Fitzgerald, BF, *Congressional Record*, August 28, 1953.
17. Culbert, ML, *Freedom, op. cit.*
18. Culbert, ML, *Vitamin, op. cit.*
19. *Ibid.*
20. *Ibid.*
21. Culbert, ML, *What the, op. cit.*
22. *Ibid.*
23. *Ibid.*
24. *The Choice*, IV:2, March 1978.
25. Culbert, ML, *What the, op. cit.*
26. Cason, James, in *Vortex*, American Chemical Society, June 1978.
27. *Response of the Committee for Freedom of Choice in Cancer Therapy, Inc., to the Publication of the National Cancer Institute 'Amygdalin (Laetrile)Clinical Trial'*. Los Altos CA: Committee for Freedom of Choice in Cancer Therapy, Inc., Jan. 29, 1982.
28. Moertel, *op. cit.*
29. "Dr. Nieper assails the NCI 'laetrile trial.'" Rochester MN *Post-Bulletin*, Feb. 8, 1982.
30. Heikkila, RE, and Cabbat, FS, "The prevention of Alloxan-induced diabetes by amygdalin." Pergamon Press Ltd., *Life Sciences* 27, 1980.
31. *Diet, Nutrition and Cancer*. Washington DC: National Academy Press, 1982.
32. Bradford, RW, et al., *Amygdalin: Its Nature, Biological Interactions, Implications for Therapeutic Use in Cancer, and Quality Control*. Los Altos CA: Bradford Research Institute, 1981.
33. Tatsumura, T, et al., "4, 6-0-benzylidene-D-glucopyranose (BG) in the treatment of solid malignant tumors." *Br. J. Cancer* 62, 1990.
34. Talalay, Pawel, et. al., *Proc. Natl. Aca. Sci.* April 12, 1994.
35. *The Choice*, XX: 2-3, 1994.

XIII
AIDScam and CFSide:
Immune dysregulation — end of humanity or end of allopathy?

"Even if you accommodate [HIV] virus with all sorts of absurd and paradoxical hypotheses that doesn't get you around the solid number of 4,621 HIV-free AIDS cases. Here we have a real cover-up."
— **Molecular biologist Peter H. Duesberg PhD, 1993**

"Our national pride is at stake. We claimed that the US discovered the cause of AIDS, and we would develop a vaccine and some antiretroviral drugs. The government has literally funded nothing but HIV research for years, and it's very difficult for any bureaucracy, especially the federal government, to admit that they were wrong. I suspect what's going to happen is they will continue to say that HIV is the cause of AIDS, but the entire rest of the chapter will be about how 'co-factors' are necessary, and so forth."
— **Michigan State medical researcher Dr. Robert S. Root-Bernstein, 1993**

"The mystery of that damn virus has been generated by the $2 billion they spend on it. You take any other virus, and you spend $2 billion, and you can make up some great mysteries about it, too."
— **Kary Mullis PhD, Nobel Prize for Chemistry, 1993**

"Although HIV is universally accepted as the cause of AIDS, the evidence is still not all that compelling. In fact, HIV infection is not even required for a diagnosis of AIDS, according to the Centers for Disease Control and Prevention. The current definition of AIDS is any one of 27 different diseases accompanied by low numbers of CD4 cells in the immune system. Thus the causal agent (HIV) of a disease (AIDS) is not required to cause the disease. Is this a bit of scientific legerdemain or what?"
— **Dr. Gordon Edlin, professor of biochemistry and biophysics, University of Hawaii, 1993**

"The results of Concorde do not encourage the early use of zidovudine [AZT] in symptom-free HIV-infected adults. They also call into question the uncritical use of CD4 cell counts as a surrogate endpoint for assessment of benefit from long-term antiretroviral therapy."
— **The Concorde (European AZT assessment study) Coordinating Committee, 1994**

AIDS as apocalypse
Only superlatives have been used to define the pandemic of AIDS:

It is variously described as an unprecedented threat to world health, a Black Death of the late-20th century, even as an end of civilization provoked by nature, manmade errors or biological warfare.

Never before in medical history has such a massive global effort been mounted in such a short time, and never before has so much money in research funds been raised in such a short time, to stop or at least slow down a menace which in its first 14 years (1981-1995) had thwarted every effort at cure — if agreement is reached on the meaning of the word "cure" (let alone agreement on the word "AIDS.")

In spring 1994, repeating earlier official statements of gloom and doom, Michael Merson, director of the "Global Program on AIDS" of the World Health Organization (WHO), synthesized: "The end is nowhere in sight. The pandemic is certain to continue well into the 21st century. There is no breakthrough and I do not think one is imminent. We will not have a magic potion for AIDS before the year 2000."[1]

This was also the WHO's message to the gloomier-thanever Tenth International Conference on AIDS meeting that year in Yokohama, Japan, and in January 1995, when it was claimed that 19.5 million people were presumed to have been infected by the alleged causative agent of AIDS, HIV, and that some three million people had developed "full-blown" AIDS — however defined —since the syndrome was first defined in 1981.[2,2a,2b]

As in all previous conferences, actual rates of infection and caseloads were thought to be severely underreported due to poor statistics-gathering in many countries. Some estimates have it that the HIV infection rate could reach or surpass 50 million by the end of the decade, with the actual number of AIDS cases continuing to balloon exponentially by then.

It was estimated in 1994 that "full-blown" AIDS had killed or would be killing at least 60 percent of AIDS cases. By that year the United States accounted for 40 percent of reported cases (though only 13 percent of the estimated total), down from 50 percent a few years earlier. It was assumed — based on projections of HIV incidence — that a wide swath of central Africa and a substantial portion of Asia would eventually succumb to AIDS. There was no truly useful drug — or vaccine — to stop the slaughter.

The 1994 Tenth International Conference, which gathered more than 11,000 researchers, journalists and AIDS activists from 128 countries, received less press coverage than its nine predecessors, primarily because it had less to report and largely synthesized the findings of the ninth conference — that the figures were getting worse, there was no effective treatment, and no vaccine.

In fact, as the message of doom developed over the years — following the headier days of the early 1980s when the alleged "cause" of the syndrome was said to have been found and antibody tests developed to find it — international AIDS conferences had become biennial rather than annual events as an embarrassing paucity of research progress was turning up every 12 months.

In the United States, the AIDS-monitoring Centers for Disease Control and Prevention (CDC) in spring 1994 reported[3] a doubling of AIDS cases primarily based on yet another broader definition of just what AIDS is. It was also estimated that at or around one million Americans were "carrying" HIV, consistently reported in the United States as "the AIDS virus" (although this ironclad description was frequently less ironclad outside the USA). Some 400,000 US AIDS cases had been logged by CDC as of 1994, with upwards of 250,000 having died.

The million-infectee figure had been holding steady for several years, and was actually a compromise between some estimates which placed infection levels as considerably smaller or even greater. No one knew for sure just how many people were infected with "the AIDS virus," let alone what it really meant to be infected with it.

AIDS had also become a political and social phenomenon in the US, frequently enmeshed with and tainted by the politics of organized homosexuality and civil rights. By being incorrectly described since the outset as a "gay disease," it had provoked as much sociological as medical concern and had lulled the non-gay world into a protracted period of feeling somehow immune to a multifactorial disorder which, as it turned out, might take many years to appear (if it appeared at all) and then could kill in a combination of gruesome ways.

AIDS also became a gigantic new industry, rapidly gaining on cancer, and by 1993 as much federal research funding was being dumped into the hunt for an "AIDS cure" as for a "cancer cure," even though cancer was still killing far more Americans than was AIDS (and, of course, almost a quarter of AIDS is, by definition, cancer). This was a result of political organizing and deft media manipulation. The projected federal AIDS bill for 1994, involving research, "education" and prevention, was $6.2 billion — but even that was only an estimated 35 to 45 percent of total HIV-related spending.[4]

For by then, both domestically and worldwide, AIDS had become a major moneymaker: billions of potential dollars loomed in the ownership and use of "AIDS tests" (primarily antibody tests but also various higher-tech methods to capture HIV or parts of it) and, more important, the enormous profitability in developing either drugs designed to trick, thwart or inhibit "the AIDS virus" or to attempt to manage any of the multitude of "opportunistic diseases" which came about *because* of the alleged "AIDS virus" and actually did the killing and crippling. It was obvious even after the first few years of AIDS that insurance policies, and even some whole insurance plans, were being wiped out simply by the patient's attempting to pay for one or more "AIDS drugs" — none of which "worked" in the sense of stopping HIV, if that were even an appropriate target.

The demographic aspect of AIDS was changing going into the mid-nineties:

Worldwide, AIDS is *far more* a heterosexual disorder than

it is a "gay disease" and, as this writer had argued for a decade, more related to drug abuse than to sexual habits even though sexual promiscuity remains highly correlated with AIDS. In areas of the world allegedly facing mass extermination because of presumed widespread infection by HIV, which in turn is presumed to develop at some point into "full-blown" AIDS for a majority of people, the sexual deployment of the syndrome is almost equally between men and women, with an apparently easier likelihood of transmission *to* women.

Even in the United States, whose CDC first characterized the "gay" nature of the original infectees (though many printed lines down from the first paragraph it was also revealed that the first infectees also were drug abusers), new infections among homosexual males were beginning to level off with the highest increases noticeable among women (primarily "minority"), intravenous drug abusers of both sexes and children born to infected women. A majority of hemophiliacs were thought to be infected by "the AIDS virus," yet — intriguingly — nowhere near a majority had "died of AIDS."

There also were increases in "no identifiable risk" cases of HIV infection where there simply was no clear reason (some of the victims, including children, were not practicing male homosexuals, some "practiced" no sex at all, had had no blood transfusions or blood products, were not hemophiliacs, were not intravenous drug users, and were not the sexual partners of any of the above). Such cases called into question the reliability of HIV antibody tests in general, the nature of HIV itself — and the entire HIV theory of AIDS causation.

The course of the syndrome also seemed to be changing:

While there still were "fast" AIDS cases where death seemed to ensue a few months to a few years following diagnosis, the syndrome was increasingly seen as a long, lingering, up-and-down affair, almost an Allopathic Industrial Complex (AIC) delight since it meant extensive periods of ultimately unsuccessful therapies which seemed to be extending death rather than prolonging life. Since a variety of its various opportunistic diseases and cancers could be temporarily "managed," the syndrome became more chronic than acute. The parallel reality was that just as many hospitals were emptying the endless assortment of lingering "AIDS" conditions appeared in time to fill some of them up again.

Common sense vs. panic

With the world facing what seems to be an imminent catastrophe of mind-numbing proportions over AIDS, it is necessary to bring some doses of common sense to the fore while by no means denigrating the reality that AIDS is and will continue to be a significant medical problem. But there is this startling reality:

• Almost everything originally said about AIDS (including its mostly being a "gay disease") has turned out either to be all wrong, mostly wrong, or misleading.

On the ever-growing bill of particulars:

— The word itself: *a*cquired *i*mmune *d*eficiency *s*yndrome (AIDS) is a syndrome — that is, a combination of symptoms, diseases and disorders — and not *itself* a disease. Hence, nobody has truly "died of AIDS."

— The definition of elements of this syndrome has been both "officially" and "unofficially" altered so many times that AIDS is not easy to define. As this was written (1995), an individual "presenting with" any one or a combination of (by my count) 34 ("officially," 27) "opportunistic" fungal, parasitical, bacterial, mycoplasmic or viral infections and/or "forms" of cancer and who had a "count" of 200 or fewer "helper" (that is, CD4 or T4) cells per cubic millimeter of blood, and who was positive for antibodies to the HIV (human immunodeficiency virus types 1 or 2), was an "AIDS case."

— As I pointed out in an earlier book,[6] definitions of AIDS are now allowable even in the absence of blood tests — that is, simply from clinical signs and symptoms and a physician's merely guessing at the patient's presumed "lifestyle." What this may mean, some of the dissidents to the key theories of AIDS and HIV have stressed, is that a significant amount of diagnosed "AIDS cases" might not be AIDS cases at all!

— Even if the theory that a "new" virus, HIV, is the single "cause" of AIDS, and that antibody tests somehow remain the gold standard in spotting presence of the pesky virus, there exists the irritating reality that an individual with virtually *any* disorder may be classified as "AIDS" simply on the basis of a positive antibody test. What this means, for example, is that a tuberculosis patient who is antibody-positive for HIV automatically becomes an *AIDS* case. The list of conditions gathered under the AIDS umbrella has grown so swiftly that it became a funereal joke among some researchers in the mid-1990s to wonder if a big toe infected by a rusty nail on which it stepped should be classified as an opportunistic AIDS symptom if the stepper should turn out to be HIV antibody-positive.

— By 1995, or some 12 years after the alleged "cause" of the syndrome had been breathtakingly announced to the world, despite billions of dollars of research efforts it was still not clear just exactly how HIV "works" — that is, how it actually "causes" AIDS. (And at least three HIVs - 1, 2, and "1-subtype O" — or was this really HIV-3?) — were thought to be threatening the human population.)

— In the earlier days of AIDS, the most common deadly sequelae were either *Pneumocystis carinii pneumonia*, (PCP), variously described as a fungal or protozoal infection primarily of the lungs, and Kaposi's sarcoma, an often hideous skin cancer — or cancer-like condition — which, like melanoma, can become lethal, particularly if it internalizes. For a time, PCP alone was accounting for approximately 60 percent of the deaths of American AIDS patients. Yet, PCP — as is true for all the 33 (26?) other presentations and forms of AIDS — is not a new disease, and was last encountered *en masse* among immune system-depressed German children and infants at the end of World War II. And the medical establishment had a hard time figuring out whether KS, thought to be a "form" of cancer, was truly a part of AIDS, a parallel infection, or an expression of the syndrome occurring toward the beginning, rather than the end, of it.

(— Our own research group suggested in 1986 that KS might be a parallel viral infection, particularly since on an experimental blood test "AIDS" patients presenting only with KS were exhibiting a viral-infection pattern, not a cancer one, at least in earlier stages.

(A year earlier, research in *Human Pathology* strangely not followed up on with much vigor indicated[6a] that KS was much more widely distributed in patients than earlier suspected. Such investigations drew a distinction between "typical" KS and "inflammatory" KS. When aspects of "inflammatory" KS were considered in an "autopsy series" involving Haitians of both sexes, IV drug users of both sexes, gay males, hemophiliacs and three with "unknown risks," the disease was found to be widespread.

(Our group's view that Kaposi's might be a parallel viral infection was strengthened in late 1994 when a Columbia-Presbyterian Medical Center team announced discovery of yet another human herpesvirus which it found highly correlated with KS.[6b]

(As information developed that increasing numbers of KS patients even in the United States [it has long been common in North Africa and parts of the Mediterranean as a relatively unimportant skin cancer] were *negative* for HIV antibodies [as was also true for a small but growing number of PCP patients — the PCP having been *induced* in some cases by chemotherapy drugs for cancer![7]] — then it became obvious: neither PCP nor KS alone should always be considered to be AIDS. If, of course, PCP and KS were removed from the combination of AIDS diseases, then the *true incidence* of AIDS deflates on a monumental scale.)

— Data continued to surface that the vaunted HIV "antibody tests" — the primary ways to detect the alleged "AIDS virus" — were not always reliable.[8] While the standard ELISA (enzyme-linked immunosorbent assay) and the allegedly "confirmatory" Western Blot tests were conceivably error-prone themselves, information developed that *other* infections and conditions could cause "false positives" on such antibody tests.[9] It also became increasingly clear, particularly among healthcare workers exposed to possible HIV infections, that there could be actual infection, however transient, which the antibody tests would not "pick up." Adding these realities to the continually disturbing ones concerning difficulties both in isolating whole viruses or parts of whole viruses, let alone how to interpret such findings, it is now obvious that there *is* no single guaranteed blood test which actually tells an individual he or she *has* AIDS. There simply are tests (including, as of late 1994, a saliva test) to indicate exposure to HIV.

—At the same time, research, though much of it regarded as "anecdotal," continues to surface that even the traditional disturbances in immune function (namely, precipitous declines in the CD4/T4 "helper" colony, precipitous rises in the CD8/T8 "suppressor" colony, causing the customary "inverted ratio" between both, immunologically a kind of hallmark for alleged AIDS), may not always be specifically related to AIDS, may be linked to other conditions and other viruses, and may occasionally not be relevant at all. That is to say, *neither* a "positive" HIV antibody test nor a disturbance in immune function as measured primarily by the CD4/CD8 ratio can be used to prove absolutely either that the person has, or soon will have, AIDS!

— It was also more evident to researchers — and our own research group could take some credit for earlier observations thereof — that critically low CD4/T4 "helper" cells did not always spell imminent doom for the patient, particularly if he or she had highly abnormal levels of CD8/T8 "suppressor" cells. Our medical team noted a small but growing segment of AIDS cases ("full-blown" by definition only) who had extremely low "helper" cell levels but remained essentially free of clinical disease as long as the low "helper" level was matched by huge increases in "suppressors." All were on "unorthodox" therapies of one kind or another. Several ranking American AIDS researchers also observed this phenomenon and one of them, San Francisco's Jay Levy, has long proposed a possible viral-killing or other control factor from a subset of CD8/T8 cells.[11,12]

— It was obvious enough so that I could recount the data in two AIDS studies in the 1980s that the following observations could be made concerning the conventional wisdom about AIDS: increasing numbers of patients with immune disturbances and HIV antibody positivity were either only minimally ill or not ill at all; increasing numbers of patients ill with one or more AIDS-related illnesses had little or no immune perturbation and some were negative for HIV antibodies; increasing numbers of patients who were HIV-positive and with hematological signs of immune disturbance were essentially healthy and had remained that way for years.

— By the 1990s, these earlier observations were now becoming far more commonplace, and they led to three startling sets of data which, together, influenced increasing numbers of well-credentialed independent AIDS researchers (about 500 in the USA by 1994, including two Nobel Laureates) to question the key premise put forth by the orthodoxy about the syndrome (namely, it is singly caused by HIV):

• First, it had become ever clearer, primarily from studies of long-followed "cohorts" of potential AIDS patients tracked for their HIV "seropositivity," as well as a rising wave of anecdotal data and some from statistical extrapolations, that a significant number of HIV-infected individuals were living well over a decade — perhaps a *third* up to 14 to 15 years (based on backtracking their blood tests) — without developing even significant immune disturbances or any clinical signs and symptoms of AIDS.[13] (Many, but by no means all [and there was no way to determine this fully] were on "unorthodox" preventive therapies).

• Second, information developed that there might somehow be "milder" strains of HIV which, while infecting a given group of people, provoked no significant disease. Australian research was particularly precise on this point.[14] And the aforementioned surveys of healthcare workers who had had known exposures to HIV through needlestick injuries and other treatment accidents pointed both to very low infection rates of HIV and cases in which there was "transient" infection — that is, the virus "hit," but it was overcome by body defenses before antibodies formed.

• Third, and more astounding for defenders of the HIV theory, it was increasingly being reported in both the "standard" literature and more widely in "unorthodox" circles that ever-growing numbers of patients were "presenting" with terminal, full-blown AIDS symptoms and their concomitant immune system disorders assessable in blood tests without *ever* having had either antigens (actual pieces of) HIV or antibodies to them! One estimate by 1993 was that there were at least 4,621 "HIV-negative" AIDS cases in the world, with at least a third of those in the United States — and that even many US AIDS cases had been "presumptively" (rather than hematologically) diagnosed with HIV.[15]

Making the facts fit the theory

As we have seen, this nation's Allopathic Industrial Complex (AIC) is nothing if not adroit in manipulating semantics and making the facts fit the theory. We note in X how the AIC essentially invented a new disease — *hypercholesterolemia* (too much cholesterol) — as a pathology needing to be treated by cholesterol-lowering drugs, cornerstones of the cardiovascular industry.

In terms of AIDS, it became ever more obvious that numerous people — both from "risk groups" (that is, married to, or the sexual partners of, allegedly HIV-infected people) and, more importantly, those *not* from "risk groups," a reality which most damaged the paradigm — had either AIDS-related diseases and/or AIDS-like immune disturbances without ever having had any evidence of HIV. Hence, a new term was created, literally out of wholecloth, to explain what this new subset of individuals seemed to have:

"Idiopathic CD4 T-lymphocytopenia." The translation of this phrase: "helper T-cells falling for no known reason." ICL become the common abbreviation.

The questions nagged supremely: if, by 1994, there were at least hundreds (and probably thousands — maybe even millions throughout the world) of people infected with the HIV virus who had failed to come down with either pre-AIDS or AIDS conditions for a decade or more, and if, on the other hand, there were reportedly (and presumptively) hundreds to thousands of so-called AIDS patients without HIV, then:

How could it still be said that HIV is the cause, or at least the sole cause, of the admittedly devastating syndrome?

The observation that HIV is a *lentivirus* — that is, a slow developer — was insufficient as a total answer.

The American AIDS research network, originally funneled — strangely enough — through the failure-prone National Cancer Institute (NCI), continued to go to extravagant, elegant, byzantine and even outrageous lengths to explain all of this away.

The way HIV infects people and "causes" AIDS remained truly unknown as late as 1995, even though the retrovirus had been found in virtually every body fluid and numerous tissues. Abstruse theories have been adduced as to how HIV still can cause AIDS even if various antibody and antigen tests cannot find it. And, yes, by any virological definition, HIV is an unusual, seemingly clever, escape-prone virus which "replicates" and mutates so fast no two isolates from the same person are ever the same. And HIV seems to be associated with, correlated with, somehow linked to, certain aspects of AIDS and is a possible cancer factor (lymphomas) — but again, there is no smoking gun to prove the above.

Most intriguingly, almost from the moment HIV (originally baptized HTLV-III) was pronounced, in 1983, to be the "cause" of AIDS by an American medical establishment under heavy pressure to explain the nature of the seemingly new syndrome, whose numbers had been growing exponentially since it was first delineated in 1981, a few key experts begged to disagree.

The most vocal dissenter has been University of California-Berkeley molecular biologist Peter Duesberg PhD. Duesberg is not just a heretic: he is one of the fathers of retrovirology and a discover of "oncogenes" in cancer. Possessed of an innovative mind, Duesberg has argued both that it has not been specifically proven that any so-called oncogene actually *causes* cancer (*XI*) — and it has not been proven anywhere that HIV actually *causes* AIDS. He has attributed AIDS more to drug abuse than anything else and has published repeatedly and convincingly on the reasons why, drawing both professional wrath and reductions in research funds for doing so. [16, 16a, 17, 18]

Too, however fiendish HIV seems to be — able even, it would seem, to mutate in a host more rapidly than other rapidly mutating viruses, and selectively targeting the quarterback of the immunological team (the CD4 cell) — "the AIDS virus" seems almost benign alongside some other quick killers:

By the mid-1990s, perhaps the most horrific of the airborne viruses was that causing the rapidly fatal Ebola hemorrhagic fever. And there was the hantavirus, said to infest deer mice and which led to alarming numbers of rapidly killed Americans beginning in 1993 (yet, interestingly, others allegedly infected recovered), and there were "new" — or newly discovered — viruses linked to other potentially fatal syndromes. Science was hard pressed to answer: where do these things come from? Answers ranged from the overtly conspiratorial (biological warfare) to the possible-if-difficult-to-prove — that some viruses in the earth's soil had been loosed upon the planet by deforestation.

While it is not the aim of this account to become involved in all the multiple aspects of the HIV debate, suffice it to say that by the mid-1990s some 500 American scientists, researchers and AIDS investigators were on record as dissenting from the HIV-as-single-cause theory, and the list included two Nobel Laureates. One of these was San Diego's Kary Mullis, inventor of the PCR (polymerase chain reaction) test, one of the precision assays used for isolating HIV. Some of the best data gathered against the HIV theory was in print not only from Duesberg but also from Michigan State medical researcher Dr. Robert Root-Bernstein.[19]

But we should also point out that, long before it was fashionable, our own maverick Bradford Research Institute (BRI) was the first research organization to question the HIV-as-single cause theory, and I outlined the reasons why in a 1986 monograph and a 1990 book.[20,21]

With more than a decade of debate behind us, it seems likely that HIV has *some* role in AIDS and in CD4 cell depletion. It seems increasingly *un*likely that it is the single cause of AIDS.

Dissidents to the HIV theory — just as in the case of dissidents to the broadly held cancer-cause theories — found it difficult to publish their ideas and impossible to secure research funds. The hermetically sealed mind of the AIDS research apparatus, growing faster even than the cancer industry, has been no more enthusiastic about free thought or novel new ideas than the cancer industry, despite a seemingly all-out effort to study, explain and stop AIDS.

Yet the same central allopathic errors abound in AIDS:

The allopathic paradigm needs to find single causes for single diseases, and then to fashion "contraries" against the causes. This 17th-century approach dominates Western —that is, American — medicine, as we see time and again throughout this study. It is neither greater nor lesser than in the case of AIDS.

But the result in AIDS has been, proportionally, even more devastating:

For, by 1995, the 14th year of the Plague, adherence to the notion that a single virus — new, old, mutated, manmade or whatever — is the single "cause" of the syndrome; and to the notion that only devastatingly toxic "nucleoside analogue" drugs can slow down or stop the virus had failed to cure a single — that is, not one, not even the suggestion of one — case of AIDS! The research establishment could gloss over this fact, attempt to sidestep it, attempt to explain it away on a host of recondite experimental grounds and high-technology verbalese to snare the unwary, but it could not actually deny that harsh, crude fact.

Enter the 'co-factors'

By then, the complex of public and private research institutes and renowned scientists (as well as fund-raising organizations) we style "AIDS Inc." was running out of excuses. Slowly, a trend of thought introduced from within the orthodoxy was gathering steam:

If HIV *alone* is not the cause of the syndrome, then it must have help, perhaps a lot of it. The term "co-factors" surfaced even by the middle 1980s among some scientists who were beginning to suspect that, however interesting HIV was, it could not be doing its devastation all by itself. Only a few on-line physicians (such as Joseph Sonnabend MD, New York, who was among the first to suggest "multifactoriality" both in AIDS causes and treatments[22]) had voiced their suspicions of the establishment "line."

So the HIV dissidents split into two general camps: a few, as headed by Duesberg, suggesting that HIV is a totally irrelevant retrovirus playing no meaningful role in AIDS at all, and the bigger group, believing that HIV might be a "sentinel" or "marker" virus for something else or at least be contributing in some way to the syndrome. (Widely disseminated photos from the scanning electron microscope did, in fact, display HIV seeming to invade its target of choice — the regulating CD4/T4 "helper" cells of the immune system, surveillant over viral infections and hence a vital target for a weapon which seemed aimed at provoking immune collapse.)

While numerous researchers found likely co-factor viruses from the better-known families (particularly the herpes family, headed by Epstein-Barr [EBV] and cytomegalovirus [CMV]), none seemed to fit the mold as probable "catalyst" or "trigger" viruses.

By the late 1980s, even researchers within the orthodox camp were beginning to talk about "co-factors" (the last redoubt, as one dissident scientist told me, when one cannot consistently fit the pathology with the etiology) to HIV. By then, even Robert Gallo, the National Cancer Institute (NCI) investigator who allegedly co-discovered HIV and originally claimed that any dissent from the notion that the retrovirus was the cause was "crazy," had begun to talk of "co-factors."

And the Pasteur Institute's Luc Montagnier, who actually was the first scientist to isolate the alleged "AIDS virus," broke ranks earlier — he insisted that although HIV must be involved, surely a tiny structure called a *mycoplasma* must be a "co-factor." Independent research by US Army Institute of Pathology scientist S-C Lo, somewhat ignored at first, even showed that it was a kind of mycoplasma which, when injected into test animals, could sicken and kill them with AIDS-like diseases while HIV remained unable to do significant damage to any non-human species.[23,24]

(In October 1994, *Science* reported[24a] that an "AIDS-like" condition had been induced in baboons by a strain of the "second AIDS virus," HIV-2. The fact that six test baboons had "sero-converted" following infection by this particular strain, that four developed swollen lymph nodes, while three had immunological features similar to "AIDS infection" and one was killed after developing significant disease, was broadly parroted by the media[24b] as a sign that, finally, test animals had developed "full-blown AIDS" apparently from an HIV virus. Yet there was no way to know how the animals lived or were fed or what other infections they might have had — and the HIV-2-UC2 strain is not the virus commonly said to be infecting humans.)

But by the time AIDS Inc. began talking "co-factors," at least in the United States, there were enormous industrial considerations at stake: HIV as the cause, and only toxic nucleoside drugs, led by Burroughs Wellcome's AZT (Retrovir, zidovudine, azidothymidine), and possible "protease inhibitors," able somehow to "slow down" what was still widely called "the AIDS virus." The HIV-as-single-cause theory was the central excuse for the entire federal (and interconnectedly private) research effort. The mass testing of the population (leading, in

Cuba, to the actual quarantining of "AIDS carriers") with HIV antibody tests was itself a new industry. Between billions dumped into research on "the AIDS virus" and development of antibody tests as well as a spate of far more precise virus-isolating assays, and multi-billions more in toxic drugs, AIDS research and propaganda seemed to take off wildly on a course of their own; anyone who stood in the way would not be taken seriously.

For the medically (in distinction to the biochemically) minded, questions arose early over why so much research was directed at HIV when, by any valid assessment of the syndrome, it was *other* viruses, bacteria, parasites, yeasts, fungi and probably mycoplasmas that were doing the actual sickening and killing of patients.

At some point in the AIDS infection curve, rampant yeast infection, elevated "titers" of Epstein-Barr Virus (EBV) and cytomegalovirus (CMV) occurred, yet little was done to curb these pathogenic conditions in terms of fresh research. Some older drugs, essentially antibiotics, were found to slow down or even prevent PCP, but these often were also toxic and sagged in efficacy over time.

Intense diarrhea and a multiplicity of pulmonary disorders were killing AIDS patients, along with rare "forms" of cancer, but research seemed strangely not to concentrate on these truly lethal diseases. The AIDS research establishment remained obsessively focused on HIV.

As the second decade of the Plague Era began it was ever more obvious that allegiance to HIV as single cause and the hopes pinned on AZT as some kind of pharmaceutical white knight were probably misplaced. There also loomed, as we shall see, nettling possibilities that, if in fact there is a single catalyst for AIDS and it is viral, that orthodox research may have focused on the wrong virus.

Aside from ominous hints of conspiracies and coverups including everything from a global conspiracy to wipe out a segment of humanity to institutional efforts either to hide biological warfare research or simply to paper over a series of shocking laboratory blunders, there also arose the terrible consequence of misplaced faith in nucleoside analogue drugs — that they might be *causing* AIDS symptoms in and of themselves (a point made by Duesberg and a growing band of observers) and also killing patients. (As we have seen in cancer, this would be nothing new — toxic chemotherapy [which AZT was originally developed to be] is a "cure" often worse than the disease and may kill directly or indirectly a significant portion of patients said to have died from "complications of cancer.")

And what has been so far the abject failure of AIDS Inc. to get to grips with mankind's fastest growing menace is turning out to be the final rapier thrust to finish off the allopathic paradigm in medicine, a key element in the revolution of medical paradigms now underway.

Some historical background is necessary if one is to attempt to make any kind of sense of the AIDS disaster.

Cancer Inc. joins AIDS Inc.

It should be remembered that the ever-more-funded National Cancer Institute (NCI) was the federal conduit through which, President Richard M. Nixon hoped, a hugely financed "Conquest of Cancer" program would wipe out this greatest of the diseases of civilization. Raise enough money, open enough labs, and cancer will be wiped out the American way, the citizenry was assured.

It should also be recalled that for decades of the post-WWII era, and in sound alignment with the linear, monofactorial allopathic paradigm which controls the chief concepts of American-led Western medicine, the "viral theory of cancer" was paramount. Billions of research dollars were spent publicly and privately to find cancer-causing human viruses let alone ways to "inhibit" (but not truly kill, since viruses are not actually "alive" in a biological sense) the same. Decades came and went, and though some viral activity might be inferred in some "tumor systems," rare was the virus that could be isolated which absolutely and irretrievably could be said to have "caused" a malignancy.

By the time the first few years of the "Conquest of Cancer" program were assessed, in the 1970s, it was clear that there were more cases of, and fatalities from, cancer in the United States than ever before in our history. The massive campaign to track down a cancer-causing virus and then stop it, thus vanquishing cancer, was plainly failing. If anything, the NCI, by the latter 1970s, was a good example of the institutionalization of error as funded and refunded by taxpayers and propped up by politicians. In the private sector, such bungling would have, and should have, led to enormous job layoffs. But federal employment, just as federal agencies, endures. And endures.

Suddenly, in 1981, there was AIDS — a term settled on after some earlier unwieldy acronyms (even GRID, as "gay-related immune deficiency") were dropped. No doubt about it: something seemingly new and menacing had broken out along the socially-perceived pestilential soft underbelly of the population: promiscuous male gays and intravenous drug users were coming down in ever spiralling numbers with a variety of conditions and diseases hitherto seen only in chemically or nutritionally immune depressed people. They had somehow "acquired" an immune depression. Hence the evolution of the concept of the acquired immune deficiency syndrome.

For whatever reason, the major research effort to halt a rapidly developing new plague was handed to the NCI, the very same apparatus which had so miserably mismanaged the "war on cancer." And the NCI was still guided by 17th-century allopathic beliefs about single causes for diseases and still entranced with the endless hunt for viruses, around which so many other industries (particularly the development of "immortal cell lines," and several early waves of genetic technology) were already flourishing. The unstated mandate was *find the virus*.

By 1993, France's legendary Institut Pasteur and the American NCI seemed to be racing neck-and-neck to determine which would "find the virus." It is now clear — despite a rather childish, testy and potentially expensive dispute between the Americans and French that took years to settle and involving patents on test kits which ultimately enriched both countries and several researchers, including the US' Robert Gallo to the tune of $100,000 a year[24c] — that the French got there first, but close enough in time so that both could take credit for "co-discovering" what at first was more correctly called "the virus most often associated with AIDS." That is, a majority of persons who had developed full-blown AIDS were thought to be harboring this agent, and it had been isolated in most of them.

The hasty announcement by the US government that the AIDS "cause" had been found seemed to be a payoff for American research and sound scientific technology. With the "etiological agent" now identified, the next phase would be to research its structure and fashion weapons to knock it out or a vaccine to prevent it. Sound allopathic thinking.

Indeed, over the years more money was raised to study the HIV virus than had ever been raised in medical history for any virus — and more is known about it than any other virus in history. All of which makes the lack of full evidence that it is *the* cause, or possibly *any* cause, of AIDS so triply frustrating and humiliating.

As more data continued to come in worldwide, it seemed that Africa might have been the source of the virus which the NCI's controversy-plagued Robert Gallo and associates originally called "HTLV virus type three" (from earlier descriptions of a presumed family of "human T-cell-lymphotropic" structures). Travel patterns between AIDS patients and Africa suggested such an origin, even though outbreaks of AIDS seemed spontaneously to have occurred in three separate geographical areas, all at the same time — central Africa, the Caribbean and the gay enclaves of New York and San Francisco.

Since HTLV-III, later to be rechristened HIV-1, seemed to be a blood-borne virus and so many American victims were male homosexuals or intravenous drug users or both, it seemed a safe assumption that HIV was essentially a blood-and-semen-carried virus and that AIDS, hence, must be a kind of venereal disease. The "gayness" of the syndrome dominated the American response, primarily due to the Centers for Disease Control's 1981 definition, a move which arguably set back AIDS research and muted effective social response to it for the better part of five years.

AIDS in Africa: horror and hoopla

But questions rose fairly early: the Africans said either to be infected by HIV or dying from AIDS or both were overwhelmingly heterosexual and were not IV drug users. In southern Europe and the Mediterranean, AIDS was considered — and by the mid-1990s was still considered — to be more an intravenous drug user's disease than anything else.

How research on AIDS got off on several wrong feet and ran smack into the vested interests of ego and misplaced research was recounted by the late Randy Shilts (himself an AIDS victim) in *And the Band Played On* (1987), one of the first popular works which helped to galvanize American awareness of the onrushing syndrome.

The international viral research community held to the notion that somehow a mutated simian virus had "jumped species" into man some time in Africa as the origin of the syndrome, and it spread outward in a pattern similar to that of an allegedly related virus, HTLV-I. But was it new or old? Ultimately, it was found that AIDS-like conditions had killed at least one American in 1968, one Englishman in the 1960s and that HIV-like antibodies had been traced back to *healthy* Amazonian Indians in the 1960s and to Africans in the late 1950s. The research establishment was agreeing, by the 1990s, that HIV was new but not terribly new — no older than 100 years, maybe only a few decades. It must have mutated from lower animals, ran the thinking. Perhaps it did.

Throughout AIDS' first meteoric decade, AIDS Inc. kept informing the world that in the "AIDS belt" of central Africa (some nine countries in the sub-Saharan part of the continent) a whole population was about to be wiped out, and that HIV infection and AIDS cases there would dwarf anything seen in the USA. Even so, during most of that time at least half the world's reported AIDS cases were in the admittedly more statistics-and-quantification-obsessed USA than in Africa.

Nonetheless, since "the AIDS virus" was said to have originated there, had been incubating there longer, and had infected so many, droves of people should in fact be dying of AIDS in Africa. And, indeed, some television and even print media reports did find some terrible examples of people in AIDS-like death throes.

Even so, journalists who took the trouble to visit Africa in the 1980s began questioning just how many people were dying of AIDS. The syndrome in Africa was, primarily, an urban calamity in countries which are essentially rural. A media investigation in 1987 cast doubt on just how many Africans were truly dying of AIDS.[25]

Later, AZT-baiter John Lauritsen, one of the few cool heads in the AIDS catastrophe, quoted from Richard and Rosalina Chirimuuta (*AIDS, Africa and Racism*) about what had really gone on in the "AIDS belt:"

> *"[Western doctors] conducted small and unreliable seroepidemiological surveys that 'proved' that millions of Africans were infected with the virus. (One Belgian team spent three weeks in Kinshasa, diagnosed 38 people as having AIDS), 'then figured out how many cases this would amount to in a year's time, divided that by the total population of Kinshasa and estimated an annual rate of developing AIDS in that country to be about 17 per 100,000.'"*[26]

Yet, when West German researchers examined thousands of serum samples from central Africa, they found only four contained HIV antibodies. Their findings, noted Lauritsen, were ignored because they did not fit the "AIDS plague myth."

And the "AIDS belt" countries involved contain roughly

only about 10 percent of the population of Africa.

Seeming virtually to be fighting back to convince the world that there *is* a major AIDS plague in Africa, Centers for Disease Control (CDC) officers editorially described as "confirmed and quantified" in 1994 a rather strange report on "two-year HIV-1-associated mortality" in an area of rural Uganda. It was said to be "the largest prospective study of its kind in sub-Saharan Africa."[26a, 26b]

True, Daan W. Mulder *et al.*, in assessing 9,389 individuals, found 89 deaths in individuals seropositive for HIV (as opposed to 198 who were seronegative), including 64 adults. Of these, only five were said to have died of AIDS by a *pre*-1987 definition thereof called the "Bangui case definition"; 31 had "one or more major symptoms" and 28 "no major symptoms." Overall, disease progression to death in general was higher among those infected with HIV. The highest mortality rates were for children under 5 and adults over 55 whether they were positive for HIV or not.

The report discussed "excess mortality" as a statistical correlate of those with HIV. It did not prove HIV causes AIDS. Since it is not clear exactly what these individuals died of, or whatever else they may have been positive for, such research raised more questions than answers.

By late 1994, the Ivory Coast, in w*est* Africa, was reporting among the highest rates of HIV infection and AIDS cases, with prostitution considered a major "vector."[26a]

But what also is true about Africa — where the main presenting feature of AIDS was long reported to be "slim disease," the gradual wasting away of the body accompanied by intense diarrhea?

The same "AIDS belt" countries said to be awash in AIDS are also countries which have long had galloping rates of amoebic dysentery, other protozoal diseases and parasites of all kinds, malnutrition, malaria, yellow fever, leprosy, tuberculosis, syphilis, yaws, pinta and a galaxy of other bacterial and viral infections. Blood samples from such chronically diseased people are "interesting," to say the least.

In 1993 and 1994, studies by well-credentialed scientists and researchers, in part based on African "AIDS," began to raise the question of usefulness of HIV antibody tests to ever higher octaves: Zairian officials, working with US AIDS expert Max Essex, found that certain bacterial infections (leprosy and tuberculosis among them) could cause up to an astounding 70 percent of "false positives" on HIV tests![27]

Earlier, an Australian research team, going so far as to argue that such tests might be "counterproductive," suggested that the assays, far from detecting the presence of a virus, might simply be reacting to cellular proteins — in which the blood of multiply infected people is noticeably aswarm. Such observations strengthened the thinking of others that retroviruses themselves might be artifacts — that is, results of, rather than causes of, disease.[28] (Retroviruses are viruses which must "replicate" by "transcribing" the reproduction-capable amino acid combination RNA to DNA, the catalyst of cellular growth in normal cells.)

The new attacks on HIV antibody tests, particularly those run on the blood of multiply infected people, of course throw into doubt all assessments based on generalizing just how much HIV is present in any population. Antibody tests, at best, measure responses to something, and not the *somethings* themselves.

In Africa, the possibility has thus been raised that one of two things or both might be occurring: that great numbers of diseased people (that is, diseased with tuberculosis, malaria, yellow fever, syphilis, amoebic dysentery, leprosy, gastrointestinal parasites), are being "transferred" to the AIDS column because either HIV antibodies are found or are presumed to be found in them; or that great numbers of people carrying proteins produced by disease states (tuberculosis, leprosy, for example, whether they have any clinical signs or symptoms of these diseases) — are showing "false positive" on HIV tests.

Either reality greatly inflates both the AIDS and the AIDS-prone categories and nourishes the belief in the worldwide mass infestation of HIV as a global threat to the human population.

As of 1994, at least from reviewable records from admittedly backward countries, it could not be demonstrated that the population of central Africa was being wiped out by AIDS (birth rates were rising) even though — of course — the ever-lengthening incubation period of the all-purpose killer virus could indeed simply mean that the wipeout was taking far longer than expected. We cannot discount this possibility — only call it into question.

But even assuming the worst about African AIDS, there also developed a ray of optimism which, if extrapolated to humans as a whole, bodes well:

At the end of 1993, 25 Nairobi female prostitutes were under "intensive scientific study" because, although some of them had had repeated, unprotected sexual activity for up to 13 years, not only did none of them have AIDS conditions, neither were they "positive" for HIV. This group of sex workers in a high-AIDS area, together with groups of both promiscuous male homosexuals and hemophiliacs all of whom allegedly must have been exposed to HIV but developed neither antibodies nor any other reaction to it, seemed to provide, as *Time* put it, "the strongest evidence yet that that people can have a natural immunity to AIDS."[29]

From either the HIV theory point of view or the general assumption of the venereal-disease nature of AIDS, that was, at the very least, good news.

And, in early 1995, scientists who studied prostitutes in Gambia reported that in at least three cases "killer cells" called "HIV-specific cytotoxic T-lymphocytes" had been able to kill HIV-infected cells, a possible reason the trio had not developed any sign of "HIV infection." The same cells have also been found in other AIDS-less HIV-infected people — another sign of a a possible fall-safe element of immunity.[29a]

An oriental conundrum

AIDS surveillance in other "third world" countries also

undercut certain beliefs about the syndrome while strengthening others:

Two points in passing are Thailand and the Philippines.

In the former, AIDS has been traced since 1984.[30] Ten years later, it was estimated that the country had at least 700,000 HIV-infected people, proportionally the highest infection rate in the world, even though — while 1,600 had died from 8,000 cumulative cases of the syndrome — most people had still not developed symptoms.[31,31a]

In the latter, AIDS has been traced since 1985 — beginning with outbreaks among "sex workers" at the American Subic Bay Naval base (highly suggestive of a port of entry from US servicemen). Yet nine years later, even though officials generally agreed the numbers were probably underestimated, an incredibly tiny amount of 475 HIV infections had been reported, and only a little more than 100 full-blown AIDS cases had occurred. Even projections for the syndrome for the year 2000 were far under anything estimated for nearby Thailand.[32]

As a frequent traveller in both countries, I was fully aware of the intensely promiscuous, socially bisexual nature of both Thai and Filipino societies. Sex was, and is, easy, casual, and omnipresent. Prostitution of women *and* men is common, and, in both countries homosexual or bisexual sexual activity is far less shameful or restrained than in the Western countries, particularly the farther one moves away from the highest social classes. Hence, the statistical correlate of sexual promiscuity is significant in both countries.

Yet, as we have seen, incidence of both HIV infection and actual definable AIDS represents a chasm of difference. In both countries, claimed heterosexuality is a far greater correlate than claimed homosexuality (though part of this may be due to social convention and an obscuring in such societies of what is meant by such frankly idiotic words as "straight" and "gay"). In both, as of 1994 AIDS cases were roughly divided equally between the sexes.

There is a difference, however, in one key factor between

the two societies, particularly in the earlier years — drug abuse, particularly intravenous drug abuse, was far more common and of easier access, and remained so throughout the early AIDS years, in Thailand than in the Philippines. In the latter, the authoritarian regime of Ferdinand Marcos, ending in 1986, had virtually, but not totally, eliminated drug abuse.

If AIDS is primarily a venereal condition, incidence of infection and actual cases should at least be proportionally similar in both countries. But if — as some of us argued in the early AIDS years — drug abuse *of all kinds* has a higher correlation with AIDS than does sexual promiscuity, then such noticeable differences may be explained.

This does not militate against the reality that sexual promiscuity and specific sexual acts (particularly insertive anal intercourse) are strongly related to AIDS, but it does suggest that substance abuse directly (through injection and possibly through other routes) and indirectly (by altering immune function over time) plays larger roles than does sexual activity itself.

HIV: the ever-lengthening incubation

In the earlier years AIDS — defined substantially more narrowly than now — survival was measured in months to a few years. By the time HIV antibody test kits were available, the time between alleged infection by HIV and the onset of symptoms of AIDS began a dizzying ascent. The "incubation period" was stretched from three to five to seven years — indeed, with each passing year of AIDS and the accumulation of computer printouts from ELISA and Western Blot test kits, it became apparent that another 12 months of incubation could safely be ascribed to a virus which seemed to lie in wait (save in some spectacular cases of "fast AIDS" when it seemed to kill within a matter of a few months to years after exposure).

By the end of the 1980s, the ever-lengthening incubation period was not only fortifying the position of Duesberg and others that HIV, at least by itself, could not possibly be the cause, but provoking grumbling even from the informed public.

By the 1990s, it was becoming established doctrine that HIV might incubate for anywhere from 10 to 15 years before striking — if it ever struck at all. A review of AIDS patient "cohorts" led to the conclusion that at least some AIDS-prone people might be "HIV-positive" for the whole of their lives and escape "full-blown" AIDS.[33]

And, a general pre-AIDS syndrome loosely called "AIDS-related complex" (ARC) had been added to the picture: in many cases, long before any of the (was it two dozen, 30, 32, 34?) "opportunistic diseases" and "forms" of cancer appeared, allegedly due to HIV-induced immune depression, there might be long periods of non-fatal general malaise, joint and bone pains, headaches, respiratory distress, extreme fatigue, swollen glands, rashes, gastrointestinal disturbances, nightsweats, spiking fevers, some diarrhea and weight loss.

Without HIV antibodies such a profile could be described as mononucleosis, secondary syphilis, endocrine imbalance and a dozen other things. But should the patient "test positive" for HIV it automatically became "AIDS-related" and the patient was informed he — or she — would be counting the weeks, months, years until "full-blown" AIDS took over, at which time 100 percent fatality was predicted.

The pattern slowly emerged that, as HIV took longer and longer to wend its evil way, more and more conditions could be lumped together as ARC, or pre-AIDS. This pattern was developing just as the "standard literature" was beginning to take note of AIDS-like cases in HIV-negative people and the press was reporting on more and more seemingly healthy people known to have had HIV antibodies for years who had failed to develop AIDS.

There was, as I noted whenever possible, the possible scenario of a virus in search of a disease. Just as, in the early times of Western medicine when it had been faced with "the great imitator," it was easy to dismiss all otherwise inexplicable symptoms as syphilis, and as, in later times, to attribute many of them to mononucleosis, it now became equally easy to blame everything on HIV/AIDS. Even forgetfulness and occasional mood swings on the part of a carrier of HIV antibodies became not simply empty-headedness but "AIDS dementia" — and, yes, it could be demonstrated that HIV was present in the central nervous system, as it was everywhere else.

But arithmetic was beginning to mount inexorably against the key AIDS concepts: estimates of the people in the world said to be carrying HIV ranged into the millions, while actual definable AIDS cases remained, until the mid-1990s, essentially in the thousands. The CDC several times redefined what AIDS was, automatically adding diseases to the syndrome, just as some diseases seemed ready to be leaving the standard definition (old standbys PCP and KS among them).

(So convinced were some researchers and physicians that HIV not only was not the cause of AIDS or anything else that they offered to drink or inject themselves with HIV. At least one American, Robert Willner MD PhD, did so very publicly in Spain in 1993, in the USA in 1994, and wrote an impassioned attack on the basic AIDS premises.[33a]) *See Note, page 538*

HHV-6: riddle within an enigma

So, "co-factors" inexorably began to catch up with AIDS Inc., which was never any more likely to admit basic error than Cancer Inc. — with which it is so intimately interlocked — has been.

In what was an astounding change of gears, yet not originally presented this way — the original comments coming not in American but British journals — the key American AIDS explicator, Robert Gallo, who had for so long promoted the HIV-only theory, added his name to some new research. It found that, at the very least — above and beyond other possible "co-factor" viruses and the Montagnier/Lo mycoplasmas — yet *another* virus, HHV-6 (human herpes virus number six), might be a "co-factor." [34,35,36]

The virus was conveniently said to have been isolated in Gallo's National Cancer Institute (NCI) laboratory and, shortly after its delineation, was found to be infecting very broad sectors of the human family without, in most carriers, seeming to "cause" anything. But it also became apparent that HHV-6 had at least two "strains" and one of them might be truly lethal to man.

The AIDS research community was "officially" informed (though some dissidents were previously theorizing the connection) that HHV-6 contributed to "the striking depletion of CD4 cells seen in patients with AIDS" and that HHV-6 was found to be active in autopsy studies of dead AIDS patients — that is, it was detected in all lung, lymph node, spleen, liver and kidney tissues "obtained at necropsy."[37] The infection rate was far higher than for CMV, a "co-factor" virus which, in or out of AIDS, can be the most damaging of all human viruses — and of course far more active than HIV, which is often not found in dying AIDS patients at all.

As the middle of the decade approached, the stream of research implicating HHV-6 — be it variant A or B or combinations thereof — as playing an ever-greater role in multiple AIDS pathology seemed to be reaching torrential proportions.

With HHV-6 known to be infecting natural killer cells — considered to be key in the immune response to cancer — the apparently higher rates of certain "forms" of cancer in patients classed as AIDS (and Chronic Fatigue Syndrome) could be (allopathically) explained. One of AIDS Inc.'s ever-trickier explanations for HIV latency in seemingly healthy people has been the supposition that the virus is "hiding" in lymph tissue. But no sooner had this research approach settled in than Italian research indicated that HHV-6 is "hiding" there too — and that "variant A" HHV-6 has a high frequency of occurrence in cases of Kaposi's sarcoma, a role earlier attributed to HIV.[37a]

Research has also linked HHV-6 with such potentially lethal complications of bone marrow transplants as pneumonitis (a severe lung disease) and the immunological disorder called GVHD — graft-versus-host-disease.[37b]

And, perhaps even more intriguingly, German research found that HHV-6 could be detected in the blood of blood donors — a conceivably chilling reality which could mean that HHV-6 is as easily transmissible by blood (and perhaps saliva and urine) as HIV allegedly is — and that blood supplies are at risk.[37c] As of 1994, the US was not screening the blood supply for HHV-6.

In fact, somewhat like Mary and the little lamb, everywhere that HIV went, HHV-6 was sure to follow. Or, possibly, vice-versa.

The AIDS Inc. research establishment was not saying, by 1994, that HHV-6 was the *real* AIDS virus, since such a 180-degree angle turn might paralyze the whole research effort. The admission, however, that a seemingly "new" virus was so strongly present in AIDS patients (and, as we shall see, in *many others*) that it was *the* likely "co-factor," opened the door to possible abandonment of the HIV-only theory and an industrially acceptable gradual transfer of research tools and test kits to a whole new dimension of thought still slavishly in keeping with the precepts of allopathy.

The NCI could and did take credit for the discovery of HHV-6 (and HHV-7), originally dubbed HBLV — for human B-cell lymphotropic virus — but it could not easily answer the questions of from whence that virus sprang and why hadn't the world known of it before.

Conspiracy theories arise

The "new" virus has thus found itself the centerpiece of one of the more sinister of the various sinister conspiracy theories surrounding the origin of AIDS.

We have reprised the AIDS conspiracy theories elsewhere.[38] Abstracting them:

— Information developed by Glendale CA gastroenterologist Robert Strecker MD and his late attorney brother Ted (a "suspicious" suicide) suggested that "the AIDS virus" is a manmade splice-together of two bovine viruses — *Visna maedi* virus in sheep (VMV) and the bovine leukemia virus (BLV) in cattle — "evolved upward" in humans, and that World Health

Organization (WHO) and other documents can be interpreted as "calling for" creation of just such an experimental virus with which to suppress the human immune system(s).

— Information developed by British venereologist John Seale that HIV is a tampered-with version of the visna virus and available as a biological warfare weapon among the superpowers for years.

(The Strecker thesis held that the "manmade virus" probably was a product of Soviet biological warfare aimed at the United States. Seale has been quoted as variously saying that both the Americans and Soviets developed the virus for biological warfare.)

— The vaccine theories. These hold that manmade experimental viruses were "tested" on Africans and on male homosexuals by inoculating both populations with vaccines — the smallpox vaccine in central Africa, a special hepatitis B vaccine in New York. They are paralleled by the idea that a mutated simian virus causing human AIDS was spread through an earlier form of the injectable polio vaccine. Various subtheories hold that these inoculation programs were either purposeful experiments, laboratory mistakes, or one or more parts of a coordinated conspiracy to reduce the human population. (Dr. Alan Cantwell's *AIDS and the Doctors of Death* and *Queer Blood* make strong cases.)

In truth, a case can be made for them all to some extent:

That there has been international research into immune-suppressing viruses is a fact. This in itself need not be sinister (a primary problem in the failure of organ transplants, for example, has long been how to overcome the human immune system attack on foreign tissue). That the superpowers, despite signing anti-biological warfare treaties, engage in and have engaged in biological warfare for decades is an essentially open secret. That many countries have the technological knowhow to manipulate, alter, splice together or semingly create "new" viruses is also true. These realities may encompass both human conspiracy (what better weapon than a virus which wipes out an immune system and is thus killing millions of people before its presence is even detected?) as well as human foibles (errors in high-tech gene research, gene-splicing and viral manipulation have been widely reported. In an era of petri-dish "immortal cell lines" and the exchange of active viral strains between laboratories and scientists, an "Andromeda strain"-like disaster is waiting to occur at any time).

The timeframes for the seemingly sudden appearance of AIDS in Africa and among male homosexuals in the United States neatly coalesce with the smallpox and hepatitis B vaccine theories, each of which has some other intriguing twists and turns which could either lead to chilling new revelations or go nowhere. The widespread appearance of AIDS in "third world" countries also neatly dovetails with polio inoculations.

An African swine fever connection?

Another theory, part of which may — or may not — fall into what international spy network participants class as "disinformation," holds that "AIDS" is really what arrived in the United States in lieu of "swine flu" — an alleged epidemic warned about during the Gerald Ford presidency (1970s) and for which a vaccine was developed which killed several people and sickened others while no epidemic appeared.

Part of this theory is that African Swine Fever Virus (ASFV), an extremely lethal structure which can wipe out entire pig populations and antibodies to which have been found in human AIDS patients (among others), has long been an American biological warfare research item and was in fact deployed against Cuba to wreck the island's pork production. Part of the theory also holds that ASFV, man-mutated for human inoculation, became the true "AIDS virus."

There should be more than passing interest in the latter statement.

As I noted in 1986, researcher Jane Teas originally proposed[39,40] that ASFV might be the real "cause" of AIDS — that is, the catalyst virus. Later, researcher John Beldekas argued that ASFV is in reality HHV-6, and that the virus was pirated by the NCI, which provided its present name and description.[41]

It is thanks to the persistent reporting of Neenyah Ostrom, a writer for the gay-activist *New York Native* weekly, that the theory of ASFV-as-biological-warfare-weapon-transmuted-to-HHV-6 as the "cause" of AIDS has reached out to many minds. It is true that the AIDS Inc. orthodoxy has denied any connection between ASFV and HHV-6, yet that very orthodoxy at this writing was yielding to the rising importance of HHV-6 in AIDS.

Parallel to this, as I reported both at an international seminar and a controversial book in 1993,[42] and very much in keeping with the conclusions of research reported by Ostrom and in other places, HHV-6 is also prominent in the most rapidly developing of the Western world's immunological disorders — so-called Chronic Fatigue Syndrome (CFS).

The biological warfare component in "new" viruses is a question too loud to ignore, and no amount of wishing it would go away will make it do so.

In 1994, Michigan Senator Donald Riegle testified before congress on a followup to his own investigation into the strange malady called "Gulf War Syndrome," which was afflicting hundreds, and possibly thousands, of US troops who had returned from the Gulf War of 1990 which essentially pitted Iraq, a former ally, against the United States.

The multiple symptomata of many of these veterans closely mimicked elements of either the ARC level of AIDS or the CFS syndrome. In testimony Feb. 9, 1994, the Michigan Democrat stated he had uncovered the fact that between 1984-1989 the United States had shipped various potential biological warfare agents to Iraq and that his staff researchers had made the "disturbing proposal" that some of these agents had been used *against* American troops in the Gulf War.[43]

When a reporter asked a US Department of Agriculture official: "Can M1-AL Abrams tanks or Bradley fighting vehicles carry hoof-and-mouth disease, African swine fever, or the anthrax bacteria?" the answer was yes.[44] Did US troops return from the Middle East suffering from the effects of biological warfare weapons which had originated in the USA?

Or even from experimental vaccines provided US troops upon the outbreak of the Gulf War?

Karl Grossman, a reporter for a Long Island newspaper, has long studied what he called "the mystery-shrouded island" — Plum Island, at the east end of Long Island, New York — as a long-time center of closely-guarded biological warfare (described by the military establishment as "defensive") research and at which, he and others have asserted, African swine fever virus (ASFV) has been actively studied for years.[45]

Grossman quoted *Newsday* in 1993 (*Newsday* having already reported in the 1970s on an alleged CIA plot to weaken Cuban pig herds through ASFV inoculations):

"A 1950s military plan to cripple the Soviet economy by killing horses, cattle and swine called for making the biological weapons out of exotic animal diseases at a Plum Island laboratory, now-declassified Army records reveal . . . Documents and interviews disclose for the first time what officials have denied for years: that the mysterious and closely guarded animal lab . . . was originally designed to conduct top-secret research into replicating animal viruses that could be used to destroy animal livestock . . . While officials say any such research was short-lived and ceased when the lab was turned over to the Agriculture Department in 1954, two of the diseases targeted by the military — hoof-and-mouth disease and African swine fever — remain top-priority research projects on Plum Island today."[46]

Supposing, for a moment, that Teas, Beldekas and some others are right, that African swine fever virus is somehow the "cause" of AIDS let alone a major catalyst virus in immune dysregulation in general, what do we know about ASFV?

Interestingly, in its natural state it seems to be as tricky and evasive as AIDS orthodoxy says HIV is.

In a 1987 textbook on the subject, researcher Eladio Vinuela was quite specific:

The presence in African swine virus DNA of several multigene families, a finding not reported for any other virus, may be related to the ability of African swine fever virus to evade the immune system . . . The virus . . . changes easily and different virus isolates produce diseases with different clinical symptoms or no disease at all.[47]

The very least that can be said of the startling emergence of HHV-6 as a major factor in AIDS is that part of the hype, hoopla and outright scamming that has gone on in the ranks of AIDS Inc. has been devastatingly wrong: if HHV-6 or any virus or anything other than HIV is shown to be the major "cause" (or possibly, *any* cause) of AIDS, then billions of dollars of research funds have been wasted, and lives lost to a wrong theory (including those individuals who committed suicide upon learning that they were "positive" for HIV antibodies).

By the mid-1990s AIDS Inc. had painted itself into an ever dwindling corner with allegiance to allopathy, to single viruses, and to HIV. All the while, it had denigrated, blocked, thwarted or remained oblivious to other ideas and approaches — an intellectual crime of Nuremberg War Crimes Trial dimensions.

Along with the possibility that the Allopathic Industrial Complex (AIC), AIDS Inc. subdivision, may have missed the boat about the real single cause — if there is one — of the ever-changing, multifactorial syndrome that is AIDS, its mad race to embrace AZT (and, later, didanosine [ddI], Bristol-Myers Squibb's Videx; zalcitabine [ddC], Roche Laboratories' Hivid; and stavudine (d4T, BMS' Zerit, in 1994) as "drugs of choice" in attempting to stop HIV may constitute an even greater disaster.

Indeed, the all-encompassing notions of the "single cause" and the "single cure" are the flaws of allopathic thinking which, as applied to AIDS, have accounted for the so far total failure of

Western medical orthodoxy to curb the killer. They constitute allopathy's twilight of the gods, a global death throe of an outmoded thought system for which the world population has paid and continues to pay an awful price.

Yet, it was to be expected:

If the AIDS Inc. research establishment — so overlapped with Cancer Inc. — had suddenly found the "cause" of the new killer syndrome, then it was only a matter of months, or perhaps years, before it would announce at least the first optimistic therapeutic approach.

The sorry saga of AZT

And, or course, this first optimistic therapeutic approach came from the Cancer Inc. apparatus. It was Burroughs Wellcome's AZT (Retrovir, zidovudine, azidothymidine), an old (1964), highly toxic (and highly dangerous) cancer chemotherapeutic drug which had been shelved years before because of both its overt toxicity and lack of efficacy in cancer.

The story of how AZT was literally rushed onto market in terms of a truncated "clinical trial" has been gone into great detail elsewhere,[47,48] and there is no part of that story which does not vibrate between the murky, the greedy, and the dubious.

It can be synthesized that AZT was found to kill some of the target cells that "the AIDS virus" ostensibly infects. As time wore on, it became clear that AZT and the whole family of nucleoside drugs killed more than HIV-infected cells — they set into play a chain reaction to eliminate certain cells in general since they strike at the very essence of cell reproduction (DNA chains) itself. Like most chemotherapeutic agents, AZT and its similars were/are immune suppressing themselves and capable of doing widespread damage to the host.

But because an early study seemed to show that AZT slowed down the course of AIDS — while never "curing" it — the AIC swiftly announced that the resurrected failed cancer agent should be immediately legalized for use in the new syndrome.

In 1993, ABC's "Day One" television program interviewed Dr. Itzhak Brook, a member of the 11-scientist FDA panel which approved AZT. As a scientist who disagreed with the use of AZT from the beginning, Dr. Brook said the committee had never had a way of scrutinizing the data properly and that the drug had been rushed to capture the market quickly. He was also quoted as saying, "I felt we compromised science and compromised safety."[49]

(Even Burroughs Wellcome would later concede that "the drug has been studied for limited periods of time and long-term safety and efficacy are not known."[50])

So AZT was literally sped to public acceptance based primarily on research largely paid for, and later defended by, the company. It was also evidence of the FDA's yielding, as usual, not only to the drug interests which essentially control the agency, but to organized gay activism, which politically clamored for the government to "do something."

In fact, the well-intentioned efforts of gay activists to pressure the federal research octopus into "doing something" often was nothing more than a playing into the hands of the AIC. The international drug trust was all too happy to see speedier approval for experimental toxic compounds from which millions could be gleaned.

When it was re-introduced for AIDS, AZT was for a time the most expensive drug ever marketed. It was, also, as such dissenters as California's Bruce Halstead MD[51] and Peter Duesberg PhD would keep pointing out, also among the most dangerous. By 1993, AZT was fetching $400 million in annual profits.

The outrageous costs of AZT — as well as of several older drugs "approved" for the treatment of PCP and other "opportunistic diseases" said to be part of the syndrome (see *VIII*) — led to congressional surveillance, public outcries, and the "compassionate" dropping of prices by drug companies to meet the propaganda challenge. AZT, and later the workalikes ddI and ddC (some others having failed to make it even through FDA's "fast track" approval system designed exclusively for AIDS and at the behest of AIDS activists) were held to be signs that the American medical/pharmaceutical research complex was truly "doing something."

At first, it seemed that at least in some cases AZT could "slow down" AIDS infections. But it was also becoming apparent that many patients, up to a third, could not tolerate the drug in *any* dose. There were some suggestions, mostly muted, but occasionally very vocal (Duesberg) that the AZT assault on host defense actually *caused* AIDS — particularly when given to individuals who were essentially free of symptoms but bore the tell-tale markers of HIV antibodies and/or inverted T4/T8 ratios.

As years passed, a troubling question arose: was AZT more often helping or hurting AIDS-prone patients?

Some celebrated AIDS patients — Florida co-ed Kimberly Bergalis, who went through the rapid stages of alleged HIV infection to ARC level to full-blown AIDS to death all within some three years; tennis player Arthur Ashe, who had said he had wanted to give up AZT but didn't want to offend his doctors; and ballet star Rudolph Nureyev — were all AIDS victims but they also may have been AZT victims, since their rapid descent seemed to follow the beginning of their use of the drug.[52]

Frighteningly, AIDS orthodoxy began to argue that AZT should be prescribed as early as possible — and even prophylactically! If there were antibodies to HIV and a sign of immune system disturbance let alone any of the 27 to 34 clinical signs and symptoms of overt pathology, it was argued, AZT should be given right away — though perhaps at more tolerable lower doses. The widely disseminated use of a toxic agent to prevent a disease remains, as we have seen in cancer, a centerpiece of allopathic thought, and is utterly logical if one cedes the premise.

By 1993/1994 AZT was headed both for a nosedive and a last-minute reprieve.

The nosedive came primarily in preliminary results, and then final results, of a large three-year clinical trial in the United

Kingdom, France and Ireland called the Concorde Study — in which Great Britain-based Wellcome PLC, the parent of Burroughs Wellcome, took no part.

The early results were bad enough since, among other things, a spinoff was that reliance on the CD4/T4 "helper" cell count as a guide as to when to initiate antiretroviral therapy was found to be misleading.

The key result, however, was that AZT did not slow down the advance of AIDS in asymptomatic people infected with HIV. The authors concluded: "The results of Concorde do not encourage the early use of zidovudine in symptom-free HIV-infected adults."[53]

In the midst of the two Concorde reports, a 1994 Harvard School of Public Health study of 1,338 HIV-infected people likewise found that whatever "slight benefits" there might be from taking AZT were often cancelled by the drug's side effects.[54]

All that could be said for switching patients from AZT to either ddI or ddC was that when tolerance for one developed, a physician might try another — but evidence was lacking that the AZT workalikes were any more efficacious than AZT and sometimes they caused just as many, if not more, side effects.[55]

A month after the Concorde trial was published, two other key studies weighed in to put further nails not only into the coffin of AZT but into the whole area of "retroviral therapy with nucleoside analogue drugs":

First, an AIDS in Europe Study group analysis of 4,484 patients at 51 treatment centers in 17 European countries showed that "when initiated after the time of AIDS diagnosis," AZT was "associated with improved prognosis but for no more than two years after starting therapy." And, worse, "for patients surviving more than two years since starting [AZT], the death rate was greater than for *untreated* [*emphasis mine*] patients who had developed AIDS at the same time." This was at least a statistical suggestion that AZT had worsened the condition of treated patients.[56]

Second, a nine-year followup of 761 "HIV-positive homosexual and bisexual men" in San Francisco found that there had been a one-year increase in survival times for patients classified as AIDS by the 1987 CDC definition thereof — but the small increase was due more to increased "prophylaxis" (prevention of initial or secondary PCP attacks) than to "antiretroviral therapy."[57]

This was clear evidence that some of the antibiotic therapies aimed at PCP were "working" at least for awhile (perhaps the single ray of good news in "AIDS" treatments) — but there was no evidence that the "antiretroviral drugs" were associated with increased survival.

The last-minute reprieve for AZT came in 1994 with the ongoing "Pediatric AIDS Clinical Trials Group Protocol 076 Study Group" in the US — and it of course raised more questions than answers.

In a study of infants born live to 477 women, with HIV infection status known in 363 births, it was found that in "women with mildly symptomatic HIV disease" and no prior treatment with antiretroviral drugs during pregnancy, AZT administered before and during birth and to newborns for six weeks reduced the risk of maternal-infant HIV transmissions "by approximately two thirds."[57a] This study did not offset other data suggesting that mother-to-infant transmission of HIV occurs a minority of the time whether AZT is administered or not.

While the news gave a slight lift to Burroughs Wellcome following the battery of devastating earlier research, Centers for Disease Control and Prevention (CDC) physicians editorially noted that "the long-term effects on both mother and infant are unknown" from using a drug as toxic as AZT. Too, "zidovudine-resistant virus might emerge during a short course of zidovudine during pregnancy and might affect the mother's subsequent response to zidovudine therapy."[57b]

For AIDS Inc. AZT propaganda received a boost: HIV-positive pregnant women should be treated with a potentially dangerous toxic drug to reduce chance of transmitting "the AIDS virus" to the fetus, and newborns of infected mothers should also be so treated. To medical dissidents, however, the spectre of mass prophylaxis with a toxic drug whose long-term benefits were murky at best, and possibly dangerous in the long run, was simply horrifying.

So, in the 13th year of the Plague, and despite a multi-billion-dollar research investment precariously balanced on two rickety pillars (the HIV theory of AIDS and the launching of AZT and similar drugs to attack "the AIDS virus,") AIDS Inc. had mostly come up a loser.

All of which, in 1993, led the non-profit, Los Angeles-based Project AIDS International (PAI) to submit to the United Nations Commission on Human Rights in Geneva a request for an international review both of the HIV theory of AIDS causation and the continued use of AZT against the syndrome. It asked for action to ban AZT and all "non-selective analogue-DNA chain terminating drugs."[58]

In an often startling review of data PAI had gleaned from various sources, the organization pointedly claimed that — quite distinct to AIDS Inc.'s general considerations — the "normal range" of CD4 "helper" cells in humans is far wider than usually thought: 237 to 1,817, and that

> *... in tests completed on US Olympic athletes in 1984, the average range of CD4 helper cells was between 400 to 600. Certainly, the US athletes were not considered to be unhealthy; yet these are markers used to instill fear and manipulate HIV-positive persons into taking toxic chemotherapy when they are not otherwise unhealthy.*[59]

As a science writer, I also found it difficult to find, at least at any point before AIDS, just how the general notions of what constituted "normal" CD4 and CD8 cells had originated. The simple reality is that, before the AIDS era, such lymphocytes were not being looked at in broad sectors of the population.

Even AIDS researchers began noting that T-cell counts could "go up, down and sideways" due to many factors over long periods of time — and that five different T-cell tests done from the same patient at five different laboratories on five different days could produce five different widely varying results.

PAI also claimed that although there were over two thousand cases of HIV-free AIDS known to the CDC such "information was (and is) embargoed" (!) and that, even so, by Dec. 31, 1992, the CDC admitted to knowledge of 97 such (American) cases.

It also quoted a statement by two London microbiologists in 1990:

> *"It would be irresponsible to produce guidelines on AIDS until an infectious organism is identified and the means by which it causes disease are understood.*
>
> *"It is only now becoming obvious that infection with HIV does not usually give rise to AIDS."*[60]

AIDS theory: failing on all fronts

So by the mid-1990s, AIDS Inc. had failed in virtually all of its premises:

— It remained unclear that HIV was the single cause, or possibly any cause, of a syndrome whose definition had grown to cover more than 30 infections, conditions, and "forms" of cancer. In fact, the wrong virus — if in fact there is a single viral cause — might have been targeted in the first place.

— Reliance on antibody tests to detect HIV was increasingly called into question.

— Reliance on the standard immune system markers (falling CD4s, advancing CD8s, inversions between both) as a way to "stage" the syndrome was also questionable.

— Drugs aimed at halting HIV through terminating DNA chains or interfering with two enzymes essential to HIV activity were failing to slow down the course of disease.

The American public, American science, the Western world, the world in general had been sold a nasty bill of goods which, for whatever reasons, turned out to be questionable at best.

Clearly, new thought was called for.

From the beginning, a number of innovative physicians were willing to try creative approaches to AIDS, and usually but not always these were the same kinds of men and women who, at however great a risk to their careers and professional standing, tried novel therapies against cancer and other "incurable" disorders.

With AIDS, both doctors and patients had a clearer certainty of the correctness of opting for "alternative" treatments: AIDS had no known effective treatment, no known cure and allegedly was always fatal.

AIDS medical innovators were faced by the same stone walls which faced cancer and cardiovascular innovators: how could they quantify their results, particularly if they were multifactorial, and who would publish them? Most knowledge of "alternatives" in AIDS therapy arose in the mostly-gay "AIDS underground" and in journals and publications in no way connected with the Allopathic Industrial Complex.

Just as breakthroughs in American cancer alternatives had often had to be found in such girlie magazines as *Penthouse*, such magazines and counter-culture publications also became clearing-houses for the latest ideas in AIDS treatments.

By the end of the 1980s, although American AIDS patients constituted a much smaller population than American cancer patients, a much higher percentage of them, though still in the minority, were willing to try "alternatives." This was primarily because the cancer "cure" rate in advanced disease, depending on the definition of "cure," was at least 8 to 10 percent, however discouraging such a number. But this was in contrast to 0 percent in AIDS.

Hope from the unortho-docs

Hence, increasing numbers of doctors, some as much informed by their patients as anyone, struck out on their own. On both coasts, primarily, a handful of physicians began implementing ideas of holism — detoxify the body, promote overall host defense, change diets, encourage healthy lifestyles, experiment with regimens of vitamins, minerals, enzymes, amino acids, essential fatty acids, herbs, "unapproved" but promising drugs, oxidative therapies, attitude-changing exercises.

(Included was the small group which our own research/medical team began seeing on a limited and intermittent basis beginning in 1983 — those who had the funds to seek out a foreign clinic. Following them through therapies and results allowed us to develop some early conclusions: just as in any other allegedly "terminal," multifactorial disorder of a chronic or acute nature, it made more sense to work with diet and natural factors, occasionally blending them with standard modalities, than to pursue allopathic approaches alone).

Going into the 1990s, it could be said of "unorthodox" approaches in general that long-term AIDS survivors — that is, persons either with diagnosed full-blown disease or ARC-level symptoms or even early-stage asymptomatics — had the following things in common:

— First, they had either abandoned, or never were involved in, standard therapies at all.

— Second, they were using one or several "alternative" approaches (in which diet and supplements played central roles); and/or they blended occasional "standard" therapies with such "alternatives." And

— Third, there was something different about their mental outlook: most of these patients saw themselves as "living with AIDS" rather than "dying from" it. Some had made victory over it a challenge which they faced exuberantly, and sometimes even joyously. They simply did not expect to die from the syndrome.

It also became statistically apparent that there was another cluster of patients difficult to quantify: those with no known treatments who were surviving in good condition for no known reason. These mainly involved early asymptomatics and their presence usually strengthened the idea that HIV antibody positivity did not necessarily mean the acquisition of an AIDS-related illness.

It is true that in AIDS, as in cancer, there has been a field day for charlatans as well: "magic bullet" cures of all kinds have flourished in the AIDS world. But many of these approaches have at least some rationale empirically or in biological theory.

The experience has been that, whatever temporarily exciting results an herb tea, or any herb, or a vitamin, or a serum of some kind, or a machine, or anything else, may have had, there is no single "magic bullet" against a syndrome of multifactorial causality. Rather, AIDS, perhaps even more dramatically than cancer, has presented an archetypal condition in which individualized, integrated protocols alone offer hope.

The unorganized, poorly reported, anecdotal but gathering information on "alternatives" in AIDS led to various realizations:

— That suppressing HIV, or any other virus, did not effect a "cure" and that a vast array of substances (mostly natural and from the plant and mineral kingdoms primarily) could play roles in both immune system modulation and stimulation, even though such factors did not absolutely "cure" AIDS.

Long-term survivors continued to be reported, and the better known of them continued either to have no "orthodox" therapy or to have long since abandoned it. It is also true that this multitude of "unorthodox" approaches had often simply lengthened the lives and reduced the suffering of AIDS patients so that they eventually succumbed to some complication of the syndrome — yet the months and years of unexpected, against-the-odds survival were precious to them and their families and slowly, but firmly, made the case for nutrition-based, individualized therapies based not on demolishing pathogens but on enhancing overall health.

Aside from our own surveys of our patients in Mexico, other practitioners went public with their theories, approaches and results.[61,62]

More affluent AIDS patients would try anything anywhere — they might gravitate between intravenous megadose Vitamin C therapy to treatments of the blood by ozone, from gobbling Japanese mushrooms and copious amounts of antioxidant-containing pills and foods to taking injections of live embryonic cells. What worked for one might or might not work for another — but, in sum, the multitude of mostly-natural approaches was proving that disease progression and suffering could be reduced, slowed, mitigated, if not stopped.

Interestingly enough, even establishment research was backing up at least some of the "unorthodox" findings by 1993.

In September of that year, a Johns Hopkins University study showed that some 15 percent of drug-using HIV infectees developed Vitamin A deficiency and that such a lack of a key nutrient might shave a year of life expectancy off infected individuals, of particular importance in "full-blown" cases.[63]

More impressively, none other than the National Institutes of Health (NIH) announced on Nov. 11, 1993, that antioxidants "might" help keep HIV-infected patients from getting sicker.[63a] Mentioned in this respect were Vitamins A, C and E. While it had taken cancer decades before US orthodoxy would admit the slightest possibility that vitamins, particularly antioxidants, might somehow help out against malignancy, it had taken AIDS only 12 years before orthodoxy got the picture.

In 1994, University of Georgia research added another bit of news pleasing to metabolic therapists — that depletion of selenium, a major antioxidant, might be playing a crucial role in the progression of AIDS.

The U of G study, whose authors admitted that they did not know what the mechanism might be, suggested that somehow HIV causes selenium deficiency by producing proteins which consume the body's supply of the mineral — which is often depleted in the American diet anyway.

The Associated Press quoted University of Georgia College of Pharmacy's Dr. Will Taylor:

> "... *the length of time it took to deplete the body's store of selenium could help account for HIV's latency period, which can last for years ... If this is true, then selenium biochemistry may be the key to understanding the control of the life cycle of*

HIV and perhaps some of the pathology of AIDS . . . Many AIDS patients lack selenium and have taken supplements on their own. For several years, some researchers and doctors have recommended selenium as part of the patient's dietary supplements. "(63b)

The growing connections between antioxidant vitamins and minerals speak to the revolution in *oxidology* (See *XIV*), which has added a new dimension to medicine and in which our own research entities (Bradford Research Institute/American Biologics) have played some pivotal roles.

Earlier, Australian researchers had argued that "oxidative stress" — in essence, more reactive oxygen toxic species (ROTS) and "free radicals" (toxic oxygen breakdown products) than the body knows what to do with — induced by AIDS "risk factors" might be the primary cause of the syndrome!

Among the "risk factors" described as "potent oxidizing agents" were the inhalant nitrate drugs ("poppers"), Factor III (the blood product used by hemophiliacs) — and sperm.[63c,63d]

Despite information available parallel to the outbreak of the AIDS pandemic that elements *other than* viruses might have a great deal to do with the syndrome, the AIC and its rapidly developing AIDS Inc. subdivision were not about to turn loose of the HIV theory of causation, whatever other lines of research begged to be looked at.

The syphilis connection

One such line of research, although it did not originate with him, was pursued by a heroic Manhattan physician with a high caseload of AIDS patients and who himself was infected with HIV — the late Stephen Caiazza MD, who in the midst of his investigation became a friend of mine.

Following up on German leads, Dr. Caiazza, and a small collaborating group around him, had found (as had investigator Joan McKenna in Berkeley and writer Harris Coulter[64]) that the parallels and overlaps between AIDS and late-stage syphilis were far too vast in number to be coincidental. Such probers found that the protean symptomatology of AIDS had a nearly equal relationship to the vast symptomatology of syphilis in an earlier era. Indeed, Dr. Moritz Kaposi, for whom Kaposi's sarcoma was named, was a syphilologist.

Scattered European research suggested that a good deal of what was being called AIDS (including the purplish lesions of KS and various pulmonary calamities being attributed to PCP and other microbes) were really manifestations of advanced syphilis that had invaded the central nervous system — that is, *neurosyphilis*. The same research argued that because late-stage syphilis, let alone neurosyphilis, was not ordinarily seen in young people, and had rarely been clinically seen in the Western world (since earlier in this century anyway), younger physicians who had not been trained in the multiple sequelae of "the great imitator" were simply unaware that they were often looking at syphilis.

Moreover, research suggested that the syphilitic treponeme plays numerous tricks on human immune systems — and that positivity for syphilis on a standard syphilis blood test (particularly the VDRL, as favored in the USA) could obscure HIV infection while positivity for HIV could obscure syphilis. This reality led to a strange meeting at the Centers for Disease Control (CDC) in Atlanta in 1988.

A two-day conference of experts agreed that both disease states altered each other's outcomes (a nightmare for patients "co-infected" with syphilis and the "AIDS virus"), that confirmatory blood tests for either could in effect be "thrown off" by the other, that co-infection seemed to help both infections advance, that sexually active syphilitics should be screened for HIV, that HIV patients infected through sexual intercourse or IV drug abuse should be treated for syphilis, that neurosyphilis should be considered in the diagnosis of neurological diseases being ascribed to AIDS, and that the standard treatment of choice for early syphilis, benzathine penicillin, should not be used in the treatment of neurosyphilis in either symptomatic or asymptomatic HIV-infected individuals. Rather, old-time (and patent-expired) crystalline or aqueous penicillin or procaine penicillin should be used.[65]

While it should also be added that the AIDS-syphilis link never received much orthodox attention and that even the CDC's meeting on the same failed to capture much publicity and that other scattered research was said not to confirm the most stunning possibility of all (perhaps AIDS *is* syphilis), a handful of doctors who used crystalline penicillin as a drug of choice were reporting some promising results.

Dr. Caiazza had used himself as his own guinea pig: already infected with the alleged "AIDS virus" but essentially healthy, he inoculated himself with enough syphilis to make sure he became massively infected, as he recounted in his own little-known book.[66] He described advancing from a mildly symptomatic stage to fully advanced, near-terminal conditions in a matter of days, and how using mega-infusions of aqueous penicillin restored him to mostly good health in a short period of time.

Believing he had a tiger by the tail, Dr. Caiazza began treating more and more patients with crystalline penicillin and followup antibiotics, reporting on some spectacular successes, at least over the short term. He instantly fell under attack by New York state medical authorities, and was under investigation when, several years later, he died — allegedly of complications of his disease.

Dr. Caiazza had never believed in nutritional or other supplements as a necessary part of an AIDS protocol and, good allopath that he was, wanted to prove his point with single-shot modalities — antibiotics in general, and old-time penicillin in particular, could manage AIDS, he believed.

(Since much of AIDS is indeed bacterial, and also because mycoplasmas, though not viruses, are open to attack by antibiotics, there is an implied role for the limited use of antibiotics in an integrative, mostly-natural protocol).

Parallel to his work was that of others, who claimed that

administration of the typhoid vaccine could "unmask" previously "hidden" syphilis and that aqueous penicillin could then reduce the syphilis load by crossing the blood-brain barrier. The underlying assumptions, never sharply challenged by orthodoxy, were that the standard VDRL test is not a reliable screen for neurosyphilis (that is, a negative result will occur from screening the blood but this does not mean treponemes have not already invaded the central nervous system) and that the common benzathine penicillin used in early syphilis is mostly useless in neurosyphilis.

But Dr. Caiazza had other things to report to me intermittently. The most chilling was the warning he received while in the Germanies that he should be less vocal about his theories since he was in a country which was a major headquarters of world pharmaceutical interests — and two apparent attempts on his life, one in an automobile near-accident and the other in a beating by thugs in which nothing was stolen.

It dawned on Dr. Caiazza over time that he, and indeed all proponents of the syphilis connection to AIDS, if any, were playing with fire: syphilis is an altogether "curable" bacterial disease and a primary agent in "curing" it is an essentially inexpensive form of penicillin without patent protection.

Our own medical group saw several dramatic cases in which megadoses of crystalline penicillin, accompanied by hefty infusions of Vitamin C and an oxidative agent (Dioxychlor), produced relatively rapid and spectacular decreases in several AIDS "opportunistic infections." But the syphilis-AIDS link remained heretical and, by the mid-1990s, had not seriously been followed up on.

Positivity in negativity?

Other novel magic-bullet AIDS approaches were anecdotally reported but supportive data were hard to come by. One reason was the confusing nature of the AIDS definition itself — if blood "turned negative" for HIV, did this mean that both antigens and antibodies were gone (virologically not necessarily a desired outcome) or simply that HIV was no longer active? If HIV were not causing anything, what difference did disappearance of its antigens or antibodies make? If "helper" cells were elevated and the patient remained free of disease, having never had any, did this mean he was "cured" of the syndrome? If a potentially lethal "form" of cancer associated with AIDS (as in one of our group's more celebrated cases — an HIV-positive Scandinavian) was eradicated by unorthodox therapies, had the man been "cured" of cancer, or of AIDS? (In this case, a major Southern California hospital pronounced the patient "cured" — their term — of immunoblastic sarcoma. But he remained HIV-positive. He lived in ordinarily good health for several years, dying of an indirectly related malady. Since he was still HIV-positive, had he "died of AIDS"?)

Promoters of ozone gas infusions and ozone machines spoke in glowing terms of "cures" of AIDS in the US underground and in Europe. At one point I was told that "hundreds" had been "cured," though was not provided supporting evidence. Yet research does confirm that *any* oxidative agent will, at least for a time, clear the blood of cell wall-deficient structures and organisms, including virtually all viruses, retroviruses, some bacteria, mycoplasmas and yeast forms. Is clean serum evidence of a "cure"? The same had been said of the primary natural endogenous oxidative agent of all, hydrogen peroxide, and of our own research group's Dioxychlor and similar oxidative compounds. All have been useful and all have sprung from research relegated to the shadows of medicine in decades past primarily because they collided with the vested interests of the synthetic drug empire.

The use of "frequency machines" (see *XV*) also generated claims of cures. The officially harassed anti-cancer products "CanCell" (said to be a synthetic of several compounds which somehow balance energy in the body) and Essiac (an herbal tea combination a half-century old in Canada) have been among "magic bullets" said to be useful in, even "curative" of, AIDS.

What we came to call AIDS Inc. continually did not look

at particular approaches to AIDS or follow up on promising leads developed outside the AIC, as I saw time and again.

Should an "outsider" — outside the AIC — appear with a promising product for AIDS (as antiviral, immune modulator, specific against a disease, etc.) — he was run through very expensive hoops.

A case in point has been Solutein, the modern-era incarnation of earlier work involving the use of immune boosters made of snake venoms (and anecdotally found useful against polio and MS at an earlier time.)

A small but enterprising Utah company attempted to show Solutein useful against AIDS — that is, in helping stabilize numbers of T4 cells, hastening HIV antigen negativity or modulating the immune system and specific disease states in a multiplicity of ways. The company wished to do things "the American way" by going through the ponderous, progress-blocking minutiae of the FDA.

Before the Utah company began reaching the conclusion that the federal government seemed to have only tepid interest, if that, in Solutein — which already was checking out well in animal trials and was "anecdotally" being used in HIV cases treated in Mexico — it had spent, its chief executive told me, at least in the "high six figures" in attempts to comply with FDA procedures.

Since the hospital with which I have been affiliated in Mexico was the site of much, but by no means all, of the Solutein use in human HIV cases, I am aware that in at least several cases (and, outside the hospital, in many more) of some truly impressive results with the product.

By the time this was written, and following a full-dress hearing in Washington by the FDA's "fast track" approval committee, Solutein was still not a "legal" drug in the USA.

And this, despite an authentic effort by the company to attempt to comply with the entire FDA inanity of various animal trials followed by various stages of human ones. And the company — as a non-member of the AIC — did not have millions of dollars to play with while the FDA took its time. The matter was not over at this writing, but constitutes one more frustrating reason why so much promising American research has had to be conducted outside of the USA, despite whatever utility it truly has.

Perhaps more than anything else, AIDS has focused on mental and emotional aspects of healing — and this may turn out to be another blessing from this curse of the late-20th century alongside its manifest victory in breaking asunder the allopathic paradigm in medicine.

So AIDS has understandably made news by terrifying the world over a new plague seeming to be caused by an unstoppable, incurable virus, of whatever origin.

Enter CFS, the crippler

Yet a parallel disorder has also been developing, though primarily in the Western world, silently but relentlessly spreading beyond the huge shadow cast by AIDS. Its presence, and seeming incurability, is adding a whole new dimension to the menace of man-caused or man-altered disease and stimulating the new medical approaches which must be mounted to meet the challenge of our species' very survival.

AIDS was several years old when Western medical journals began reporting cases of individuals who seemed to have AIDS-*like* conditions, but not full-blown diseases. Such patients were instantly assumed to be in no way associated with AIDS because they were not, in the main, from the "AIDS risk groups" — that is, they essentially were not promiscuous male homosexuals, intravenous drug users, hemophiliacs or receivers of tainted blood products, or the sexual partners of any of the above.

Yet they were "presenting with" a mind-boggling constellation of symptoms (up to 60 separate ones) redolent of what came to be called the ARC stage of AIDS — swollen glands, nightsweats, spiking fevers, muscular, bone and neurological complaints, gastrointestinal and respiratory stress, sensitivity to light, occasional weight loss, sore throats, earaches, headaches, mood swings, short-term memory disturbances, and, almost always, yeast infection and long periods of debilitating, extreme fatigue. The latter could last days to months — and even, in some cases, years.

But standard blood and other tests failed to reveal anything particularly wrong with these patients. Since the first cluster of them was reported in the resort area of Lake Tahoe, on the Nevada-California border, they were called sufferers of the "Lake Tahoe Syndrome." Since other clusters broke out among younger, more affluent and usually Caucasian people, they were also called victims of the "yuppie flu." The mild ridiculing of them in the media and even in the first few reports of their malady in the "literature" was excused by the fact that whatever was going on seemed to be transitory and nobody died.

Yet, the syndrome had been noted even earlier in other areas of the English-speaking world, where the countries in question equally had a difficult time finding a phrase to define what surely was yet another syndrome. But this one, if anything, seemed more associated with *activated* than *depressed* immune systems. And in all areas it seemed to be more prevalent among women than men — a reason, feminists might argue, among several to explain why it received so little attention.

Even by the time (1988) the US officially took note of this combination of symptoms and baptized them Chronic Fatigue Syndrome (CFS), a significant number of clinicians and researchers were of the opinion this was essentially an all-in-your head version of schoolgirl panic attack among adults, a kind of "in" hypochondria. At the very worst, it seemed that it might be an extreme form of yeast infection, since the general syndrome provoked by the human cohabitating yeast *Candida albicans* was also coming into its own as a pathology about whose parameters medical orthodoxy did not agree. It also had to be distinguished from mononucleosis, thyroid disorders, general endocrine imbalances, influenza infections, occasionally secondary syphilis, hypoglycemia, the closely associated fibromyalgia, and premenstrual syndrome (PMS). All of these, along with the ARC stage of AIDS, produced a similar clinical pattern. But AIDS was already distinguishable from any such presentation of confusing and conflicting symptoms thanks to the HIV antibody test and the standard helper/suppressor immune cell inversions — though CFS patients occasionally had some of the latter.

For a time, since blood tests to determine activity for reactivated Epstein-Barr Virus (EBV) were often positive in such patients, and the patients also had diagnosable yeast infection, some physicians thought they were seeing a recurring mononucleosis infection in adults, in which the yeast problem and other signs were secondary events. But as numbers of cases came to be reported in Western medical journals, primarily though not exclusively among North Americans, inhabitants of the British Isles, Iceland, northwest Europe, Australia and New Zealand, it become evident that for numerous patients there were no elevated "titers" of EBV, even though yeast infection remained a virtual constant. This naturally gave rise to an allopathic medical industry, already obsessed with the viral connection to AIDS, to look for one in CFS.

By the early 1990s, CFS had ceased to be a laughing matter: its numbers anecdotally growing much faster than AIDS, some patients seemed to be permanently disabled, and some were forced to stay in bed for years at a time.

Yet by mid-decade it was difficult to get an "official" feel for real numbes of CFS patients, if only because the multiplicity of symptoms could so easily be confused with so many other things.

By 1994, CFS prevalence data presented at the American Association for Chronic Fatigue Research showed that "as many as 500,000 Americans" might already have CFS — though many doctors and others suspected the figures were much higher. Yet the Centers for Disease Control and Prevention (CDC) claimed only 20,000 fit its case description.[66a]

The mental aspects often were as devastating as the physical symptoms: memories failed, personalities were altered, behavior patterns would swing violently, concentration diminished, IQ levels dipped, victims variously describing themselves as "unfocused," "un-wired," "coming apart." CFS caseloads and numbers grew, expanding from their younger (and even much younger) to older age brackets, and all economic levels:

The fact that the syndrome often occurred in clusters (classrooms, bands, orchestras, athletic teams, groups of nurses, any close-quarters arrangement) strongly suggested contagion, yet sexual contagion was unlikely: it became as common, if not more common, to find a mother and daughter showing symptoms as a man and a wife.

There also developed the strong possibility that CFS, whatever it was, was linked to an increased risk of some "forms" of cancer even though the syndrome itself did not seem to be killing anyone and a certain group of patients seemed to fully recover on their own while others went through frustrating, unpredictable periods of being healthy and restored or terribly ill and unable to study, hold a job or even think straight. Several physicians and patient support groups demanded to know what was going on, but it was difficult to hear their cries for help over the din caused by AIDS, held to be the great plague which had a 100 percent fatal outcome.

CFS became so variable in symptoms that it was not easy to separate it out from the earlier described fibromyalgia syndrome, and in fact the one could be part of the other. Later, as Lyme Disease broke out (a potentially devastating infection ostensibly spread by a treponemal bacterium carried by ticks), it became equally difficult to separate Lyme cases from CFS ones.[67]

Numerous physicians thought they were seeing AIDS-like conditions in an ever-growing number of people, yet conventional wisdom was that this could not be because such patients were negative for HIV antibodies and were not from the AIDS "risk groups." For many, AIDS was a "dirty," CFS a "clean" — the one was a killer, the other a crippler, and they had no real points of similarity.

Or did they?

AIDS, CFS: parts of one syndrome?

In a 1993 book,[68] based primarily on research from the first 10 years and 2,200 patients (which we originally called "no-name disease" victims) from our Mexican hospital, and at an international seminar our group presented in 1992, I outlined 14 large groups of symptoms (hematological, viral, bacterial, endocrinological, clinical) which pre-AIDS and CFS patients seemed to share. At the same time other writers, including the *New York Native's* Neenyah Ostrom, were reporting along similar lines. I asked a rhetorical final question: *"Are* these different kinds of patients?"

They could only be so on the basis of the absence of HIV in the CFS patients and the fact that pre-AIDS patients often (but by no means always) advanced into full-blown AIDS (though a few advanced CFS patients have exhibited some aspects of full-blown AIDS as well). Research from various quarters turned up some interesting items: there increasingly were thought to be aspects of "immune excitation" or "autoimmunity" in AIDS patients — and there were aspects of "immune depression" in CFS sufferers.

Our research group (Bradford Research Institutes) thus proposed[69] a new model:

A Syndrome of Immune Dysregulation (SID), which covered a broad span of *immune dysregulation,* ranging from the takeover of the host by parasites, yeasts, fungi, bacteria, mycoplasmas, viruses and cancer as was being seen in immune-depressed AIDS patients, to the over-excited immune responses of what some were calling "universal reactor syndrome" (URS). This is a condition in which the body is engaged in so many antigen-antibody immune responses and has so many confused signals it is now turning upon itself and the patient allergically reacts to everything — from all manner of food and drink to heat, cold, dryness, dampness, hair sprays, perfumes, industrial chemicals, natural and unnatural environmental allergens of all kinds, and even to the clothes on his back and bedsheets. We reasoned that URS — and/or "environmental illness" or so-called "multiple chemical sensitivity/environmental illness" — is a possible endpoint for unresolved CFS and that numerous "autoimmune" diseases, occurring in the mostly civilized Western world by the century's end, were stops along a general curve of SID.

While it seemed highly unlikely that a single factor was capable of causing the full spectrum of immune dysregulation — along whose pathological curve could be found many often new, mostly-Western "autoimmune diseases" (multiple sclerosis, scleroderma, various forms of lupus, Sjogren's syndrome, rheumatoid arthritis, possibly *all* arthritis, and various strange disorders simply never seen, or at least never adequately reported on, before this century) — it became more reasonable that a combination of ingredients was necessary in setting up a "substrate," a matrix on which a catalyst, or catalysts, might build.

(Such a matrix would contain the following elements [in no particular order of importance]: our chemically and hormonally altered food supply, particularly involving the overabundance of essentially nutritionless refined carbohydrates, known excesses/deficiencies in certain vitamins, minerals, enzymes and essential fatty acids, overuse of antibiotics and synthetic hormones [steroids], immunizations/vaccinations, overexposure to continual low-level radiation poisoning and/or low-level electromagnetic frequencies, fluoridated/chlorinated water, industrial chemicals, "recreational drugs" — and mercury amalgam dental fillings and even root canals.

(The relevance of the latter two elements was particularly brought home to me in 1993/1994 as guest speaker at meetings of patients of alleged "fibromyalgia" — and/or CFS — patients in Missoula and Billings, Montana, where large clusters of CFS-like conditions had broken out. In both meetings, of about 200 patients each, when I asked who had had a significant amount of mercury amalgam fillings prior to the onset of symptoms, 90 percent of hands went up. In Billings, when I asked who had had a root canal prior to the onset of symptoms, virtually *every* hand went up.)

(All of the above elements constitute a possible witch's brew of conceivably immune-altering substances, yet they almost certainly need, whatever their numbers or combinations, one or more "triggers" or catalysts to begin the domino-like advance to pathology.)

If catalysts were involved, and if one stood out more than any other, it was a reasonable speculation it might be found among species-jumping, easily-mutating viruses from the animal kingdom (for viral inhabitants of humankind, involving dozens of varieties, have long coexisted in man without, in the main, causing significant pathology).

HHV-6 and/or ASFV, whatever their origin, seemed to some particularly strong candidates as key viruses to initiate a series of immune dysregulating events, particularly in a vast spectrum of individuals already "immunologically compromised." The widespread presence of HHV-6 in AIDS and CFS, its affinity for some of the same key components of immunity as targeted by HIV, and ASFV's immune system-evading presence in man and other mammals, made them high-profile suspects.

There remained many other viral suspects as well. In 1994 University of Southern California pathologist W. John Martin added a "stealth" virus, which apparently caused CFS symptoms in laboratory animals, to an ever-growing list of agents listed as possible "causes."[69a]

It was observed that immunological disorders in humans are often accompanied by those in house pets or even other animals in close proximity. I pointed to the well-known statistical unusuality in which former President and Mrs. George Bush shared a single "autoimmune" disorder, Grave's disease, while their famous pet dog, Millie, had canine lupus. In 1993 I also pointed to the high prevalence of sheep (Visna virus?) in the countries which from earliest times had reported what many were calling myalgic encephalomyelitis (the equivalent of CFS in the United States) — particularly Iceland, whose clusters of

"Icelandic disease" cases dated back to the 1940s.

As of this writing, CFS remained a syndrome without an accepted "etiological cause" and still lacked a confirmatory blood test.

More diseases of civilization

While AIDS, CFS and URS represent huge clusters of cases in which immune dysregulation of some kind is going on, the Western world is also beleaguered by a raft of new disorders and conditions, some of which have no official names, and all of which involve some degree of immune-system derangement.

While it is not certain they should all be lumped under SID, certainly they should be called disorders of civilization in that they are so far essentially limited to the Western world. They include but are not limited to:

— The general constellation of conditions generally classed as "environmental illness" or "multiple chemical sensitivity" and strongly linked to exposure to organophosphates, pesticides, insecticides and an ever-lengthening list of industrial (and mostly petro-) chemicals.

— Attention-deficit disorder (ADD), afflicting untold thousands, perhaps millions, of children — and even adults — and the true extent of which is far from known.

— Silicone-induced immune disorder (among other names) — in which women, particularly in the United States, have reported an impressive series of immunological and other disturbances seemingly linked directly or indirectly to silicone breast implants, over which billions of dollars in lawsuits have occurred, and about which scientific research has been confusing.

— Agent Orange Syndrome, a constellation of symptoms strongly correlated to exposure to this Vietnam War defoliant.

— Sick Building Syndrome — a galaxy of symptoms which seem to occur in clusters among workers in particular buildings, apparently involving exposure to various chemicals involved in construction materials and air conditioning.

— Acute disturbances in behavior, including depressive

disorders and sudden acts of violence, which seem to relate to any number of synthetic chemicals both in the environment and food supply.

Diametrically opposed suppositions suggest reasons and causes. All may be involved:

The first is that man has so overchemicalized his environment that the accumulated effects of industrial molecules are now beginning to manifest themselves in a vast variety of physical and mental conditions. They are grossly akin to earlier known disasters of civilization: mercury poisoning among "mad" hatters and the long-term slow poisoning of whole populations by lead — from lead pipes, for instance, a probable contributor to the gradual deterioration of the Roman Empire.

The second is the possible immune system-altering effects of the depletion of earth's ozone layer, a kind of shield through which the sun's ultraviolet radiation is diffused. A considerable school of thought believes this depletion (the extent of which remains controversial[70] since partial depletion may indeed be transitory and normal to earth's atmosphere) is more connected with immune alteration than any other single factor.

The third, and now more historic, holds that radiation (both known and unknown, or "occult"), disturbances in electromagnetic fields and related phenomena, are primary suspects in immune dysregulation, since such energy alterations at the subcellular level (*XV*) are subtle and probably cumulative.

Since the vast amount of severe immune dysregulation occurs in more civilized nations — yet the ozone depletion effect should be planet-wide — it would seem that the chemical toxicity/ radiation views are more consistent for most expressions of immune damage among humans. Chemicalization as well as presumptive damage from ozone depletion may also account for increased evidence in the 1990s of immunological disturbances among the higher animals, some of whose species are indeed threatened by the expansion of human civilization.

As we note in *XIV*, depletion from soils of vital minerals is playing an undoubted role in mineral-deficient states in Western countries. The composite effects of reduced oxygen concentration (by some estimates down from 38 percent to 22 percent in the atmosphere since the 1940s and even lower in urban complexes[71]) are difficult to estimate, but oxygen deprivation theoretically should favor the existence of *anaerobic* life — as in cancer.

Certain medical mavericks, such as Canada's embattled Dr. Charles Reich, suggest that dietary deficiencies in calcium and Vitamin D, exacerbated by body coverings of people in cold climates (clothing as a block to already-diminished sunlight) may be major contributors to establishing a foundation for chronic disease.[72]

Whatever the root causes, mankind in general and Western man in particular may truly be reaching the end of his ecological/biological tether — unless he acts responsibly and intelligently, and the sooner the better.

Sentinels of calamity

This writer was not particularly popular in Iceland when, in 1993, examining the spiralling rates of cancer, CFS and general immune dysregulation in a tiny population 1/10th of 1 percent that of the United States — rates which are roughly the same as those in the USA, with its far greater population cushion — he warned that Western civilization faces extinction at the hands of civilization itself.[73]

In fact, civilized Iceland, far to the north; and civilized New Zealand, far to the south, with a larger but still small population; and, to some extent Australia, may be considered "sentinel countries" for the extinction or survival of the Western gene pool — and, by implication, of mankind itself.

In all Western countries, rates of chronic, metabolic disorders and immunological dysregulations match and occasionally bypass those of the United States and represent a palpable threat to the population. Complexing this situation with the rapid development of antibiotic-resistant bacteria and the presence of "new" viruses, the threat becomes one of possible extinction.

In a grim kind of way, I was intellectually satisfied to realize, following my 1993 appearances in Iceland and Canada warning of imminent catastrophe, that I was a Johnny-come-lately.

In 1982, the aforementioned combative Canadian physician/researcher Carl Reich MD, upon whom medical authorities there have not always looked kindly, wrote prophetically in an Australian "alternative medicine" magazine:

> *Two hundred years ago, while the human knew starvation and infection, the human organism was exposed to no pollution (or) drugs but the smoke of wood fires and the rare use of tranquilizing or hallucinating drugs. In contrast, in recent decades, the human has been veritably steeped in an environment which contains thousands of synthesized chemical substances . . . Most of these . . . were never present in the world prior to this decade . . . (and) are entirely foreign to the human organism.*
>
> *That the human organism has survived so well in the face of this chemical onslaught is testimony to the tremendous adaptive potential inherent in an organism that has slowly evolved over a long period of time . . . There must be a limit to this adaptive potential of the human organism, however, and I regret to suggest that the human race may soon be approaching such a limit of its adaptive potential. Once this adaptive potential of the human organism has been exceeded, one may expect that various of these adaptive physiological mechanisms may break down.*
>
> *Adaptive mechanisms, which may now be proceeding asymptomatically but which are being taxed, may therefore break down at some future date* to create disease states which are currently unknown to the human body.(Emphasis mine.)

For reason of this hazard of chemical agents, I warn the public that they not only take a new look at their chemically laden environment and chemically laden diet but that they also take a new look at the modern [medical] profession, the aim of which is to provide them with health largely by chemical means.[74]

These musings by a fiercely independent medical thinker, it must be stressed, were printed only one year into the AIDS epidemic and well before the elucidation of most of the SID-connected calamities now plaguing the Western world. Dr. Reich learned, as have so many pioneers who dared to go against the grain, that a prophet is without honor in his own country.

The holistic challenge

For the holistically inclined, it is unlikely that there is a single cause of CFS, AIDS or the full spectrum of a Syndrome of Immune Dysregulation, but even if there is, the challenge to research is the same: determining why some individuals remain essentially healthy, while others become gravely ill or even die. This holistic concern supersedes allopathic obsessions with single causes, however much viruses (new or old), uncontrolled parasites, bacteria, mycoplasmas and other elements may be involved.

The restored holistic paradigm for the 21st century is focused less on causes than on the elaboration of individualized, multifactorial treatment regimens (protocols) which already have become the only rational, workable approaches to AIDS, CFS and what lies between.

The challenge of immune dysregulation is that of human survival itself: SID is evidence of the imbalances man has largely brought about within himself and on his planet. Enmeshed with the devastation of cancer, SID represents what may be the final physiological challenge to the survival of the species itself.

In the spirit of dualism, the cancer-SID menace — threatening, as it does, the whole of the human species —

represents at the same time challenge and opportunity.

References

1. Reuters, March 7, 1994.
2. World Health Organization, January 1994.
2a. The Associated Press, Aug. 9, 1994.
2b. World Health Organization, January 1995.
3. The Associated Press, March 11, 1994.
4. Dept. of Health and Human Services, January 1994.
5. "Pneumocystis pneumonia-Los Angeles," Centers for Disease Control, *Morib. Mortal. Weekly Report* 30, 1981.
6. Culbert, ML, AIDS: *Hope, Hoax and Hoopla*. Chula Vista CA: Bradford Foundation, 1989, 1990.
6a. Moskowitz, LB, *et al.*, "Frequency and anatomic distribution of lymphadenopathic Kaposi's sarcoma in the acquired immunodeficiency syndrome: an autopsy series." *Hum. Pathol.* 16, 1985.
6b. Yuan Chang, *et al.*, "Identification of herpesvirus-like DNA sequences in AIDS-associated Kaposi's sarcoma." *Science*, Dec. 16, 1994.
7. Sepkoviz, KA, *J. Am. Med. Assn.* Feb. 12, 1992.
8. Papadopoulos-Eleopulos, Eleni, *et al.*, "Is a positive Western blot proof of HIV infection?" *Bio/Technology* 11, June 11, 1993.
9. Kashala, Oscar, *et al.*, "Infection with human immunodeficiency virus type I (HIV-1) and human T cell lymphotropic viruses among leprosy patients and contacts: correlation between HIV-1 cross-reactivity and antibodies to lipoarabinomanan." *J. Infect. Dis.* 169, 1994.
10. Clerici, Mario, *et al.*, "HIV-specific T-helper activity in seronegative health care workers exposed to contaminated blood." *J. Am. Med. Assn.*, Jan. 5, 1994.
11. Levy, JA, "Human immunodeficiency viruses and the pathogenesis of AIDS." *J. Am. Med. Assn.*, May 26, 1989.
12. Horton, Richard, "'Renegade' HIV immunity hypothesis gains momentum." *Lancet* 342; Dec. 18/25, 1993.
13. Haney, DQ, The Associated Press, Jan. 30, 1994.
14. *Brit. Med. J.* and Reuters, March 25, 1994.
15. Peter Duesberg interview, *Spin*, September 1993.
16. Duesberg, PH, "Human immunodeficiency virus and acquired immunodeficiency syndrome: correlation but not causation." *Proc. Natl. Acad. Sci.*: 86, February 1989.
16a. Duesberg, PH, "Retroviruses as carcinogens and pathogens: expectations and reality." *Cancer Res.* 47, March 1, 1987.
17. Duesberg, PH, "HIV is not the cause of AIDS." *Science* 241, July 20, 1988.
18. Miller, Jeff, "AIDS heresy." *Discover*. June 1988.
19. Root-Bernstein, Robert, *Rethinking, AIDS: The Tragic Cost of Premature Consensus*. New York: The Free Press, 1993.
20. Culbert, ML, *AIDS: Terror, Truth, Triumph*. Chula Vista CA: Bradford Foundation, 1986.
21. Culbert, ML: *AIDS: Hope, Hoax and Hoopla*. Chula Vista CA: Bradford Foundation, 1989, 1990.
22. Sonnabend, JA, *et al.*, "A multifactorial model for the development of AIDS in homosexual men." *Ann. NY Acad. Sci. V*, 1984.
23. Lo, S-C et al., "Identification of mycoplasma incognitus infection in patients with AIDS: an immunohistochemical, in situ hybridization and ultrastructural study." *Am. J. Trop. Med. Hyg.*, November 1989.
24. Lo, S-C *et al.*, "Fatal infection of silvered leaf monkeys with a virus-like infectious agent (VLIA) derived from a patient with AIDS." *Am. T. Trop. Med. Hyg.*, April 1989.
24a. Barnett, SW, *et al.*, "An AIDS-like condition induced in baboons by HIV-2." *Science*, Oct. 28, 1994.
24b. "Baboons with AIDS spur hopes for tests." (Reuters), *San Diego Union*. Oct. 28, 1994.
24c. *USA Today*, cited in *The Choice*, XX: 2-3, 1994.
25. Konotey-Ahulu, FJ, "AIDS in Africa: misinformation and disinformation." *Lancet*, July 24, 1987.
26. Lauritsen, John, *The AIDS War: Propaganda, Profiteering and Genocide from the Medical-Industrial Complex*. New York: Pagan Press, 1993.
26a. Dondero, TJ, and Curran, JW, "Excess deaths in Africa from HIV: confirmed and quantified." *Lancet*, April 23, 1994.
26b. Mulder, DW, *et al.*, "Two-year HIV-1-associated mortality in a Ugandan rural population." *Lancet*, April 23, 1994.
26c. Vigniel, Corinne, Reuters, Dec. 12, 1994.
27. Kashala, *op. cit.*
28. Papadopoulos-Eleopulus, *op. cit.*
29. Purvis, Andrew, "Cursed, yet blessed." *Time*, Dec. 6, 1993.
29a. Rowland-Jones, Sarah, *et al.*, *Nature Medicine*, January 1995.
30. *Philippines Star*, Feb. 23, 1994.
31. "AIDS: the third wave." *Lancet*, Jan. 22, 1994.
31a. Cohen, Jon, "The epidemic in Thailand." *Science*, Dec. 9, 1994.
32. *Manila Bulletin*, Feb. 21, 1994, and author interviews with Philippine health officials.
33. Culbert, *AIDS: Hope, . . ., op. cit.*
33a. Willner, RE, *Deadly Deception*. Peltec Publishing, 1994.
34. Lusso, Paolo, *et al.*, "Infection of natural killer cells by human herpesvirus 6." *Nature*, April 1, 1993.

excess ROTS or free radicals. Western diets are laden with "oxidized" fats and inadequate amounts of antioxidants.

— The implication that oxidative mechanisms are involved throughout the full spectrum of disease has become stronger each passing year. The Bradford Research Institutes (BRI) did ground-breaking research in this area, establishing the "ROTS theory of health and disease" as well as developing a specialized test and microscopy system to examine metabolic products in coagulated blood to detect oxidative stresses and reactions in the body.[43]

— Increased interest in the use of o*xidants* (that is, purveyors of atomic oxygen, such as hydrogen peroxide, ozone gas, Dioxychlor and similar products) and even hyperbaric oxygenation, as acting *similarly* to free radicals as a way to assault key elements of the infective process: cell wall-deficient microscopic and submicroscopic structures (viruses, retroviruses, some bacteria, mycoplasmas, yeasts and parasites). The rediscovery of the effective use of oxidative agents against a broad spectrum of pathogens has led both to new therapeutics and new controversies, particularly over the utility and/or overuse of hydrogen peroxide.[44]

By 1994, the usefulness of many of the common supplements in their roles as antioxidants was too overwhelming to be debated by serious people:

A non-profit public-interest group called the Alliance for Aging Research called for both FDA and Congressional action to speed the approval process for nutritional health claims and urged Americans to add antioxidants to their diets at levels far above those recommended by the government.

The media noted that the recommendations were based on information from more than 200 studies over the prior 20 years.

Said Jeffrey Blumberg, professor of nutrition and associate director of the USDA Human Nutrition Research Center on Aging, Tufts University:

We don't have the kind of definitive, unequivocal evidence that some people are calling for, namely the medical evidence required for the approval of new drugs. But is that the right standard when we're talking about vitamins that we have decades and decades of information on? These are not some new chemical(s) that the body has never seen before. These are things that have been in the diet since prehistoric man.[45]

He was essentially talking about Vitamins C, E and beta-carotene — which the surge of new information was already considering, along with (interestingly enough) aspirin, as blockers of "heart disease," stroke and cancer.

The call for governmental approval of higher levels of natural antioxidants was accompanied by research on fruit flies reported in *Science* which stressed (as earlier studies had suggested) that free radicals are prime causes of the aging process and that neutralizing excess free radicals or ROTS prolongs life.

Drs. Rajindar Sohal and William Orr claimed that by providing fruit flies extra copies of genes which protect against free radicals the flies' lives were extended by 30 percent.[46]

The fruit fly studies (and laboratory tests on sub-mammalian species need always to be viewed with a touch of skepticism as to relevance) were simply more precise definitions of research conducted in large (human) population-based studies which, as it was abstracted in 1994, "reported reductions as high as 40 percent in coronary artery disease among people taking antioxidants, and some clinical studies have produced similar results."[47]

The Club co-opts

It is instructive to note that even as both public and private research exploded in the 1980s and 1990s tracing the connections between dietary factors and nutrients to health and disease, the hard core of the AIC had a significant problem in how to integrate the rapidly onrushing new information with the established medical model and the pharmaceutical hydra which suckled it.

For, as Dean Burk PhD had observed in the matter of laetrile, once a chink in the armor of orthodoxy had appeared, it would widen: the aphorism that "that which prevents, also cures" would not be lost on rank-and-file physicians facing a tidal wave of chronic, systemic, metabolic dysfunctions and immune challenges for which the allopathic armamentarium offered little in the way of cures. The spectre of *disease prevention* through nutritional changes (and lifestyle alterations) loomed, and with it the implied threat to the need for a gigantic AIC and the international drug cartel which nourished and sustained it. How work the new knowledge into the old system?

The AIC turned to co-optation and semantical manipulation, its long-time *modus operandi* in dealing with inexorable forces.

Bowing to the growing evidence that nutritional supplements and nutrients themselves might indeed play a role in thwarting disease, yet not wanting to turn loose of the medical lexicon which protected old ideas, the AIC or Club concocted the word "chemoprevention" — as hilarious a co-optation as we had seen in decades of doctor-watching. "Chemo" retains the *chemical* nature of medicine (as in toxic *chemo*therapy, a rapidly failing cancer therapeutic approach) but adds on "prevention" — so that the subliminal phrase "chemicals used to prevent" might flourish in the psyche.[48]

As we noted, the drug industry, whose $65 billion gravy train (as of 1994) was substantially threatened by the $4 billion a year industry in food supplements, swiftly sought to accommodate unwanted new information while grabbing a share of a swiftly developing pie — so that major drug companies, by the late 1980s, increased their line of vitamin/mineral supplements, basing the same on random establishment research on animals which seemed to "suggest" that such supplements could, for example, positively impact on immunity.

This was, of course, rank heresy to the allopathic thinking of recent decades, but did underscore the genius of the marketplace: despite "quackbuster" attacks on vitamin pills, the people were going to have their pills, so why should the drug giants be left off the bandwagon even while running a distant risk that adequate supplementation might ultimately hinder the need for many, if not most, of the expensive medications in which the pharmaceutical market was awash?

The research establishment, still allopathic in tone, almost always accompanied every new disclosure of a nutrient being found successful against a disease or a condition with a "cautionary note," usually from an appropriately allopathic medical school researcher at a major university or within the federal research community, warning against "pill-popping" or simply taking supplements on a routine basis.

The pill-popping medics

But by the early 1990s, even this ploy was beginning to fail — many doctors, some of them originally anti-vitamin, were gobbling vitamin pills and admitting it.

Even by 1990, a survey showed[49] that an amazing 87 percent of family practitioners were recommending or prescribing vitamin and mineral supplements to some 25 percent of their patients, and that 28 percent of the medics were taking the food supplements themselves. And, as a "quackbuster" journal reported,[50] citing the American Dietetic Association, of a group of cancer patients studied, 92 percent of the women and 63 percent of the men admitted that, whatever other therapy they were on, they were taking vitamin supplements.

In 1993, the *Wall Street Journal* quoted an octogenarian nutrition expert and professor emeritus of the University of St. Louis School of Medicine, who was said to regularly rail about "the over-feeding of vitamins" to Americans but who was taking Vitamin E himself: "I'm ashamed to do it because of my attitude toward taking vitamins," he said, as he honestly admitted the explosion of studies on the vitamin's positive effects could no longer be overlooked.[51] (The *WSJ* reported that just in an initial three-month period ending Feb. 28 of that year, Vitamin E sales had totalled $27 million, up 31 percent from 1992).

Two major studies in the *New England Journal of Medicine (NEJM)* in May 1993 made the case for a significant reduction in the risk of coronary heart disease with Vitamin E (Shute brothers vindicated at long last), yet the reports were coupled with the usual admonition that the general public should not start dosing themselves with Vitamin E pills. Angry doctors balked.[52]

Wrote Dr. James O'Keefe, Kansas City MO:

A substantial number of physicians . . . are sufficiently convinced of the potential benefits and nontoxic nature of Vitamin E to supplement their own diets with it. If Vitamin E is good enough for doctors, should it not be good enough for our patients?[53]

In 1993 *USA Today* reported galloping increases in profits from the sales of Vitamins E, C and beta-carotene — antioxidants all and the subjects of intense public/private investigation — and it noted that Dr. Walter Willett, Harvard School of Public Health, was taking one multivitamin tablet and one Vitamin E capsule a day, while relying on food for Vitamin C and beta-carotene.

It quoted antioxidant expert Jeffrey Blumberg of Tufts: "We're at an admittedly frustrating stage, where I think one well-informed, rational person would decide to take a supplement, and the other could decide not to."[54]

This was a hedging-of-all-bets assessment made in the midst of the continuing outpouring of new information, and certainly an honest viewpoint.

Cancer Inc. does an about-face

By 1992, in what was the biggest shift of its gears in a decade or more, the American Cancer Society (ACS), for prior decades an impassioned foe of the notion that diet had much to do, if anything, with cancer, announced the start of a mammoth survey of middle-aged American dietary habits. It was launched just as the governmental National Cancer Institute (NCI) released results of *156* studies which linked cancer with diet — a sweeping review which forever ended any debate about whether nutritional factors have at least a role in the malignant process.[55] [*XI*]

Gladys Block, University of California-Berkeley School of Public Health and lead author of the study/survey, found "extraordinarily consistent scientific evidence" of dietary connections though the survey did not pinpoint a single vitamin or food factor as the Holy Grail of cancer prevention.

Virtually all the 156 studies confirmed the connection between eating more fruits and vegetables and lower cancer rates.

Peter Greenwald, chief of the NCI's cancer prevention and control branch, said the findings constituted part of the basis for the agency's recent recommendation that everyone eat five servings a day of fruits or vegetables.[56]

The survey was "so compelling," said analysts, that it meant that even cigarette smokers who also ate large amounts of fruits and vegetables derived major anti-lung cancer benefits.

The same year, the largest and most detailed study ever carried out to measure the effects of Vitamin C and death rates concluded[57] that the vitamin helps both sexes live longer — but only if taken in amounts far above those recommended by the federal government.

Among findings, reported Dr. James E. Enstrom:

Men whose Vitamin C intake was the highest — the equivalent of two oranges plus a 150-milligram Vitamin C tablet per day — had a 42 percent lower risk of death from heart disease and a 35 percent lower risk of death from any cause than the population of white men as a whole.

In continuing mixed-results research in 1993, a *New England Journal of Medicine (NEJM)* study of 89,494 nurses tracked over a nine-year period beginning in 1980 showed[50] that the consumption of foods rich in Vitamin A (particularly spinach and carrots) seemed to reduce the risk of breast cancer.

It was only one of many studies trying to get to grips with a pandemic which even by that year was killing 46,000 women per year and affecting 1 out of 9. Scattered research was indicating connections between breast cancer and a high-fat diet — though it should be noted that in the "unitarian" theory of cancer (it is a single disease) connections between excess fats and excess animal proteins in *general* seem to correlate with cancer as a whole.

Victory for the concept that the better-known vitamins and minerals might after all be truly connected with health and disease opened the door to the examination of many other food factors (as indoles, flavones, and phenols in cancer) and, much to the consternation of the "quackbuster" elite, to a reexamination of the role of herbs and their components.

The dam bursts

What was largely the province of folk medicine and alleged unabashed quackery in North America increasingly came under scientifically acceptable scrutiny: useful ingredients were found in garlic and chaparral, among many others, which vindicated the empiricism of the use of these herbs over centuries. The rediscovery by the West of ancient Chinese herbalism, and the plodding efforts of America's embattled naturopaths, brought to the fore some "scientifically" acceptable rationales for everything from spirulina, blue-green algae and wheat grass to aloe vera, herbal teas of all kinds, and such folkloric herbal war-horses as echinacea and goldenseal.

By the mid-1990s, research with and interest in herbs and their multitudinous compounds was growing as fast as the concepts of oxidology and multivitamin therapy — a dam had burst whose floodwaters would not be stanched by the AIC, whose major concern going into the end of the century is how to co-opt the research and provide synthetic look-alikes of natural products in order to enhance profits. Mimicry is, after all, the highest form of flattery.

As the plague of AIDS reached terrifying dimensions in the

1990s, and as other immunological disturbances became apparent, it was part of the standard allopathic "line" that while a healthy immune system was the best defense against such modern killers and cripplers, there was no known way to "enhance" immunity other than through the mixed results and often dangerous administration of synthetic interferons and interleukins.

Yet "metabolic" or "holistic" medical practitioners had long argued that overall host defense — including all aspects of what is meant by the misleading general term "immune system" — could indeed be increased or modulated through nutrition and dietary supplements, however "quackish" such an idea seemed to the AIC.

And as we have seen, as late as 1988 even the *Harvard Medical School Health Letter* was deriding the claim that nutritional factors could bolster immunity as "simply not supportable" and that

[T]he use of herbs or nutrition to stimulate or strengthen the immune system is a nonsense claim . . . and to the extent that people wind up believing such claims, we can say that their brains are damaged.[59]

This typically arrogant AIC point of view came acropper in 1992, though, when *The Lancet* reported research by Dr. Rajit K. Chandra, School of Hygiene and Public Health, Johns Hopkins, on the "effect of vitamin and trace-element supplementation on immune response and infection in elderly subjects."

In this study, it became obvious that even "modest" vitamin and trace-element supplementation positively affected the "immune systems" of the elderly and that the herb ginkgo biloba (extract from the leaf of the maidenhair tree) positively helped in cases of "mild to moderate symptoms of cerebral insufficiency."

Results were said to be "impressive" in immune enhancement even with admittedly "modest" doses of Vitamin A, beta-carotene, thiamine, riboflavin, niacin, Vitamins B6 and B12, Vitamin C, Vitamin D, iron, zinc, copper, selenium, iodine, calcium and magnesium.

Conclusion: "Supplementation with a modest physiological amount of micronutrients improves immunity and decreases the risk of infection in old age."[60]

By that time, of course, thousands of AIDS and pre-AIDS patients, often supported in their efforts by well-meaning, if incredulous, MDs, were finding that supplementation with a huge array of vitamins, minerals, enzymes, amino acids, herbs and other substances conclusively or suggestively linked to "non-specific immune enhancement" were seeing immune system improvements and life extension.

While attention was now given to many other factors of civilization and how they might be aiding or abetting the end-of-century plagues of cancer, AIDS and immune dysregulation (see *XI* and *XIII*), the killer diseases, by emphasizing the reality of dietary connections to health and disease, had helped correct medicine's major error, abandonment of the holistic concept.

More than any other maladies, cancer and AIDS — examples of near to total disaster on the part of the AIC — have provoked new thought and a paradigm shift to the holistic concept. And within this framework, eating habits and dietary elements play the primary *physical* roles.

The popular revolt against orthodoxy and pressure for paradigm shift *within* orthodoxy also point to a probable fail-safe mechanism within the human makeup: since survival of the species is the first and primary mandate of its existence, the species will creatively find ways to survive despite the challenges before it — and despite the entrenched bureaucracies and economic/ego vested interests which are in the way.

References

1. *The Choice*, XVIII:3, 1992. Also, Committee for Freedom of Choice in Medicine Inc. statement to National Institutes of Health, June 2, 1992.
2. *New England Journal of Medicine*, Jan. 28, 1993.
3. *The Choice* XIX:1, 1993.
4. Sampson, WI, "AIDS: frauds, finances and fringes." *New York State J. Med.*, February 1993.
5. Statement of US Council on Pharmacy and Chemistry, *J. Am. Med. Assn.*, Jan. 8, 1949.
6. *The Choice*, II:1, 1976.
7. Shute, WE, *Wilfrid Shute's Complete Updated Vitamin E Book*. New Canaan CT: Keats, 1975.
8. Wallach, JD, "The NBA: an endangered species?" Private publication; also printed in *The Choice*, XIX: 3-4, 1993.
9. Wallach, JD, address to annual convention, American Naturopathic Medical Assn. (ANMA), Albuquerque NM,

	1993.
10.	"Hard facts about chemically dependent farming." *Health Foods Business.* July 1991.
10a.	Wiles, Richard, *et al., Tap Water Blues: Herbicides in Drinking Water.* Washington DC: Environmental Working Group/Physicians for Social Responsibility, 1994.
10b.	Culbert, ML, *AIDS: Hope, Hoax and Hoopla.* Chula Vista CA: The Bradford Foundation, 1990.
10c.	Culbert, ML *CFS: Conquering the Crippler.* San Diego CA: C & C Communications, 1993.
11.	*Ibid.*
11a.	"After Silent Spring," Natural Resources Defense Council, June 1993.
11b.	Goldin, Greg, "Cancerous Growth." *LA Weekly,* May 6, 1994.
11c.	"The theft of the ark." *Seeds of Change* Catalogue, 1994.
11d-11f.	*Ibid.*
12.	"Hard facts," *op. cit.*
13.	Kesteloot, Hugo, in *J. Cardiol. and Pharm.* 6: 1984.
14.	*J. Food Quality* 9: 1987.
15.	*The Choice,* XIX:1, 1993.
16.	Harper, H, and Culbert, M, *How You Can Beat the Killer Diseases.* New Rochelle NY: Arlington House, 1977.
17.	Brennan, RO, *Nutrigenetics.* New York: M. Evans, 1975.
18.	McGee, CT, *Heart Frauds.* Coeur d'Alene ID: MediPress, 1993.
19.	Fredericks, Carlton, *Low Blood Sugar and You.* New York: Constellation International, 1974.
20.	Yudkin, John, *Sweet and Dangerous.* New York: Bantam, 1972.
21.	Culbert, ML, *What the Medical Establishment Won't Tell You that Could Save Your Life.* Norfolk VA: Donning, 1983.
22.	Cited in *The Choice,* XVI:2,3, 1990.
23.	Culbert, *What the, op. cit.*
23a.	Palma, Dick, Knight-Ridder News Service, June 18, 1994.
24.	McGee, *op. cit.*
25.	Price, Weston, *Nutrition and Physical Degeneration.* Santa Monica CA: Price Pottenger Foundation, 1945.
26.	Cleave, TL, *The Saccharine Disease.* New Canaan CT: Keats, 1974.
27.	Culbert, *What the, op. cit.*
28.	*Ibid.*
29.	McGee, *op. cit.*
30.	Culbert, *What the, op. cit.*
31.	*Feeding at the Company Trough.* Washington DC: Center for Science in the Public Interest, 1976.
32.	Culbert, *What the, op. cit.*
33.	Culbert ML: *AIDS: op. cit.*
34.	Culbert, ML: *CFS: op. cit.*
35.	The Associated Press, May 16, 1994.
36.	Rath, Matthias, *Eradicating Heart Disease.* San Francisco CA: Health Now, 1993.
37.	Beisel, WR, "The history of nutritional immunology." *J. Nutr. Immun.,* I:1, 1992.
38.	Roe, DA, *Drug-Induced Nutritional Deficiencies.* Westport CT: Avi Publishing, 1976.
39.	Bradford, RW, *et al., Oxidology: The Study of Reactive Oxygen Toxic Species (ROTS) and Their Metabolism in Health and Disease.* Los Altos CA: The Bradford Foundation, 1985.
39a.	Cerutti, PA, "Oxy-radicals and cancer." *Lancet,* Sept. 24, 1994.
40.	McGee, *op. cit.*
41.	Cathcart, RK, *et al., J. Leukocyte Biol.,* 38, 1985.
41a.	Witztum, JL, "The oxidation hypothesis of atherosclerosis." *Lancet,* Sept. 17, 1994.
42.	Jenner, P, "Oxidative damage in neurodegenerative disease." *Lancet,* Sept. 17, 1994.
42a.	Grisham, MB, "Oxidants and free radicals in inflammatory bowel disease." *Lancet,* Sept. 24, 1994.
43.	Bradford, *op. cit.*
44.	Bradford, RW, *Hydrogen Peroxide: The Misunderstood Oxidant.* Chula Vista CA: Bradford Research Institutes, 1987.
45.	McVicar, Nancy, "Vitamins against aging, disease." *Orange County Register,* Mar. 22, 1994.
46.	Sohal, Rajindar, *et al., Science,* Feb. 25, 1994.
47.	McVicar, *loc. cit.*
48.	*Science,* August 1991.
49.	*The Choice,* XVI:4, 1991.
50.	*Ibid.*
51.	Cited in *The Choice,* XIX:2, 1993.
52.	*Ibid.*
53.	McVicar, *loc. cit.*
54.	*USA Today,* June 2, 1993.
55.	*The Choice,* XVIII:3, 1992.
56.	*Ibid.*
57.	Enstrom, JE, *Epidemiology,* May 1992.
58.	*The Choice,* XIX:2, 1993.
59.	Cited in *The Choice,* XV:1,2, 1989.
60.	Chandra, RK, "Effect of vitamin and trace-element supplementation on immune response and infection in elderly subjects." *Lancet,* Nov. 7, 1992.

XV
TOWARD THE MEDICINE OF THE 21ST CENTURY:
A new paradigm in healing emerges

"All healing is magic. The Indian healer and the western healer have a common denominator — the trust and confidence of both the patient and the healer. They must both believe in the magic or it doesn't work. Western doctors make secret markings on paper and instruct the patient to give it to the oracle in the drug store [and] make an offering in return for which they will receive a magic potion."

— **Irving Oyle DO**

"I don't know what you learned from books, but the most important thing I learned from my grandfathers was that there is a part of the mind that we don't really know about and that it is that part that is most important in whether we become sick or remain well."

— **Navajo medicine man Thomas Largewhiskers**
(in *Imagery and Healing*)

"... Psychoimmunology ... will become a vitally important clinical field — perhaps the most important field in the 21st century — supplanting our present emphasis on oncology and cardiology. Healthy thinking may eventually become an integral aspect of treatment for everything from allergies to liver transplants. What all this means is that our present concept of medicine will disappear ... Medicine will change its focus from treatment to enhancement, from repair to improvement, from diminished sickness to increased performance."

— **Michael Crichton MD**

"... Regular medicine ... likes to call itself scientific and imagines that its exclusive attention to the physical reality of bodily mechanisms is in the best spirit of twentieth-century science. What most medical doctors do not know is that the scientific model of reality has changed radically since 1900 and no longer views the universe as an orderly mechanism independent of the consciousness viewing it."

— **Andrew Weil MD** (in *Health and Healing*)

". . . From a fundamental physics viewpoint, it's just about all electromagnetics anyway, at the most fundamental level. But the quantum physicists are . . . totally unaware that the physical structure, genetics, biochemistry, etc., of the living cell can in fact be directly engineered with the strange 'new' kind of electromagnetics."

— **Nuclear engineer Thomas Bearden, Lt. Col. USA (Ret.)**

New Medicine — or extinction

Hurtling toward the end of the century, the Allopathic Industrial Complex (AIC), educationally and philosophically enshrined in the AMA, is faced with its gravest of challenges: apparent inability to stave off the looming extinction of the human species.

Reminiscent of Hitler hallucinating in the bunker toward the end of World War II and still imagining that new weapons breakthroughs and nonexistent troops would somehow rescue the Third Reich at the last minute, the AIC is counting on biotechnology to save the day.

Perhaps it will — and certainly genetics and all it implies will be part of the medicine of the future — but at the present time there is little of merit in hoping the AIC will fend off the combination plagues of new and old — cancer, AIDS, immune dysregulation in the West, infections and parasites in the Third World (and the spiraling levels of antibiotic-resistant bacteria everywhere).

But because the prime directive of human biology seems to be one and one only — survival — and because *Homo sapiens* is nothing if not supremely clever when faced with extinction, as it now is, there logically is room for optimism.

Part of our species' survival is intimately involved with the rise of a new paradigm in healing — the New Medicine — which is developing as a collective mandate as the old structure dies, however brontosaurian its death throes may be.

Thomas Alva Edison was, as usual, ahead of his time with the prophetic and oft-quoted observation that "the doctor of the future will give no medicine but will interest his patients in the cure of the human frame, in diet, and in the cause and prevention of disease."

He was, after all, paraphrasing the ancients and, to some extent, Paracelsus.

His view foreshadowed by a century the disaster of the standard medical model which is now evident.

The primary medical concept of the 21st century must be

promotive health, rather — even — than preventive medicine. For the promotion of health relegates medicine to a secondary position and implies that the individual rather than the physician or the state will take upon himself the primary responsibility for what many now call "wellness."

Yet, assuming a role for medicine as long as the species exists, the new medical paradigm must be holistic and integrative — a return to the original mind/body/spirit concept of the ancients accompanied by the technological advances of our times.

The New Medicine should be a union of the composite experience of the past fused with the technology of the present — it should take from the best of all worlds (allopathy, homeopathy, naturopathy, meditation, energy medicine, etc.)

True, an integrative holistic model is revolutionary and necessarily will ruffle many feathers — those who believe that all that is natural is good and all that is manmade or synthetic bad, that there are no good drugs of any kind and that all invasive procedures are violations of the temple always to be avoided, will not enjoy making common cause with allopaths; and diehard allopaths, long trained to perceive the back-to-nature musings of the opposition as quaint at best, charlatanry of a high order at worst, will be loath to join forces with those who believe natural therapies and even attitude changes are superior to drugs and surgery.

Yet both extremes will be missing the point: it is what "works" that counts, what is best for healing to occur. No single school of medical thought has a monopoly on this.

Such integrative models are already developing. They were referred to at the precedent-setting meetings in 1992 which led to the formation of the Office of Alternative Medicine (OAM) within the allopathy-enshrining National Institutes of Health (NIH) and in which I was pleased to play a modest role.

Among attention-getting comments then were those which came from Dr. Majid Ali, a Columbia pathologist who also uses nutrition and fitness programs in environmental therapy.

Tackling the question of how the outmoded standard or allopathic model could possibly be used to evaluate multifactorial therapies against the modern disease calamities, particularly when individualized for the patient, the gifted practitioner/author said:

". . . We are incarcerated in the double-blind, crossover model. It is not appropriate for holistic therapy, in which there are many variables and neither the practitioner nor the patient can be blinded to the treatment."[1]

In these impressive gatherings of proponents of all forms of medicine, ranging from diehard allopaths to Indian tribal medicine men, from promoters of Ayurvedic medicine to chiropractors, from homeopaths to naturopaths, and from well-credentialed researchers who dabbled in all medical areas, several were in agreement about the need for a new evaluative medical parameter to be able to measure the efficacy of multi-variable therapies:

End results — i.e., "outcomes."

The only real way to assess the efficacy or lack thereof of multifactorial treatment models (protocols) is indeed the final result — how long did the patient live and in what state of health? That is, after all, the true stuff of medicine, not a workout in "science".

Establishment of a new evaluative model is a primary challenge for the New Medicine, and it will surely be met.

Genetics as a last gasp

The allopathic paradigm (treatments by contraries, single causes of disease states) is still in power and is the dominant philosophical force behind medicine's high technology. It still is producing a last, dramatic gasp.

Just as, in centuries past, the allopathic mindset placed emphasis on surgery, bleedings, purgings, and intoxications; and, in generations past, it relied upon the microbial theory of disease causation, leading to its brightest moments; and, within the past decades, it refined the latter down to the viral theory of disease as the seeming end-all of therapeutic experience, it has come up with its final card:

Genetics.

If in fact, after all, burning or poisoning out the bad humours was mostly in error and even if defining much of disease as the work of devilishly clever, invisible, not-really-alive particles (viruses) has turned up few real advances, then genes — "smaller," even, "more invisible" than, viruses — must hold the clue.

The American commitment to high technology — carrying with it an almost myopic embrace of not only not seeing the forest for the trees but actually being blinded by leaves and stems — will be part of the medicine of the Twenty-First Century and will provide useful areas of human understanding.

Most medical universalists, eclecticists and integrationists would no more deny the possible gains of genetic knowledge and its application to a new medical model than would an athlete question that performance is enhanced with a better athletic shoe.

But the reliance on genes as the over-arching, all-encompassing solution to medical problems is fraught with the same perils that have haunted all prior efforts at unilateral, linear thought: the snag is in the details and the exceptions.

By the mid-1990s, a veritable flurry of discoveries produced evidence of possible genetic "causes" for a growing number of diseases, including various "forms" of cancer. The deeper scientists probed into the stuff and nature of biology the more they dredged up those wonderful replicatory particles, genes, whose alteration or absence seemed to equate with diseases and to explain why some conditions seem to "run in families."

The road to medical Nirvana will not be paved with genes — but high tech's increasing interest in the invisible will ultimately force it into new understandings of reality which transcend medicine and biology.

The rediscovery that food (and the many elements of food) have something to do with health and disease — an idea as ancient as the holistic paradigm itself — has been the first major chink in the armor of the AIC. In less than two decades, medical practitioners who once obediently followed the AIC propaganda notion that what we eat has little to do with health and disease now agree that food is important — perhaps vital. The old medical aphorism which states that that which prevents also cures inexorably led to the idea that various nutritive factors not only prevent disease but can be used to manage and treat them. We have assigned a Marine Corps-like role to laetrile ("Vitamin B17") in helping stimulate this shift in concepts (*XII*).

As the new paradigm develops, simply at the physical level, certain approaches to health and disease quietly abandoned before or blatantly and at times ruthlessly suppressed are being looked at in a whole new light.

Oxygen therapy returns

One of these is oxygen therapy (or, more properly, oxidative therapy), whose resurgence has paralleled the gradual embrace by medical/pharmaceutical orthodoxy of its flip side — antioxidant (or "free radical") therapy. Both are pillars of what our own research group has styled *oxidology* (*XIV*).

The current medical era has witnessed what seems to be a "new" concept — the use of oxygen-based products (hydrogen peroxide, the endogenous oxidative agent par excellence; ozone gas; intermediate oxygen structures) as useful against disease primarily because of their ability to release atomic oxygen which in turn scavenges cell wall-deficient microscopic structures and thus constitutes a seemingly natural weapon against a host of viruses and microbes.

Claims for hydrogen peroxide and ozone have, like all other outside-the-pale procedures, varied from the sublime to the ridiculous, yet the persistence of what orthodoxy dismisses as "anecdotal evidence" for their use is so strong as not to be happenstance.

Yet there is little that is actually new here: as Elizabeth Baker has described[2] in a history of oxygen treatments, since the

the 20 to 40 animal and insect species which rely on it.[11c]

While industrial defenders of the chemicalization of the food supply tend to pooh-pooh such potential ecological disasters by painting a brave new world of better living through chemistry — as, of course, mandated by some kind of super-international governmental/corporative combine which already is germinating — they at least should pay glancing attention to Harvard biologist E.O. Wilson, who wrote:

Biological diversity is responsible for the maintenance of the world as we know it. This is the assembly of life that took a billion years to evolve. It has eaten the storms, folded them into its genes, and created the world that created us. It holds the world steady.[11d]

But such steadiness is now under undoubted threat by civilization — even if such threat should properly also be seen as an opportunity for civilization to work with, rather than against, nature.

Destruction of the planetary habitat is, however, only one of the major problems which threaten plant-based food as we know it — the international, corporative, transnational control over the ever-more-hybridized seed industry is the other.

Kevin Watkins, in a study by the Catholic Institute of International Relations (England), observing potential profits by transnationals from "intellectual property rights" accruing through patents on genetic mutations of seeds from crop materials selected and developed for ages by native farmers (who, one might think, should have first crack at any such profits), noted:

The main beneficiaries will be the core group of less than a dozen seed and pharmaceutical companies which control over 70 percent of the world seed trade.[11e]

Seeds of Change observed that:

In the last 20 years, more than a thousand

independent seed houses have been acquired by major chemical and pharmaceutical companies such as Monsanto, Lilly, Dow, International Chemical Industries (ICI), and Royal Dutch Shell. These corporations — the major players in synthetic fertilizers, pesticides and agricultural chemicals — view the seed acquisitions as vertical integration, from the gene to the bank. Today in Europe, the corporations have instituted the Common Catalog, which restricts the marketability of seeds to those that are patented or registered. As a result, three quarters of traditional European folk varieties are under threat. Biology does not favor centralization, and this corporate vector of concentration may well end in vertical disintegration of incomprehensible proportions.[11f]

So there are stark warnings concerning the chemicalized future of the food supply.

But, happily, there are counter measures already forming to at least broaden the dialogue. They range from the industrial production of hormone-less beef to the tidal wave of organic farming in general.

At least a little more attention is being paid to Sir Albert Howard, pioneer of "natural farming" earlier in the 20th century, one of the first voices raised against chemically-dependent farming methods. Such farming, he said, is

based on a complete misconception of plant nutrition. It is superficial and fundamentally unsound. It takes no account of the life of the soil . . . Artificial manures lead inevitably to artificial nutrition, artificial food, artificial animals and finally to artificial men and women.[12]

By some estimates, man's ancestors derived somewhere between a fourth to a third of their nutritional minerals from the water they drank. Modern research has found that populations which consume water rich in magnesium and calcium — minerals often lacking or severely depleted in modern man's polluted and/or tampered-with supply — have lower rates of cardiovascular disease, heart attack and high blood pressure.[13]

While industrial propagandists and "quackbusters" routinely sneer at the notion of "organically" grown (that is, naturally cultivated *without* synthetic chemicals) fruits and vegetables as being somehow healthier than the chemically-altered varieties, considerable observation over time, as well as competent research such as that at the universities of Maine and Vermont, have demonstrated the superiority of the organics. The latter research showed higher levels of beta-carotene, Vitamin C, magnesium and calcium in organically grown vegetables.[14]

Western civilization is hence increasingly confronted by interlocked problems involving food production methods: a considerable amount of water has been polluted as an offshoot of such methods, leading to decreased minerals; this depletion could be compensated for by nutrients in fruits and vegetables but they, too, are deficient due to commercial cultivation methods.

These are problems apart from the dangers to the water supply from fluoridation and chlorination and from the over-chemicalization through food processing of fruits, vegetables, fibers, grains and meats for storage, transportation and marketing.

The connections, thus, between dietary/nutritional/food elements (deficiencies, excesses, chemicalization) and health problems have accumulated over the years.

And, now, scandalously, it is clear that the US government knew early in the 1970s about such connections — and chose to cover them up.

Uncovering a coverup

It was not until 1993, and then thanks primarily to a health-freedoms group (Citizens for Health) that it could be reported that a long-suppressed US government report assessing $30 million worth of research had found — in 1971 — that the nation's major health problems were related to diet, that the solution to illness may often be found in nutrition, and that dietary improvement may defer or modify the course of many diseases.

The document, a US Department of Agriculture publication called *Human Nutrition Report No. 2, Benefits from Human Nutrition Research*, was a referenced, 129-page report, ostensibly suppressed by then Secretary of Agriculture Earl Butz at the behest of the food-processing industry.

Said CfH's executive director, Alexander Schauss, after the organization reprinted the "one copy which mysteriously missed confiscation and recently surfaced:"

The government has known for 21 years that such illnesses as heart disease, many types of cancers, and other serious degenerative diseases can be prevented by diet . . . It is inexcusable that they have kept this information from the public all these years.

Had this information been made available in 1971 we would have been ten years ahead of where we are today in our knowledge of the role nutrition [plays] in the prevention and treatment of disease. The loss of lives and suffering of two generations of citizens denied this information should go down in history as one of the greatest tragedies of modern medicine . . .[15]

Because the government destroyed copies of the 1971 document, it was not until the 1977 *Senate Select Committee on Nutrition and Human Needs, Diet Related to Killer Diseases* report that the public was made aware of the amount of supportive evidence of a role for diet in the prevention of disease.

Yet due to the destruction of the 1971 report, even the 1977 Senate committee was unaware of the wealth of evidence available from our own government agencies.

By then, more researchers were drawing links between excess chemicalized processed foods, excess animal fats and proteins, the enormous consumption of refined sugar in the USA and the Western world, and the ever-more-noticeable deficiencies in essential nutrients, ranging from Vitamin C to magnesium, selenium and other minerals.

A carbohydrate calamity

A former co-author of mine, the late Harold W. Harper MD, probably did as much as anyone to rivet national attention on the refined sugar problem, arguing that the excess of refined sugars and starches (carbohydrates) in the civilized Western diet was, above and beyond all other problems with the food supply, the fundamental basis — as the cause of glucose metabolism dysfunction (GMD) — of much chronic, metabolic disease.[16]

His arguments, echoed by other researchers and current investigators[17,18,19,20], were that refined carbohydrates, particularly refined sucrose, act as "metabolic thieves" in depleting the body's store of B vitamins and other nutrients. GMD led ineluctably to hypoglycemia, a condition possibly affecting a majority of Americans, and over time hypoglycemia could lead to diabetes; in turn, the connections between diabetes and cancer were strengthened year by year. GMD's contribution to atherosclerosis was an early counter to the rapidly growing "cholesterol theory of heart disease" (X) and was frequently overlooked in the industrial race to develop ostensibly cholesterol-lowering drugs and cholesterol-lowering foods. If the proponents of GMD as a "substrate" for chronic, metabolic diseases are anywhere near the mark, "heart disease" is far more apt to be due to too many refined carbohydrates than simply to fatty and meat-oriented diets.

But awareness of the refined carbohydrate problem was just the beginning:

Western scientists looked ever more closely at non-Western eating habits to find clues between chronic metabolic disorders and food, endeavors which could only be viewed as threatening to significant sectors of the food-processing industry, the chemical industry, and, ultimately, to the pharmaceutical industry. This was because of industrial group-think which rightly perceived the chain of thought: if dietary elements were central to chronic diseases, if chemicalization of the food supply were a considerable portion of the problem of chronic diseases, and if the management (rather than the prevention of) chronic diseases were the central concern of the pharmaceutical cartel, then too much probing into worldwide eating habits represented a thinly veiled economic menace.

But clues everywhere abounded:

The Los Angeles Basin might be among the most atmospherically polluted areas in North America, yet one group of residents there, not definable by race or sex, was consistently reporting lower rates of cancer, heart disease and metabolic disorders in general. Exposed to the same polluted air and water, the Seventh-Day Adventists were (are) simply healthier overall. This is not due to genes but to habits: professed SDAs are essentially vegetarians and eschew nicotine and alcohol. Similar cases have been made over time for Utah's Mormons, but the analogy is less precise because Utah is generally healthier than the LA metropolitan complex to begin with.[21]

The early results of a huge collaborative study between Cornell University and mainland China on the relationship between diet and disease risk in 1990 provided more solid information between the two. Summarized the New York Times News Service: the initial 920 pages of data, "the Grand Prix of epidemiology," in fact "paints a bold portrait of a plant-based eating plan that is more likely to promote health than disease."[22]

There had been many other clues, particularly in the connections between diet, cancer and longevity, with laetrile proponents (including ourselves) noting how little cancer existed in populations (Vilcabamba Indians of Ecuador, Hunzakuts of Pakistan, Arctic Circle Eskimos of an earlier era, southern and non-urban Filipinos, Abkhasians of the former Soviet Union, and others) who consumed diets very high in plants, grains, fibers, vegetables (and natural laetriles). (See *XII*).

A US Navy study of American pilots shot down and captured during the Vietnam War and who underwent years of dietary privation as contrasted with pilots who were not captured and whose health/disease components were studied years later made it dramatically obvious that the mostly-meatless, essentially vegetarian, minimal-portion subsistence diet of captivity was strongly related to less chronic disease later — assuming the pilots survived at all.[23]

In 1994, Knight-Ridder News Service reported on "some of the bleakest health statistics compiled in the Western world" — those of Scotland, already known to have the highest concentration of cancer spread across its population.

In a two-year study by the Scottish government, a panel of experts found that Scots have the highest mortality rate from coronary heart disease in the world, are more likely to die before age 69 than the citizens of any other Western nation — and that 20 percent of men, 13 percent of women and nearly 20 percent of children never eat vegetables and that the sale of fruit and vegetables actually fell in the country from 1990 to 1992.

The Scottish diet has long been extremely high in fats and animal proteins but almost entirely devoid of fruits and vegetables, the latter — if apparent at all — more apt to be utilized as decorations than foods.

Part of the problem is political and economic — new Scottish eating habits took root after the disruptive era of World War II, when Britain evolved a mass food distribution system and stores became dependent on processed and packaged foods from England while local vegetable farmers were given incentives to switch to meat and dairy foods.

Even in the 1990s, reported Knight-Ridder, Scots who still were growing produce were compelled by the European Union to destroy crops to keep prices down.[23a]

Indeed, the general overview from many angles of research is decisive:

Populations which consume more unrefined grains, more

fruits and vegetables in as natural a state as possible, and which consume fewer or no refined carbohydrates, stimulants and drugs and less animal fats and animal proteins, and by sheer dint of poverty eat smaller portions, in general have far less chronic metabolic disease than do those of the more "civilized" world, whatever other pathological problems they may have.

McGee, also citing Price, Cleave, McCarrison and others,[24,25,26] has pointed out how the introduction of modern refined foods (refined carbohydrate products so often leading the pack) was followed by the development of chronic, degenerative diseases — an outcome which occurred *regardless* of the fat content of native diets, other lifestyle variables, and even prior genetic dispositions.

Problem one: the food business

While this reality has been obvious, thus, to hundreds of researchers for decades, the answer to why Western populations, particularly Americans, have for so long been unaware that what we might call the primitive, poor people's diet correlates with an essential absence of major chronic diseases is to be found in politics and economics — and naturally leads the unwary straight into the vested interests of the enormous food-processing industry, quite aside from the Allopathic Industrial Complex (AIC).

For years, America's views as to what constitutes "proper diet" (and the vaunted, if changing, "food groups"), let alone the government's various efforts in at establishing "recommended daily allowances" (RDAs) of nutrient supplements, have been dominated by the food-processing industry and, to a lesser extent, the drug industry.

As early as 1983, in a survey of the above problems I reported[27] that the medical/pharmaceutical/nutritional establishment — even in the face of growing evidence to the contrary at that time — continued to tell Americans we were the best-fed people on earth and that there was no need for vitamin and mineral supplementation as long as we ate a "balanced diet."

There might be some substance in this claim if the components of such a diet in themselves were either balanced or natural. But this is hardly the case. Even if an American of adequate economic means consumes the presumed proper amounts of leafy greens, fruits and vegetables and their juices, meat, eggs, and carbohydrates, he is absorbing foods the great majority of which have been tampered with in some way. This would include the thousands of chemicals (estimates range from 1,500 to 10,000) with which foods have been prepared, stored, treated, preserved, colored, buffered, and so forth.

A century ago, Americans were consuming wheat with a protein count of up to 20 percent, untampered-with meat and organically grown fruits and vegetables. The balancing of that diet was in fact something worth defending. But even by 1983, American bread was 9 to 12 percent protein, meats were often artificially colored and came essentially from artificially fattened and hormone-and-antibiotic-laden cattle, hogs, and poultry, and rare indeed was the table set with natural fruits and vegetables.

Americans were already brainwashed by the US Department of Agriculture and the FDA into believing that the MDRs (minimum daily requirements) and RDAs on nutrients were sufficient. I pointed out in 1983 the lack of logic: surely the allowable amounts of certain nutrients vary greatly between a Swedish longshoreman, an African pygmy, a ninety-pound octogenarian retiree and a 19-year-old fullback. Indeed, such recommended amounts had been based by the official Food and Nutrition Board on what it called the "reference man and woman," described as being of "normal" height and weight, living in a temperate zone, and being 22 years old!

It was Senator William Proxmire who did most to take on the notion of the RDAs and the food industry's influence on government, as he warned that

> *. . . at best the RDAs are only a "recommended" allowance at antediluvian levels designed to prevent terrible disease. At worst, they are based on conflicts of interest and self-serving views of certain*

parts of the industry . . .

The [Food and Nutrition Board of the National Research Council] *is both the creature of the food industry and heavily influenced by the food industry.*

. . . The RDA standard is established by the Food and Nutrition Board of the National Research Council, which is influenced, dominated and financed in part by the food industry. It represents one of the most scandalous conflicts of interest in the Federal Government.[28]

It should be realized he made these remarks in Congressional testimony in 1976. Even then, of course, total profit-taking from the totality of industries and companies comprising the food industry constituted the number-one stock investment in America, with the drug companies in number-two position. (By 1993, the total food industry was estimated at about $280 billion per year.[29])

I reported in 1983 that at the time

. . . most loyal AMA physicians and dedicated readers of the Journal of the American Medical Association *will readily admit they know little about nutrition and had no more than one or two hours of nutrition in their medical school courses.*

When they need information about nutrition, they turn to the few "A-Okay-" stamped nutritionists who are supposed to be worthy of the name, including — sometimes first and foremost — those of the Department of Nutrition at the Harvard University School of Public Health. Yet this school has accepted millions of dollars in grants from such food giants as General Foods, Kellogg, Nabisco, the Sugar Association and the International Sugar Foundation. One of the school's foremost professors of nutrition has been a consultant to the sugar and drug industries as well as a member of the Continental Can Company board of directors. It is an honest exercise to speculate about how fair and objective food science instructors can be when linked one way or another to the food industry.[30]

As early as 1976, Congressman Benjamin S. Rosenthal brought part of the problem to light as he and a consumer group claimed that some of America's eminent nutritionists had traded independence for industry favors and that some of the nutritionists who were making public analyses of consumer products were on the boards of, or otherwise had ties to, major food companies.[31]

Rep. Rosenthal found that the Harvard Department of Nutrition had received $2 million in donations from the food industry between 1971 and 1974, some of them coming from Amstar, Beatrice Foods, Coca-Cola, Kellogg, Gerber, and Oscar Mayer. Harvard vehemently denied, of course, that much contributions in any way influenced research.

Things have changed only slightly since then, although more physicians receive slightly more education in nutrition than before.

In the meantime, parallel to the organized "quackbuster" attack on nutritional therapy, metabolic treatments, holistic medicine, etc., a coordinated campaign has developed over several years around the co-opting of the term "dietitian" — only individuals said to be board-certified or otherwise sanctioned are to be allowed even to *discuss* nutrition and health with the public. This AIC state-by-state tactic, which ran into increased opposition by the 1990s, was a way, among other things, to stop proprietors and employees of healthfood stores and/or other informed laymen from even making nutritional supplement suggestions to consumers.

Yet the past decades have only served to shore up the connection between diet and health, nutrition and disease. They constitute belated conceptual victories for such progressive thinkers as the National Cancer Institute's Dr. Gio B. Gori, who ran into severe institutional opposition after he testified in 1976 that:

... Until recently, many eyebrows would have been raised by suggesting that an imbalance of normal dietary components could lead to cancer and cardiovascular disease. Today, the accumulation of epidemiologic and laboratory evidence in man and animals makes this notion not only possible but certain.[32]

But at that time, as even in its earliest days, the industry-dominated NCI was not ready to shift much interest into the food-cancer connection. Perhaps that was because it had its propaganda hands full at the time staving off the Laetrile Revolution, which was making precisely such a connection.

Making the dietary connection

The relentless rise in cancer incidence and mortality, suddenly accompanied by exponential increases in AIDS — almost a quarter of which is, by definition, cancer — has caused many researchers to look elsewhere for answers, very much including dietary/nutritional links.

As the AIDS crisis grew, more research funds were dumped into studies of immunology during the plague's first decade than in all prior years combined. Areas of research linking nutritional factors to immune depression, about which we have gone into some detail in other publications,[33,34] included these:

• Deficiencies in zinc leading to PEM, or protein-energy malnutrition, an immune system-altering condition well-known in the impoverished Third World but unexpectedly cropping up in the "civilized" Western world as well.

• The introduction of "plastic fats" into the American diet, primarily through margarine, refined vegetable oils and many products developed thereafter. The alteration of essential fatty acids (EFAs) by a food processing technique called hydrogenation caused the addition of abnormal EFA variants or *isomers* into the food chain. Scattered but growing research has implicated deficient or altered EFAs in the imbalance of the hormone-like substances called prostaglandins, at least one variety of which is strongly implicated in immune function.

(While some maverick medics and researchers had warned about the addition of industrially produced *trans* fats into margarine and certain vegetable oils decades before they were, as usual, ignored by the AIC.

(Yet, in 1994, in what The Associated Press called a "startling new report," Harvard University nutritionists found that diets high in margarine and similar foods could double the risk of heart attack and lead to as many as 30,000 of the nation's annual heart disease deaths.[35]

(At the root of the controversy is — as metabolic doctors had argued for decades, usually preaching only to the choir — the hydrogenation process for the solidifying of liquid oils. Hydrogenated or partially hydrogenated vegetable oils are used to make margarine, shortening and a wide range of cookies, crackers, chips and other processed foods — i.e., elements abounding in "civilization" while mostly unknown among primitive peoples.)

• Vitamin C deficiency. While the late two-time Nobel Laureate Linus Pauling PhD did yeoman research in elevating ascorbic acid to a prominent role against the common cold, cancer and disease in general, important research had gone on earlier by Vitamin C's delineator, Albert Szent-Gyorgyi, and the indefatigable Irwin Stone. The latter argued that man's inability to produce his own ascorbate, when accompanied by a lack of sufficient Vitamin C from the food chain, produced a state of "chronic, subclinical scurvy" which underlay much of disease. Early efforts using Vitamin C against AIDS produced considerable reduction in symptoms and seemed to correlate with longer survivals of AIDS patients.

Pauling, who died in 1994, and Hamburg cardiovascular specialist Matthias Rath MD added greatly to knowledge of how Vitamin C helps in overall heart/circulatory health and how Vitamins C and E, together with the amino acids proline and lysine, help prevent or reverse atherosclerosis. Rath has pointed out how a broad range of nutrients can successfully treat heart conditions in general.[36] [X]

By 1992, a compilation of major research from around the world proved[37] once and for all that nutritional aspects (deficiencies and excesses) are strongly linked to the body's innate defense system, so that immunological disturbance could have as much to do with these factors as anything else. But there was also the very understated problem of nutritional deficiencies induced by standard allopathic (that is, drug-based) medicine — medications and drugs of all kinds given for reasons of all kinds could, whatever else they might be doing of a therapeutic nature, cause wholesale deficiencies of all manner of nutrients, a situation which could worsen an organism which was already nutrient-depleted due to the nature of (and the alterations in) the food being consumed daily (*immunotoxicology*).[38]

The oxidology revolution

Among conceptual breakthroughs which accompanied the diet/nutrition revolution was the ever-more-abundant evidence that the way in which the body utilizes (metabolizes) oxygen is of primary importance in disease induction, prevention and management.

Our own research group (Bradford Research Institutes), looking into this problem since the the latter 1970s, became aware that there was no word to define such an important medical subspecialty, so we coined one: *oxidology* — the study of oxygen breakdown products (metabolites) in both health and disease.[39]

By the late 1970s only a handful of scientists in the world were obsessed with the importance of what usually were being called "free radicals" or more precisely "oxygen free radicals" as inducers or enhancers of disease processes. Our group looked at the broader field of "reactive oxygen toxic species" (ROTS) of which free radicals are the more prominent members in ongoing efforts to correlate ROTS in both disease *and* health.

The research establishment began widening its interest in

"antioxidant" substances — that is, compounds which had the capacity of "scavenging" or inhibiting ROTS and free radicals. To the seeming chagrin of some allopathic thinkers, it turned out that some of the commonest vitamins and other nutrients — beta-carotene ("precursor" of Vitamin A), Vitamins C and E, certain B vitamins, enzymes and minerals, particularly selenium — were "antioxidants." And, as it became increasingly clear that a good deal of chronic disease — the modern "killer diseases" of the Western world — were intimately involved with free radicals, the role of antioxidant substances took on a research life of its own.

The relationship between cancer's ability to spread (metastasize) and the production of the "ROTS/free radical cascade" became a research effort worthy of its own study — and it opened the door to antioxidants against the malignant process. Some 1994 research indicated that "free radical" mechanisms may be key in the transformation of cells from normal to cancerous.[39a] Even the damned "quackery" drug laetrile turned out to be, whatever else, an antioxidant. [*XII*]

The oxidology revolution was breaking full sway by the mid-1990s — and it was developing this way:

— The biochemical processes leading to chronic disease increasingly were seen to be a result of, or influenced by, or strongly related to, the inability of the body to compensate for excess reactive oxygen toxic species ("free radicals" and others). Free-radical damage — an aspect of the oxidation process — was as surely linked to the buildup of plaque in arteries as was the excess amount of carbohydrates which might comprise the sticky bedrock on which serum fats and toxic metals could accumulate. (In fact, the "oxidation theory of arterial disease," backed by consistent research in the 1970s and 1980s,[40,41,41a] holds that if cholesterol is truly implicated in arterial blockage, it is *not* the "reduced" form found in *natural* foods and fats that is the culprit. It is "oxidized" — literally rusted — blood fats which are a result of civilization's tampering with the food chain.)

— Free radical mechanisms are implicit in radiation

sickness, in the capacity of cancer to spread (metastasize), in the general overall aging process, and possibly in immune dysregulation ("self" attacking "self" may involve free radical attack). "Free radical pathology" came to be a general term defining a pathological process leading to various diseases and conditions in which toxic oxygen breakdown products were held to be catalysts or important contributors.

— British research in 1994 made the case for the contribution of increased free-radical production or defects in antioxidant defenses in amyotrophic lateral sclerosis (ALS — Lou Gehrig Disease), via superoxide dismutase (SOD) deficits, and in Parkinson's Disease, via glutathione deficits. Indeed, noted P. Jenner, such antioxidant defense problems "may be central to the neurodegenerative process."[42] US research the same year tied oxidology to inflammatory bowel disease.[42a]

— The antioxidant (that is, the free radical-or-ROTS-scavenging) capability of various nutrients was more and more held to be the central utility of such important substances as Vitamins A,C and E, beta-carotene, and a host of minerals and enzymes. There hence was a developing reason *for* the therapeutic use of such substances, even by the medical orthodoxy, against the killer/crippler "diseases of civilization" (diabetes, cardiovascular diseases, Alzheimer's, immunological disorders, cancer), and virtually always at levels far above those officially recommended by food-and drug-industry-controlled government oversight boards. Such realities led in some quarters to the concept of "neutraceuticals" — nutrients used in certain doses against deficiency states (beriberi, pellagra, scurvy, ricketts, for example) and/or higher doses which might help "control" a condition.[42]

— Oxidology can explain, to no small extent, just why certain primitive peoples may have high-fat diets and yet have no heart disease, diabetes or hypertension — first, their blood fats are natural or "reduced"; second, the other aspects of their diets (grains, fruits, vegetables) provide them with enormous amounts of antioxidants — that is, substances which "sop up" or inhibit excess ROTS or free radicals. Western diets are laden with "oxidized" fats and inadequate amounts of antioxidants.

— The implication that oxidative mechanisms are involved throughout the full spectrum of disease has become stronger each passing year. The Bradford Research Institutes (BRI) did ground-breaking research in this area, establishing the "ROTS theory of health and disease" as well as developing a specialized test and microscopy system to examine metabolic products in coagulated blood to detect oxidative stresses and reactions in the body.[43]

— Increased interest in the use of *oxidants* (that is, purveyors of atomic oxygen, such as hydrogen peroxide, ozone gas, Dioxychlor and similar products) and even hyperbaric oxygenation, as acting *similarly* to free radicals as a way to assault key elements of the infective process: cell wall-deficient microscopic and submicroscopic structures (viruses, retroviruses, some bacteria, mycoplasmas, yeasts and parasites). The rediscovery of the effective use of oxidative agents against a broad spectrum of pathogens has led both to new therapeutics and new controversies, particularly over the utility and/or overuse of hydrogen peroxide.[44]

By 1994, the usefulness of many of the common supplements in their roles as antioxidants was too overwhelming to be debated by serious people:

A non-profit public-interest group called the Alliance for Aging Research called for both FDA and Congressional action to speed the approval process for nutritional health claims and urged Americans to add antioxidants to their diets at levels far above those recommended by the government.

The media noted that the recommendations were based on information from more than 200 studies over the prior 20 years.

Said Jeffrey Blumberg, professor of nutrition and associate director of the USDA Human Nutrition Research Center on Aging, Tufts University:

We don't have the kind of definitive, unequivocal evidence that some people are calling for, namely the medical evidence required for the approval of new drugs. But is that the right standard when we're talking about vitamins that we have decades and decades of information on? These are not some new chemical(s) that the body has never seen before. These are things that have been in the diet since prehistoric man. [45]

He was essentially talking about Vitamins C, E and beta-carotene — which the surge of new information was already considering, along with (interestingly enough) aspirin, as blockers of "heart disease," stroke and cancer.

The call for governmental approval of higher levels of natural antioxidants was accompanied by research on fruit flies reported in *Science* which stressed (as earlier studies had suggested) that free radicals are prime causes of the aging process and that neutralizing excess free radicals or ROTS prolongs life.

Drs. Rajindar Sohal and William Orr claimed that by providing fruit flies extra copies of genes which protect against free radicals the flies' lives were extended by 30 percent. [46]

The fruit fly studies (and laboratory tests on sub-mammalian species need always to be viewed with a touch of skepticism as to relevance) were simply more precise definitions of research conducted in large (human) population-based studies which, as it was abstracted in 1994, "reported reductions as high as 40 percent in coronary artery disease among people taking antioxidants, and some clinical studies have produced similar results." [47]

The Club co-opts

It is instructive to note that even as both public and private research exploded in the 1980s and 1990s tracing the connections between dietary factors and nutrients to health and disease, the hard core of the AIC had a significant problem in how to integrate the rapidly onrushing new information with the established medical model and the pharmaceutical hydra which suckled it.

For, as Dean Burk PhD had observed in the matter of laetrile, once a chink in the armor of orthodoxy had appeared, it would widen: the aphorism that "that which prevents, also cures" would not be lost on rank-and-file physicians facing a tidal wave of chronic, systemic, metabolic dysfunctions and immune challenges for which the allopathic armamentarium offered little in the way of cures. The spectre of *disease prevention* through nutritional changes (and lifestyle alterations) loomed, and with it the implied threat to the need for a gigantic AIC and the international drug cartel which nourished and sustained it. How work the new knowledge into the old system?

The AIC turned to co-optation and semantical manipulation, its long-time *modus operandi* in dealing with inexorable forces.

Bowing to the growing evidence that nutritional supplements and nutrients themselves might indeed play a role in thwarting disease, yet not wanting to turn loose of the medical lexicon which protected old ideas, the AIC or Club concocted the word "chemoprevention" — as hilarious a co-optation as we had seen in decades of doctor-watching. "Chemo" retains the *chemical* nature of medicine (as in toxic *chemo*therapy, a rapidly failing cancer therapeutic approach) but adds on "prevention" — so that the subliminal phrase "chemicals used to prevent" might flourish in the psyche.[48]

As we noted, the drug industry, whose $65 billion gravy train (as of 1994) was substantially threatened by the $4 billion a year industry in food supplements, swiftly sought to accommodate unwanted new information while grabbing a share of a swiftly developing pie — so that major drug companies, by the late 1980s, increased their line of vitamin/mineral supplements, basing the same on random establishment research on animals which seemed to "suggest" that such supplements could, for example, positively impact on immunity.

This was, of course, rank heresy to the allopathic thinking of recent decades, but did underscore the genius of the marketplace: despite "quackbuster" attacks on vitamin pills, the people were going to have their pills, so why should the drug giants be left off the bandwagon even while running a distant risk that adequate supplementation might ultimately hinder the need for many, if not most, of the expensive medications in which the pharmaceutical market was awash?

The research establishment, still allopathic in tone, almost always accompanied every new disclosure of a nutrient being found successful against a disease or a condition with a "cautionary note," usually from an appropriately allopathic medical school researcher at a major university or within the federal research community, warning against "pill-popping" or simply taking supplements on a routine basis.

The pill-popping medics

But by the early 1990s, even this ploy was beginning to fail — many doctors, some of them originally anti-vitamin, were gobbling vitamin pills and admitting it.

Even by 1990, a survey showed[49] that an amazing 87 percent of family practitioners were recommending or prescribing vitamin and mineral supplements to some 25 percent of their patients, and that 28 percent of the medics were taking the food supplements themselves. And, as a "quackbuster" journal reported,[50] citing the American Dietetic Association, of a group of cancer patients studied, 92 percent of the women and 63 percent of the men admitted that, whatever other therapy they were on, they were taking vitamin supplements.

In 1993, the *Wall Street Journal* quoted an octogenarian nutrition expert and professor emeritus of the University of St. Louis School of Medicine, who was said to regularly rail about "the over-feeding of vitamins" to Americans but who was taking Vitamin E himself: "I'm ashamed to do it because of my attitude toward taking vitamins," he said, as he honestly admitted the explosion of studies on the vitamin's positive effects could no longer be overlooked.[51] (The *WSJ* reported that just in an initial three-month period ending Feb. 28 of that year, Vitamin E sales had totalled $27 million, up 31 percent from 1992).

Two major studies in the *New England Journal of Medicine (NEJM)* in May 1993 made the case for a significant reduction in the risk of coronary heart disease with Vitamin E (Shute brothers vindicated at long last), yet the reports were coupled with the usual admonition that the general public should not start dosing themselves with Vitamin E pills. Angry doctors balked.[52]

Wrote Dr. James O'Keefe, Kansas City MO:
>*A substantial number of physicians . . . are sufficiently convinced of the potential benefits and nontoxic nature of Vitamin E to supplement their own diets with it. If Vitamin E is good enough for doctors, should it not be good enough for our patients?*[53]

In 1993 *USA Today* reported galloping increases in profits from the sales of Vitamins E, C and beta-carotene — antioxidants all and the subjects of intense public/private investigation — and it noted that Dr. Walter Willett, Harvard School of Public Health, was taking one multivitamin tablet and one Vitamin E capsule a day, while relying on food for Vitamin C and beta-carotene.

It quoted antioxidant expert Jeffrey Blumberg of Tufts: "We're at an admittedly frustrating stage, where I think one well-informed, rational person would decide to take a supplement, and the other could decide not to."[54]

This was a hedging-of-all-bets assessment made in the midst of the continuing outpouring of new information, and certainly an honest viewpoint.

Cancer Inc. does an about-face

By 1992, in what was the biggest shift of its gears in a decade or more, the American Cancer Society (ACS), for prior decades an impassioned foe of the notion that diet had much to do, if anything, with cancer, announced the start of a mammoth survey of middle-aged American dietary habits. It was launched

just as the governmental National Cancer Institute (NCI) released results of *156* studies which linked cancer with diet — a sweeping review which forever ended any debate about whether nutritional factors have at least a role in the malignant process.[55]
[*XI*]

Gladys Block, University of California-Berkeley School of Public Health and lead author of the study/survey, found "extraordinarily consistent scientific evidence" of dietary connections though the survey did not pinpoint a single vitamin or food factor as the Holy Grail of cancer prevention.

Virtually all the 156 studies confirmed the connection between eating more fruits and vegetables and lower cancer rates.

Peter Greenwald, chief of the NCI's cancer prevention and control branch, said the findings constituted part of the basis for the agency's recent recommendation that everyone eat five servings a day of fruits or vegetables.[56]

The survey was "so compelling," said analysts, that it meant that even cigarette smokers who also ate large amounts of fruits and vegetables derived major anti-lung cancer benefits.

The same year, the largest and most detailed study ever carried out to measure the effects of Vitamin C and death rates concluded[57] that the vitamin helps both sexes live longer — but only if taken in amounts far above those recommended by the federal government.

Among findings, reported Dr. James E. Enstrom:

Men whose Vitamin C intake was the highest — the equivalent of two oranges plus a 150-milligram Vitamin C tablet per day — had a 42 percent lower risk of death from heart disease and a 35 percent lower risk of death from any cause than the population of white men as a whole.

In continuing mixed-results research in 1993, a *New England Journal of Medicine (NEJM)* study of 89,494 nurses tracked over a nine-year period beginning in 1980 showed[50] that the consumption of foods rich in Vitamin A (particularly spinach and carrots) seemed to reduce the risk of breast cancer.

It was only one of many studies trying to get to grips with a pandemic which even by that year was killing 46,000 women per year and affecting 1 out of 9. Scattered research was indicating connections between breast cancer and a high-fat diet — though it should be noted that in the "unitarian" theory of cancer (it is a single disease) connections between excess fats and excess animal proteins in *general* seem to correlate with cancer as a whole.

Victory for the concept that the better-known vitamins and minerals might after all be truly connected with health and disease opened the door to the examination of many other food factors (as indoles, flavones, and phenols in cancer) and, much to the consternation of the "quackbuster" elite, to a reexamination of the role of herbs and their components.

The dam bursts

What was largely the province of folk medicine and alleged unabashed quackery in North America increasingly came under scientifically acceptable scrutiny: useful ingredients were found in garlic and chaparral, among many others, which vindicated the empiricism of the use of these herbs over centuries. The rediscovery by the West of ancient Chinese herbalism, and the plodding efforts of America's embattled naturopaths, brought to the fore some "scientifically" acceptable rationales for everything from spirulina, blue-green algae and wheat grass to aloe vera, herbal teas of all kinds, and such folkloric herbal war-horses as echinacea and goldenseal.

By the mid-1990s, research with and interest in herbs and their multitudinous compounds was growing as fast as the concepts of oxidology and multivitamin therapy — a dam had burst whose floodwaters would not be stanched by the AIC, whose major concern going into the end of the century is how to co-opt the research and provide synthetic look-alikes of natural products in order to enhance profits. Mimicry is, after all, the highest form of flattery.

As the plague of AIDS reached terrifying dimensions in the

1990s, and as other immunological disturbances became apparent, it was part of the standard allopathic "line" that while a healthy immune system was the best defense against such modern killers and cripplers, there was no known way to "enhance" immunity other than through the mixed results and often dangerous administration of synthetic interferons and interleukins.

Yet "metabolic" or "holistic" medical practitioners had long argued that overall host defense — including all aspects of what is meant by the misleading general term "immune system" — could indeed be increased or modulated through nutrition and dietary supplements, however "quackish" such an idea seemed to the AIC.

And as we have seen, as late as 1988 even the *Harvard Medical School Health Letter* was deriding the claim that nutritional factors could bolster immunity as "simply not supportable" and that

> [T]he use of herbs or nutrition to stimulate or strengthen the immune system is a nonsense claim . . . and to the extent that people wind up believing such claims, we can say that their brains are damaged.[59]

This typically arrogant AIC point of view came acropper in 1992, though, when *The Lancet* reported research by Dr. Rajit K. Chandra, School of Hygiene and Public Health, Johns Hopkins, on the "effect of vitamin and trace-element supplementation on immune response and infection in elderly subjects."

In this study, it became obvious that even "modest" vitamin and trace-element supplementation positively affected the "immune systems" of the elderly and that the herb ginkgo biloba (extract from the leaf of the maidenhair tree) positively helped in cases of "mild to moderate symptoms of cerebral insufficiency."

Results were said to be "impressive" in immune enhancement even with admittedly "modest" doses of Vitamin A, beta-carotene, thiamine, riboflavin, niacin, Vitamins B6 and B12, Vitamin C, Vitamin D, iron, zinc, copper, selenium, iodine, calcium and magnesium.

Conclusion: "Supplementation with a modest physiological amount of micronutrients improves immunity and decreases the risk of infection in old age."[60]

By that time, of course, thousands of AIDS and pre-AIDS patients, often supported in their efforts by well-meaning, if incredulous, MDs, were finding that supplementation with a huge array of vitamins, minerals, enzymes, amino acids, herbs and other substances conclusively or suggestively linked to "non-specific immune enhancement" were seeing immune system improvements and life extension.

While attention was now given to many other factors of civilization and how they might be aiding or abetting the end-of-century plagues of cancer, AIDS and immune dysregulation (see *XI* and *XIII*), the killer diseases, by emphasizing the reality of dietary connections to health and disease, had helped correct medicine's major error, abandonment of the holistic concept.

More than any other maladies, cancer and AIDS — examples of near to total disaster on the part of the AIC — have provoked new thought and a paradigm shift to the holistic concept. And within this framework, eating habits and dietary elements play the primary *physical* roles.

The popular revolt against orthodoxy and pressure for paradigm shift *within* orthodoxy also point to a probable fail-safe mechanism within the human makeup: since survival of the species is the first and primary mandate of its existence, the species will creatively find ways to survive despite the challenges before it — and despite the entrenched bureaucracies and economic/ego vested interests which are in the way.

References

1. *The Choice*, XVIII:3, 1992. Also, Committee for Freedom of Choice in Medicine Inc. statement to National Institutes of Health, June 2, 1992.
2. *New England Journal of Medicine*, Jan. 28, 1993.
3. *The Choice* XIX:1, 1993.
4. Sampson, WI, "AIDS: frauds, finances and fringes." *New York State J. Med.*, February 1993.
5. Statement of US Council on Pharmacy and Chemistry, *J. Am. Med. Assn.*, Jan. 8, 1949.
6. *The Choice*, II:1, 1976.
7. Shute, WE, *Wilfrid Shute's Complete Updated Vitamin E Book*. New Canaan CT: Keats, 1975.
8. Wallach, JD, "The NBA: an endangered species?" Private publication; also printed in *The Choice*, XIX: 3-4, 1993.
9. Wallach, JD, address to annual convention, American Naturopathic Medical Assn. (ANMA), Albuquerque NM,

	1993.
10.	"Hard facts about chemically dependent farming." *Health Foods Business*. July 1991.
10a.	Wiles, Richard, *et al., Tap Water Blues: Herbicides in Drinking Water*. Washington DC: Environmental Working Group/Physicians for Social Responsibility, 1994.
10b.	Culbert, ML, *AIDS: Hope, Hoax and Hoopla*. Chula Vista CA: The Bradford Foundation, 1990.
10c.	Culbert, ML *CFS: Conquering the Crippler*. San Diego CA: C & C Communications, 1993.
11.	*Ibid.*
11a.	"After Silent Spring," Natural Resources Defense Council, June 1993.
11b.	Goldin, Greg, "Cancerous Growth." *LA Weekly*, May 6, 1994.
11c.	"The theft of the ark." *Seeds of Change* Catalogue, 1994.
11d-11f.	*Ibid.*
12.	"Hard facts," *op. cit.*
13.	Kesteloot, Hugo, in *J. Cardiol. and Pharm.* 6: 1984.
14.	*J. Food Quality* 9: 1987.
15.	*The Choice*, XIX:1, 1993.
16.	Harper, H, and Culbert, M, *How You Can Beat the Killer Diseases*. New Rochelle NY: Arlington House, 1977.
17.	Brennan, RO, *Nutrigenetics*. New York: M. Evans, 1975.
18.	McGee, CT, *Heart Frauds*. Coeur d'Alene ID: MediPress, 1993.
19.	Fredericks, Carlton, *Low Blood Sugar and You*. New York: Constellation International, 1974.
20.	Yudkin, John, *Sweet and Dangerous*. New York: Bantam, 1972.
21.	Culbert, ML, *What the Medical Establishment Won't Tell You that Could Save Your Life*. Norfolk VA: Donning, 1983.
22.	Cited in *The Choice*, XVI:2,3, 1990.
23.	Culbert, *What the, op. cit.*
23a.	Palma, Dick, Knight-Ridder News Service, June 18, 1994.
24.	McGee, *op. cit.*
25.	Price, Weston, *Nutrition and Physical Degeneration*. Santa Monica CA: Price Pottenger Foundation, 1945.
26.	Cleave, TL, *The Saccharine Disease*. New Canaan CT: Keats, 1974.
27.	Culbert, *What the, op. cit.*
28.	*Ibid.*
29.	McGee, *op. cit.*
30.	Culbert, *What the, op. cit.*
31.	*Feeding at the Company Trough*. Washington DC: Center for Science in the Public Interest, 1976.
32.	Culbert, *What the, op. cit.*
33.	Culbert ML: *AIDS: op. cit.*
34.	Culbert, ML: *CFS: op. cit.*
35.	The Associated Press, May 16, 1994.
36.	Rath, Matthias, *Eradicating Heart Disease*. San Francisco CA: Health Now, 1993.
37.	Beisel, WR, "The history of nutritional immunology." *J. Nutr. Immun.*, I:1, 1992.
38.	Roe, DA, *Drug-Induced Nutritional Deficiencies*. Westport CT: Avi Publishing, 1976.
39.	Bradford, RW, *et al., Oxidology: The Study of Reactive Oxygen Toxic Species (ROTS) and Their Metabolism in Health and Disease*. Los Altos CA: The Bradford Foundation, 1985.
39a.	Cerutti, PA, "Oxy-radicals and cancer." *Lancet*, Sept. 24, 1994.
40.	McGee, *op. cit.*
41.	Cathcart, RK, *et al., J. Leukocyte Biol.*, 38, 1985.
41a.	Witztum, JL, "The oxidation hypothesis of atherosclerosis." *Lancet*, Sept. 17, 1994.
42.	Jenner, P, "Oxidative damage in neurodegenerative disease." *Lancet*, Sept. 17, 1994.
42a.	Grisham, MB, "Oxidants and free radicals in inflammatory bowel disease." *Lancet*, Sept. 24, 1994.
43.	Bradford, *op. cit.*
44.	Bradford, RW, *Hydrogen Peroxide: The Misunderstood Oxidant*. Chula Vista CA: Bradford Research Institutes, 1987.
45.	McVicar, Nancy, "Vitamins against aging, disease." *Orange County Register*, Mar. 22, 1994.
46.	Sohal, Rajindar, *et al., Science*, Feb. 25, 1994.
47.	McVicar, *loc. cit.*
48.	*Science*, August 1991.
49.	*The Choice*, XVI:4, 1991.
50.	*Ibid.*
51.	Cited in *The Choice*, XIX:2, 1993.
52.	*Ibid.*
53.	McVicar, *loc. cit.*
54.	*USA Today*, June 2, 1993.
55.	*The Choice*, XVIII:3, 1992.
56.	*Ibid.*
57.	Enstrom, JE, *Epidemiology*, May 1992.
58.	*The Choice*, XIX:2, 1993.
59.	Cited in *The Choice*, XV:1,2, 1989.
60.	Chandra, RK, "Effect of vitamin and trace-element supplementation on immune response and infection in elderly subjects." *Lancet*, Nov. 7, 1992.

XV
TOWARD THE MEDICINE OF THE 21ST CENTURY:
A new paradigm in healing emerges

"All healing is magic. The Indian healer and the western healer have a common denominator — the trust and confidence of both the patient and the healer. They must both believe in the magic or it doesn't work. Western doctors make secret markings on paper and instruct the patient to give it to the oracle in the drug store [and] make an offering in return for which they will receive a magic potion."

— **Irving Oyle DO**

"I don't know what you learned from books, but the most important thing I learned from my grandfathers was that there is a part of the mind that we don't really know about and that it is that part that is most important in whether we become sick or remain well."

— **Navajo medicine man Thomas Largewhiskers (in *Imagery and Healing*)**

". . . Psychoimmunology . . . will become a vitally important clinical field — perhaps the most important field in the 21st century — supplanting our present emphasis on oncology and cardiology. Healthy thinking may eventually become an integral aspect of treatment for everything from allergies to liver transplants. What all this means is that our present concept of medicine will disappear . . . Medicine will change its focus from treatment to enhancement, from repair to improvement, from diminished sickness to increased performance."

— **Michael Crichton MD**

". . . Regular medicine . . . likes to call itself scientific and imagines that its exclusive attention to the physical reality of bodily mechanisms is in the best spirit of twentieth-century science. What most medical doctors do not know is that the scientific model of reality has changed radically since 1900 and no longer views the universe as an orderly mechanism independent of the consciousness viewing it."

— **Andrew Weil MD (in *Health and Healing*)**

". . . From a fundamental physics viewpoint, it's just about all electromagnetics anyway, at the most fundamental level. But the quantum physicists are . . . totally unaware that the physical structure, genetics, biochemistry, etc., of the living cell can in fact be directly engineered with the strange 'new' kind of electromagnetics."

— **Nuclear engineer Thomas Bearden, Lt. Col. USA (Ret.)**

New Medicine — or extinction

Hurtling toward the end of the century, the Allopathic Industrial Complex (AIC), educationally and philosophically enshrined in the AMA, is faced with its gravest of challenges: apparent inability to stave off the looming extinction of the human species.

Reminiscent of Hitler hallucinating in the bunker toward the end of World War II and still imagining that new weapons breakthroughs and nonexistent troops would somehow rescue the Third Reich at the last minute, the AIC is counting on biotechnology to save the day.

Perhaps it will — and certainly genetics and all it implies will be part of the medicine of the future — but at the present time there is little of merit in hoping the AIC will fend off the combination plagues of new and old — cancer, AIDS, immune dysregulation in the West, infections and parasites in the Third World (and the spiraling levels of antibiotic-resistant bacteria everywhere).

But because the prime directive of human biology seems to be one and one only — survival — and because *Homo sapiens* is nothing if not supremely clever when faced with extinction, as it now is, there logically is room for optimism.

Part of our species' survival is intimately involved with the rise of a new paradigm in healing — the New Medicine — which is developing as a collective mandate as the old structure dies, however brontosaurian its death throes may be.

Thomas Alva Edison was, as usual, ahead of his time with the prophetic and oft-quoted observation that "the doctor of the future will give no medicine but will interest his patients in the cure of the human frame, in diet, and in the cause and prevention of disease."

He was, after all, paraphrasing the ancients and, to some extent, Paracelsus.

His view foreshadowed by a century the disaster of the standard medical model which is now evident.

The primary medical concept of the 21st century must be

promotive health, rather — even — than preventive medicine. For the promotion of health relegates medicine to a secondary position and implies that the individual rather than the physician or the state will take upon himself the primary responsibility for what many now call "wellness."

Yet, assuming a role for medicine as long as the species exists, the new medical paradigm must be holistic and integrative — a return to the original mind/body/spirit concept of the ancients accompanied by the technological advances of our times.

The New Medicine should be a union of the composite experience of the past fused with the technology of the present — it should take from the best of all worlds (allopathy, homeopathy, naturopathy, meditation, energy medicine, etc.)

True, an integrative holistic model is revolutionary and necessarily will ruffle many feathers — those who believe that all that is natural is good and all that is manmade or synthetic bad, that there are no good drugs of any kind and that all invasive procedures are violations of the temple always to be avoided, will not enjoy making common cause with allopaths; and diehard allopaths, long trained to perceive the back-to-nature musings of the opposition as quaint at best, charlatanry of a high order at worst, will be loath to join forces with those who believe natural therapies and even attitude changes are superior to drugs and surgery.

Yet both extremes will be missing the point: it is what "works" that counts, what is best for healing to occur. No single school of medical thought has a monopoly on this.

Such integrative models are already developing. They were referred to at the precedent-setting meetings in 1992 which led to the formation of the Office of Alternative Medicine (OAM) within the allopathy-enshrining National Institutes of Health (NIH) and in which I was pleased to play a modest role.

Among attention-getting comments then were those which came from Dr. Majid Ali, a Columbia pathologist who also uses nutrition and fitness programs in environmental therapy.

Tackling the question of how the outmoded standard or allopathic model could possibly be used to evaluate multifactorial therapies against the modern disease calamities, particularly when individualized for the patient, the gifted practitioner/author said:

". . . We are incarcerated in the double-blind, crossover model. It is not appropriate for holistic therapy, in which there are many variables and neither the practitioner nor the patient can be blinded to the treatment."[1]

In these impressive gatherings of proponents of all forms of medicine, ranging from diehard allopaths to Indian tribal medicine men, from promoters of Ayurvedic medicine to chiropractors, from homeopaths to naturopaths, and from well-credentialed researchers who dabbled in all medical areas, several were in agreement about the need for a new evaluative medical parameter to be able to measure the efficacy of multi-variable therapies:

End results — i.e., "outcomes."

The only real way to assess the efficacy or lack thereof of multifactorial treatment models (protocols) is indeed the final result — how long did the patient live and in what state of health? That is, after all, the true stuff of medicine, not a workout in "science".

Establishment of a new evaluative model is a primary challenge for the New Medicine, and it will surely be met.

Genetics as a last gasp

The allopathic paradigm (treatments by contraries, single causes of disease states) is still in power and is the dominant philosophical force behind medicine's high technology. It still is producing a last, dramatic gasp.

Just as, in centuries past, the allopathic mindset placed emphasis on surgery, bleedings, purgings, and intoxications; and, in generations past, it relied upon the microbial theory of disease causation, leading to its brightest moments; and, within the past decades, it refined the latter down to the viral theory of disease as the seeming end-all of therapeutic experience, it has come up with its final card:

Genetics.

If in fact, after all, burning or poisoning out the bad humours was mostly in error and even if defining much of disease as the work of devilishly clever, invisible, not-really-alive particles (viruses) has turned up few real advances, then genes — "smaller," even, "more invisible" than, viruses — must hold the clue.

The American commitment to high technology — carrying with it an almost myopic embrace of not only not seeing the forest for the trees but actually being blinded by leaves and stems — will be part of the medicine of the Twenty-First Century and will provide useful areas of human understanding.

Most medical universalists, eclecticists and integrationists would no more deny the possible gains of genetic knowledge and its application to a new medical model than would an athlete question that performance is enhanced with a better athletic shoe.

But the reliance on genes as the over-arching, all-encompassing solution to medical problems is fraught with the same perils that have haunted all prior efforts at unilateral, linear thought: the snag is in the details and the exceptions.

By the mid-1990s, a veritable flurry of discoveries produced evidence of possible genetic "causes" for a growing number of diseases, including various "forms" of cancer. The deeper scientists probed into the stuff and nature of biology the more they dredged up those wonderful replicatory particles, genes, whose alteration or absence seemed to equate with diseases and to explain why some conditions seem to "run in families."

The road to medical Nirvana will not be paved with genes — but high tech's increasing interest in the invisible will ultimately force it into new understandings of reality which transcend medicine and biology.

The rediscovery that food (and the many elements of food) have something to do with health and disease — an idea as ancient as the holistic paradigm itself — has been the first major chink in the armor of the AIC. In less than two decades, medical practitioners who once obediently followed the AIC propaganda notion that what we eat has little to do with health and disease now agree that food is important — perhaps vital. The old medical aphorism which states that that which prevents also cures inexorably led to the idea that various nutritive factors not only prevent disease but can be used to manage and treat them. We have assigned a Marine Corps-like role to laetrile ("Vitamin B17") in helping stimulate this shift in concepts (*XII*).

As the new paradigm develops, simply at the physical level, certain approaches to health and disease quietly abandoned before or blatantly and at times ruthlessly suppressed are being looked at in a whole new light.

Oxygen therapy returns

One of these is oxygen therapy (or, more properly, oxidative therapy), whose resurgence has paralleled the gradual embrace by medical/pharmaceutical orthodoxy of its flip side — antioxidant (or "free radical") therapy. Both are pillars of what our own research group has styled *oxidology* (*XIV*).

The current medical era has witnessed what seems to be a "new" concept — the use of oxygen-based products (hydrogen peroxide, the endogenous oxidative agent par excellence; ozone gas; intermediate oxygen structures) as useful against disease primarily because of their ability to release atomic oxygen which in turn scavenges cell wall-deficient microscopic structures and thus constitutes a seemingly natural weapon against a host of viruses and microbes.

Claims for hydrogen peroxide and ozone have, like all other outside-the-pale procedures, varied from the sublime to the ridiculous, yet the persistence of what orthodoxy dismisses as "anecdotal evidence" for their use is so strong as not to be happenstance.

Yet there is little that is actually new here: as Elizabeth Baker has described[2] in a history of oxygen treatments, since the

1920s H2O2 (hydrogen peroxide) and ozone were used to put into remission many a disease. The aforementioned Dr. William Koch (*XII*) was a pioneer in the oxidative area.

The utilization of either a natural substance or a portion of the atmosphere against disease swiftly ran into trouble: who could turn much of a profit using such unpatentable things? The sulfa drugs were in the wings, then came penicillin, then came other antibiotic wonder drugs, and interest in oxidative therapies was buried under a blizzard of negative propaganda.

Even so, some 3,300 cities across the world, most of them in Europe, routinely ozonate their water supplies.

Oxidative agents function as antiseptics and purifiers. In the United States, industrial chlorine oxides are used as potent antiseptics for everything from fish tanks to swimming pools.

One industrially available product, Dioxychlor, refined for human use, was literally "rescued" for utility as a broad-spectrum antiviral, antifungal, antibacterial agent. A related compound, chlorozone, added to the water supply of a Greek village, dramatically reduced an epidemic of infectious hepatitis and was successfully used in Vietnam in the treatment of civilian war casualties. Yet, neither chlorozone nor similar compounds were ever granted patents for medical uses in the United States.[3,4]

The discovery — or actually re-discovery — that oxidative agents may be among the least expensive, least dangerous and most effective antiviral agents has great relevance in the Age of AIDS. And, indeed, astonishing claims (some undoubtedly hyped beyond reason) attribute to such products some major achievements.

It is true that claims for oxidative agents may not always hold up — and that such medical approaches have been more commercialized than scientifically established. Yet the abundance of evidence in favor of their utilization far outweighs any argument about why such methods have not been pursued, particularly when viral diseases, by their nature, are inherently "incurable."

And, overzealous use of several agents as oxidative "magic

bullets" carries with it the downside of the generation of the "free radical cascade," in which harmful oxygen metabolic byproducts can wind up doing as much harm to the body as may be done by the very microbes the oxidative agents are deployed to attack. Yet the possibility of danger by overuse has never been used by the AIC as an excuse not to develop toxic drugs.

Co-opting live cell therapy

In the area of rediscovered medical approaches it became almost humorous to longtime observers how the AIC in the 1990s was attempting to co-opt a form of therapy American medicine had derided as ineffective at best, dangerously quackish at worst. But it provided another glimpse at the AIC's boundless capacity to alter semantics.

The therapy in question is what the Europeans have long called "live cell" or "cellular" therapy — the subcutaneous or intramuscular injection of cellular suspensions of living birth-related tissue (embryonic, fetal, placental), usually but not always of the endocrine glands, from animals.

While the pedigree of live cell therapy is ancient (consumption of animal organs for reasons of health and vitality are referred to in most ancient medical systems), it became particularly known in the 20th century through the long-time work of Paul Niehans MD of Switzerland.[5]

The late Dr. Niehans and a group of otherwise allopathically trained physicians and researchers demonstrated that suspensions of cells of birth-related tissues (birth-related so that immune responses from the host would not be triggered) could be used not only against problems of infertility, impotence and sterility, but to enhance vitality, lengthen lives, balance the endocrine system in general and, in many cases, revitalize or repair damaged organs and tissues.

While there is extensive research data in languages mostly other than English, live cell therapy in the United States has long been treated as a gimmick whereby elderly males hoped to restore sexual vitality. And while just such effects have often been reported, it was not the intention of Niehans or his followers to set up sexual-potency clinics but to demonstrate, along Paracelsian terms, that in fact "like cures like" — that injections of embryonic heart tissue from a sheep, for example, did in fact somehow stimulate or improve a flagging human heart (and vice-versa.)

Even though radioactive tagging of the material could "prove" what doctors had long empirically observed, just how this could be happening escaped full understanding, and American-led Western medicine mostly derided cellular injections. Even so, famous Americans from politics, entertainment and literature joined famous citizens of other countries in trekking to Paul Niehans' chateau/clinic for just such therapy.

In the early 1980s, live cell therapy made its appearance in Mexico and elsewhere in the Americas, usually as part of an "eclectic" or "metabolic" treatment program, and began turning in some exciting "anecdotes" which could not help but catch the eye of honest American scientists.

What was exciting to independent minds, of course, was the implicit concept of the universality of birth-related proteins in the mammalian and viviparous species — and possibly of all species. If animal embryonic heart and lung cellular material could really improve the function of damaged human hearts and lungs, then here was an inexhaustible source of a potentially inexpensive, and possibly highly effective, therapy.[6]

During the 1980s, several lines of research among "qualified experts" (a code for allopathic investigators) began demonstrating that *human* embryonic — and other — tissue seemed to be useful in treating such human pathologies as muscular dystrophy and Parkinson's disease. The ethical problem loomed: how to secure embryonic tissue other than through the use of aborted fetuses? While other research suggested successful trans-species use of birth-related tissues (animal to animal and human to animal), the US establishment still did not take seriously the notion of animal-to-human cellular implants. The political/social debate over abortion blunted real research along these lines for more than a decade.

With the advent of the Clinton Administration (1992) a ban on the possible use of human embryonic/fetal research was lifted. But how could the medical/pharmaceutical establishment, which had long damned the Niehans and related approaches as unproven or quackery, now espouse a similar approach without calling it by the right name?

Voila — the development of "fetal cell transplantation therapy" and/or "tissue transplantation therapy" as a clever semantical artifice to avoid saying "live cell" or "cellular" therapy.

True, the American orthodoxy seemed determined to make this investigative therapy all the more complicated and potentially dangerous: usually, as in Parkinson's, adrenal tissue either from the patient himself or from aborted human fetuses was injected directly into the brain.

To classical live cell therapists this was both risky and unnecessary:

Under the standard European model, the cellular suspensions (usually in saline solution) are injected into the fatty tissue of the buttocks. And, as our own research group long argued, there not only is no reason to use human tissue whatsoever but it may be more dangerous to do so.

Even so, the attempted co-optation of live cell therapy by the US medical establishment as "fetal cell transplantation therapy" was another landmark on the way to a new paradigm.

For, implicit in any consideration of cellular therapy is the underlying suggestion that, whatever else the cellular suspensions are doing, they clearly seem to work on — and possibly balance — the endocrine system, the complex of "ductless glands" whose secretions, the hormones, constitute the bridge between the physical and the non-physical.

While the precise methodology of how the cellular suspensions work remains to be elucidated, our own research group has made important contributions thereto.[7] And one of them involves a homeopathic principle — it may be that all that is needed to incite a chain reaction of organ or tissue regeneration or stimulation is a *single molecule* of the "foreign" protein.[8]

Whatever the final determination is as to the mechanics of cellular therapy, it indicates protein universality and a linkage between the species. It will play a role in 21st century medicine.

The rediscovery of the holistic paradigm in healing, then, is carrying with it the re-application and re-definition of healing systems either abandoned or left in limbo for any of various reasons.

Rise of the 'X factor'

The breakthroughs of nutrition, of megavitamin therapy, of continued evidence of the importance of food in health and disease, of oxidative therapies and even of live cell therapy comprise ever-more-important elements of a new understanding of the *body* part of the mind/spirit/body triad.

But for many, the totality of the physical, corporeal element within the triad is the lesser. What some, including ourselves, call the "X factor" will probably become the more important of the elements, for it speaks to *mind* and *spirit*.

Larry Dossey MD has recalled that it was a particularly well-structured (and hence, more acceptable in terms of allopathy-guided Western physicians and others asea in a world of statistics, double blinds and other aspects of quantification) 1987 study in San Francisco that changed his life.[9]

Before then, Dr. Dossey, who had practiced medicine for 20 years and had been chief of staff at a Dallas medical center, was simply a successful, if unusually insightful, physician.

What particularly struck his powers of insight was a "randomized, double-blind trial" conducted over 10 months at the University of California-San Francisco Medical School.

In this particular study, self-avowed religious volunteers, participating from outside the medical school hospital, offered prayers for about half of 393 patients in the coronary care unit.

During the course of treatment it was found that the prayed-for group had a significantly lower "severity score," with the "controls" (not prayed for) more often needing ventilatory assistance, diuretics and antibiotics.

Reported the American Medical Assn.'s weekly, *American Medical News*, investigator Randolph Byrd MD concluded that the prayers had had "a beneficial therapeutic effect."[10]

After Dossey reviewed the San Francisco study, he decided to look more closely into the effect of prayer on living organisms. He even started to pray for patients (one wonders just which statutes of which medical boards might be violated by such an effort). Explained the free thinker:

"I reached the conclusion that withholding prayer was the equivalent of withholding any other valid medical treatment."

Had a known quack from south of the border or the evangelical leader of a faith-healing service said this, the medical and research communities would probably have ignored the remark.

But in fact Dr. Dossey had tapped into a vein already being exploited: the role of the mind (of spirit, of attitudes) in health and disease, and his excellent 1993 book on the subject followed earlier blockbusters by the well-credentialed Bernie Siegel MD. The latter had scrapped simple surgery for medical intervention *plus* aspects of caring, love and good humor in the treatment of patients, certain they could receive such positive energy whether they were conscious or not.[11]

And, *AMN* quoted Jeffrey S. Levin PhD, associate professor of family and community medicine at Eastern Virginia Medical School: "There is a considerable amount of scientific evidence showing that prayer is effective." Dossey calculated that more than 130 "sound" studies exist in the English language alone which attest to the power of prayer.[12]

Lest the Allopathic Industrial Complex (AIC) trot out one of its favorite arguments to explain the inexplicable — the "placebo effect" — Dossey and others noted that the psychological support one might expect from prayer could indeed be explained by the fact a person knows he is being prayed for, and/or is praying himself — yet it is difficult to dismiss research suggesting that adult humans, children and *animals* who and which have been unaware they were prayed for experienced positive effects.

To the religious, that prayer "works" is so obvious that it needs no explanation by individuals trained in the (Western) "scientific method." For the more materialistic/agnostic segment of the Western population, quantification of the observation looms as intellectually necessary.

That "faith works wonders" was quantified before the San Francisco experiment.

Between 1954 and 1989, when the data were published, 19 out of 38 research dossiers studied by a group called the International Medical Commission of Lourdes (CMIL) — which attempts an objective overview of alleged miracle cures by religious pilgrims visiting the shrine of Saint Bernadette in Lourdes, France — were essentially accepted as legitimate cures, though medically and scientifically inexplicable. The CMIL has been described as a panel of medical doctors who are "independent of interference by outside bodies."[13]

Important to the CMIL were reliability of diagnosis, precluding of "spontaneous remission" in the known natural history of the disease, and the fact that no known medical treatment could have effected the cure.

In 1977, Dr. Charles Weinstock noted, speaking of the phenomenon of "spontaneous regression" in cancer:

> *In every single case of "spontaneous" regression where the psychosocial situation is described, a favorable change in it (or the favorable psychological change occasionally experienced on facing death) has invariably just preceded the tumor shrinkage. Some of the former include: a sudden fortunate marriage; the experience of having one's entire order of clergy engage in intercessory prayer; sudden, lasting reconciliation with a long-hated mother; unexpected and enthusiastic praise and*

encouragement from an expert in one's field; and the fortunate death of a decompensated alcoholic and addicted husband who had stood in the way of a satisfying career.[14]

Substantial evidence indicates the negative effects of mental stress on human immunity (death of a spouse, divorce, separation, for example) and that difficulty in coping with mental stress may be related to allergies, autoimmune and infectious diseases, as well as cancer.[15,16,17,18]

Evidence has also accumulated that what some have called "hardiness" has had a mitigating effect on mental stress and stress-related illness (elements — sense of control, commitment and challenge), and that a "fighting spirit" has better outcomes in breast cancer.[19,20,21]

Norman Cousins' books relating long-term controls over his own condition through a seemingly perpetual sense of humor, among other positive factors, have become classics.[22,23]

In 1993, California's pioneering Institute of Noetic Sciences attempted a "scientific-method" assemblage of phenomena related to "spontaneous remissions," which turned out to include 1,385 articles which covered 3,500 reports and appeared in 800 "standard" medical journals in 20 languages.

Of the survey, in which cancer cases represented 74 percent of the collection, investigators found widespread evidence of such "psychosocial mechanisms" as group support, hypnosis/suggestion, meditation, relaxation techniques, mental imagery, "miraculous spiritual phenomena," "faith/positive outcome expectancy," "fighting spirit," "denial," "sense of control," "sense of purpose" and "placebo effect" as correlating with many cases of remission.[24]

In 1993, the newly established Office of Alternative Medicine (OAM) began funding various projects to look into what many called "the mind-body connection." In 1994, an NIH "Reunion Task Force" actually held a "Mind-Body Interactions and Disease" symposium at which 50 researchers were gathered to address aspects of the interplay between mental states, immune function and health.

That such a symposium could be held under the aegis of federal sponsorship, let alone that the OAM could fund a tiny study at the University of New Mexico on "intercessory prayer," were — as was the establishment of the OAM itself in 1992 — landmark events.

They represented if not a coming of age then at least a successful prepubescence for a concept which had been primarily developed in the 1980s and which had finally been given its own name (perhaps as much as anything else to keep it a pristine ideology and/or an approach susceptible at some point of coverage by insurance plans).

PNI says it all

The name was *psychoneuroimmunology* — PNI, for short (to which some have already added *psychoneuroendocrinology*, PNE). The jawbreaking word said it all: mind to nerves to immunity. And not to be confused with *psychosomatic*, of a more general range.

The stage had been set in the 1970s primarily due to the pioneering work of psychologist Robert Ader and immunologist Nicholas Cohen at the University of Rochester. What they demonstrated, as other researchers also had suggested, was that the immune system (or, as we stress, systems) do not work independently of the brain and the emotions — but that they are somehow bound together.[25]

Pioneering work by Lawrence LeShan did much to suggest the role of attitude in cancer, a complicated pathology which, perhaps more than any other, provides the bridge between the worlds of the physical and the non-physical.[26]

In the 1980s, Dr. Lydia Temoshek, University of California-San Francisco, in reviewing the cases of long-term AIDS survivors, found that whatever the patients were doing mentally "may affect the immune system and survival."[27]

Another major PNI proponent, Dr. George Solomon, psychiatry professor at the University of California-Los Angeles, suggested that personality and emotions, particularly one's ability to cope with adversity, may help the immune system(s) respond to illness.[28]

Seemingly celebrating PNI's emergence, *Newsweek* devoted a "cover story" on "body and soul" and the elucidation, by PNI's main proponents, of the "feedback loop" — an intricate interplay of multi-system communication in which not only does the brain seem to speak to the immune system(s), as earlier guessed by researchers, but the latter also "talk back" to the brain.[29]

The suggestion is a language of both hormones and hormone-like substances and nerve signals in which parallel systems are somehow able to converse.

By the 1990s researchers were giving increased attention to *neuropeptides*, substances which affect nerve system function and, by implication, overall host defense, including all aspects of immunity, and to where and how they are produced and their connections to attitudes and emotion.

The breakthrough linkage was achieved by the University of Alabama's J. Edwin Blalock, who discovered that an aspect of the immune system is the production of neuropeptides (originally thought only to be produced by the brain). Thanks to this and similar research the ties between "mind" and immunity can be considered fully established.[30]

The PNI connection hence helps to explain, in however preliminary a way, the vital importance of attitude, belief, thoughts and emotions in both the induction and control of disease. It does not yet account for the next phase — the influence over physical events (mediated through thoughts and emotions) by unaware patients: e.g., for example, how prayer might provide a positive effect whether the PNI "feedback loop" is involved or not.

Aside from the relatively better-known aspect of attitude in cancer (perhaps up to 20 percent of advanced cancer cases may somehow be linked to a subconscious desire of the patient to die) doctors and healers since time immemorial have known (though not in a Western scientific sense) that the mind contributes both to *ease* and *dis-ease*. This has long been an empirical observation and it is only now that rivulets of "proof" susceptible to the Western mind-set are emerging.

In 1993, the University of California-Los Angeles (UCLA) Neuropsychiatric Institute and Hospital and Johnson Comprehensive Cancer Center released results[31] of a six-year study which examined the benefits of combining extensive psychological support with education to help melanoma cancer patients cope with their disease.

This conservative but well-constructed trial of 68 patients indicated that those who learn how "to cope" may keep a disease from recurring as rapidly. What remains to be demonstrated is whether teaching patients how to *reject* disease could be as successful.

Such experiments and the rise of PNI virtually demolish the "placebo" and "false hopes" arguments hurled by the AIC against practitioners of "holistic" medicine. This is because the "placebo effect" is clearly of demonstrated therapeutic benefit (that is, simple belief that a potion or a doctor visit will help spurs the brain to release opiate-mimicking chemicals called endorphins which, whatever else they may or may not do, allow the patient to feel better — an event often of awesome importance in such pathologies as advanced cancer) and the question is now raised: "what *is* 'false hope'?"

While it is true that the charlatan preys on the ignorant by promising miracle cures, it is now clear from virtually all sides that the injection of hope in the mind of a terminal-disease patient often correlates with life extension if not outright "cure."

By far the greater ethical crime is within the current — failed — allopathic medical mindset as the continual promotion, in one hospital or clinic or doctor's office after another, of the idea that there *is* no hope. This conclusion is usually reached after a patient has tried all conceivable allopathic approaches which, having failed, allow no room for even the faintest hint that there might be a better way.

This then leads, in case after case, to the patient's being told that "you have six months to live" or some other estimate conjured up by the perhaps well-meaning practitioner who bases such a conclusion on statistical analyses and "best" — that is, allopathic — evidence. Since the patient has usually already transferred his responsibility for health or illness to the physician (symbolically equipped as the quasi-divine arbiter of life and death) the patient may be programmed by such a statement to die in six months.

The author's two-decade experience dealing with patients who flock south of the border grasping for miracles provides copious evidence of the mind/attitude connection — as a group, "terminal" patients who outright rejected the idea that another mortal on this planet can adequately predict when they are going to die tended to postpone their "terminality," often for many years; those who ceded attitudinal terrain to the physician as authority figure tended to die on schedule.

It becomes ever clearer that ideas and attitudes help induce either wellness or illness.

By 1993, it was clear that mental depression — whatever its actual source — was itself a factor so significant in American pathology that it was costing $43.7 billion a year in treatment and lost productivity.[32]

That same year, psychiatrist James Gordon, director of the Center for Mind-Body Studies in Washington and clinical professor in the departments of psychiatry and community and family medicine at Georgetown Medical School, summarized that:

> *[T]he capacity for self-regulation that once seemed unbelievable even in Indian yogis is now commonplace in our clinics. Biofeedback, relaxation and simple visual images may enable us to change our heart rate, blood flow, urine output, brain-wave patterns and even the numbers and activity of white blood cells, often with demonstrable clinical benefits .... It has become clear too that the effect of many*

therapeutic interventions — conventional or alternative, Western or non-Western — may be enhanced by loving, individual attention from health care providers and group support from others with similar illnesses. This is true at every stage of life and in virtually every chronic illness. [33]

Holism comes West

By the 1990s, some unique societal trends had coalesced to give a boost to the Eastern concept of holism — the trinity of mind, spirit and body, the core fundamental belief of ancient and original medicine (*IV*).

First, the antiestablishmentarianism of the 1960s left, among its residue, many seedlings of conceptual change in Western minds including increased respect for Eastern religious and philosophical systems and the healing methods which sprang from them, together with reverence for ancient healing techniques among the indigenous peoples of the New World.

And the demands of world politics (America's "opening to China" among the more paramount) and the explosion of communications, through which all parts of the globe were increasingly ever more in contact with each other, caused a transfer of ideas, concepts and methods between East and West leading, as a particularly notable example, to the embrace of acupuncture by the West.

Too, the profound failures and catastrophes of Western "scientific medicine" against chronic disease led by sheer numbers to the need for an ever more open spirit of inquiry.

Within this spirit, individuals appropriately credentialed by the allopathic majority were given space to try new ideas, ranging from the sublime to the ridiculous.

Among the fusions of Eastern thought and Western methodology came aspects of using the mind against disease — for which the words "imaging" and "guided imagery" came to be descriptive. While numerous savants have entered this field, particularly solid advancement has occurred through the work of

O. Carl Simonton MD[34] and psychologist Jeanne Achterberg.[35]

At meetings in which I participated which led eventually to the formation of the OAM, more than 100 proponents of various "alternative" or "complementary" therapies heard individuals with seemingly impeccable credentials refer more and more to the mind-body-spirit connection, and to emphasize the importance of attitude in healing — not only the attitude of the patient but also that of the healer.

One such presentation referred to something new to most of us: "human intention factor" (HIF) — that is, the palpable improvement of therapy administered by a clinician if his or her *intent* were to heal (rather than, for example, simply to see the 3:15 pm patient at 3:15 pm and dash off a prescription in a lackadaisical, ho-hum manner). Interest also centered on such seemingly irrelevant areas as the cheerfulness or lack of same of the doctor's office and the color of wallpaper therein. Conversations on such cosmic subjects engaged in by multiply-degreed people appearing at government-sponsored ad hoc seminars would have been unthinkable, if not impossible, a few years before.

The respect for traditions of the East had opened up primarily because of the West's meteoric interest in acupuncture (and its adjuvant approach, acupressure), some of which doubtless accompanied the political needs of accommodating mainland China with the United States. Whatever, through acupuncture a bond between Eastern and Western healing models was firmly established.

Yet the West could not absorb the physical aspects of acupuncture (obviously useful in reducing chronic pain, reducing craving in chemically addicted individuals, in altering the moods of depressed people) without taking along some of its philosophical baggage. For acupuncture, however disciplined it may seem to be at the physical level, is an expression of a philosophical/religious system: cosmic dualism, Taoism, the concepts of the equal balance of forces, of *yin* and *yang*, of harmony/disharmony.

Not only acupuncture, but many other healing systems "rediscovered" in the West in recent years, strike at the very root of the Cartesian-Newtonian postulates which, among other things, see an endless separation between mind, body and spirit. These Eastern beliefs, consonant with those of virtually the whole world before the advent of Western allopathy, hold the mind and the body to be inseparable — just as man (they would argue) is inseparable from nature and nature inseparable from the universe.

In such systems, the ideas of *ease* vs. *dis-ease* (ill health, in the Western model) are secondary to the broader concepts of balance/imblance or harmony/disharmony.

From India, the ancient systems of yoga (not itself a medical system but impinging on medicine) and Ayurvedic medicine, enjoying a rebirth in the West largely thanks to Deepak Chopra MD, have brought insights useful to the Western mind.

Of subtle energy, prana *and* qi

Underlying these ancient systems is the concept of a vital, subtle, universal energy flowing through everything — the *prana* of the Indians, the *chi* or *qi* (in modern transcription) of the Chinese, and the alterations of which (through the meridians and pressure points of acupuncture and the *chakras* of Indian holism) may bring health or disease.

From a Western "scientific" standpoint, the *prana* or *qi* is "unquantifiable" and hence (cognitive dissonance!) non-existent. Subtle atoms of this energy cannot be gathered, studied, tested, reproduced, so therefore they must not truly *be*.

Yet such a concept is wholly redolent of the underlying nature of homeopathy, of 18th-century Western (German) inspiration, which evolved into an entire medical system which challenged allopathic concepts and posed the most serious threat to the vested and ideological interests thereof in the United States in the 19th century. [*V*]

The same essential element in the homeopathic paradigm which eludes allopathy is exactly that element in ancient Oriental medicine which the West cannot quantify:

The notion of a subtle, cosmic energy field or vital force. Homeopathy's founder, physician Samuel Hahnemann, called it the *vis medicatrix naturae*, the vital force, the disturbance in which would lead to imbalance which would lead to disease. Because Hahnemann's method utilized infinitesimally dilute amounts of natural substances to affect the vital force, and because such substances were often so dilute as not to be palpable in and of themselves, "Western science" was both taken aback by, and never could explain (other than in elegant placebo terms), the manifest victories of homeopathics over disease.

However, I (and certainly others) have argued that homeopathy, and Hahnemann, were "on to something," and that the something has to do with subtle universal energies. These energies are not now, in terms of modern physics, nearly as abstruse as they seemed in the 18th and 19th centuries — for much of physics now concerns itself with the unseen and the *presumed*.

Indeed, homeopathy may be described as quantum mechanics applied to biology: infinitesimal disturbances in an infinitesimally dilute or subtle energy field, perhaps the very stuff of the universe itself, are the root of *dis-ease*! If the universal vital force is the wellspring of all life, all vitality, in the physical universe (cosmos), then it is the ultimate expression of a single energy — perhaps, some might argue, of a single thought.

Whether one extends this vital force to its theological conclusions, it does present science — as third-dimensionally understood by hominid mammals within our own parameters of space, mass and time — with a conceptual statement: all existence is, ultimately, a reflection of energy, and there are many states of energy. In physics it can now be stated that there are subatomic forces the ultimate limit of which — if there is one — remains unknown.

Only by perceiving the possibility of an as-yet-unquantifiable subtle energy flow do such realities that "prayer heals" mean much to the rational mind.

The concept of such a universal subtle energy force,

sometimes expressible as electromagnetism, biomagnetics or some other relevant term which attempts to capture at least part of its nature, provides a possible basis for understanding of both treatment and diagnostic models which, for various reasons, have yet to be broadly accepted by mundane science.

Radionics, for example, posits that a mere part of a person as small as a lock of hair or a drop of blood emits "vibrational energies" which can be used either for diagnostics or even for healing at a distance. This approach, developed primarily in the US in the early part of this century, evolved into more modern attempts to project healing at a distance through the use of a photograph of the patient. Radionics ran afoul of the Food and Drug Administration (FDA) in the USA though various forms of the theory and practice are legal in several countries.

Homeopathy triumphant

Homeopathy, however, has surged forward on all sides and may be bringing with it a concept of ancient healing more in tune with modern physics: Hahnemann's minuscule dilutions may be operating against symptoms on the basis of *pure energy*, or at last a pure *biological* energy. That shaking (succussion) of liquids seems to enhance their potency is often observed in standard experiments — but can dilutions be literally shaken into a state of virtual pure energy where no trace of the original substance is recoverable?

This of course was the core and marrow of the 1988 Benveniste experiments, which excited an international flurry of "quackbuster" activity:

French researcher Jacques Benveniste and 11 colleagues in research laboratories in France, Italy, Israel and Canada demonstrated that an antibody solution so dilute (up to 10^{120}) that not a single molecule of the substance could be present seemed to alter the chemistry and internal structure of white blood cells. The work was presented in a major British "learned journal," *Nature*, whose reviewers had been unable to find a flaw which could be used to invalidate the results. The magazine editorially expressed both "reservation" and "incredulity" — a clear conflict of cognitive dissonance: what was reported "could not be," yet the methods followed were appropriately "scientific" and the results therefore "seemed to have been," ran the logic.

But three observers soon were found (including a magician connected with America's best-known "quackbuster" group) to go over the lengthy, multi-laboratory data. In a matter of weeks they claimed to have found that the experiments had been poorly designed and constituted a "delusion." For his part, Benveniste declared the quickly-assembled and quickly-executed investigation "a mockery" and compared it to the Salem witch trials.

Also helping stir American interest was an analysis by the *Washington Post* that

> ... *If taken at face value, the research shows that the immune system's antibodies can work even when the solution they are in is so diluted that no antibody molecules are left in it. There is no known physical basis for such action. It would mean there is some bizarre way that the solution could "remember" the presence of the antibody molecules and act as if they were still there.*[36]

This, of course, would lead both a radionics proponent and a homeopath to exclaim, "Well, yes, indeed — that's the way it works."

Benveniste stood his ground despite the inability of another team to reproduce the results.

The Benveniste matter, however, was only one in a series of seeming breakthroughs for homeopathy in the modern era.

In 1986, the British journal *Lancet* published a study of homeopathy that followed what the orthodoxy described as "the rules of proper clinical research." It compared hay fever sufferers treated with a homeopathic remedy with similar patients given a dummy pill. Symptoms improved dramatically enough in the homeopathic group that by the end of the study its members had used half the antihistamines as the control group. Yet, noted *Consumer Reports*, "the remedy they had taken was so greatly diluted that none of the original material should have remained."[37]

None, a homeopath might say, except what really counted — the remedy's own "vital force."

Since these results, and later the Benveniste experiments, seemed to say that homeopathy was worth pursuing, a team of Dutch epidemiologists then began a literature search for evidence of homeopathic usefulness demonstrated through "controlled trials."

They published their results in 1991 in the *British Medical Journal;* of 105 studies with "interpretable results," 81 appeared to show that homeopathic remedies had been effective.

While numerous trials were said to be flawed in one way or another, the Dutch team pulled out 23 of those thought to be the most "scientifically" sound — and even then 15 showed positive results.

There then entered the usual dash of negative cognitive dissonance: "Based on this evidence," they wrote, "we would be ready to accept that homeopathy can be efficacious, if only the mechanism of action were more plausible." The question was implicit: *plausible to whom?* It seemed redundant at the time to note that in 1492 what Christopher Columbus seemed to have accomplished was simply not "plausible" to nautical science as then understood.

Consumer Reports, usually thought of as a bastion of disinterested rational thought, reported in 1994 how it had asked "two scientists well versed in study design" to comment on the Dutch case review, the hay fever study and two other earlier homeopathic studies involving flu and rheumatoid arthritis in which homeopathy had seemed to have a positive effect.

One of the researchers, apparently using every acceptable technique of the "rigorous scientific method," found the flu and hay fever results had indeed been "impressive," adding that "these papers used orthodox research methods to show effectiveness, and demonstrated it soundly."[38]

Intriguingly, when *CR* asked him if he would prescribe

these homeopathic remedies for patients with hay fever and flu he delivered a resounding no. "Ultimately, it gets to the issue of plausibility and how well it fits into your scientific view of the world," he said. "It doesn't fit."[39]

"Plausibility" and "fit" are hallmarks of paradigm capture (domination by a preheld set of beliefs) and the negative aspect of cognitive dissonance (inability or lack of interest in processing new and unwanted information). They are, as we have seen, the ideological and psychological supports of the Allopathic Industrial Complex (AIC) or The Club.

Also in 1994, as "quackbusters" railed in ever higher decibels against the growing public awareness of homeopathy, another "scientifically" acceptable study of the healing approach appeared in a "standard" journal: J. Jacobs *et al.* reported in *Pediatrics* that homeopathic preparations had been beneficial in the management of acute diarrhea in Nicaraguan children.[40]

California pediatrician Carol D. Berkowitz, who wrote a "commentary" in *The Lancet* on this case, noted that the research was a "small but methodologically sound study." Moreover, she editorialized, in an embrace of honest objectivity:

> *Despite...barriers to universal acceptance of homeopathy, physicians should maintain an open mind about potential benefits. Although we have often relied on drugs such as antibiotics to manage disorders such as diarrhea, the emergence of resistant organisms may necessitate a change in strategies.*[41]

Given the rapid and ominous spread worldwide of antibiotic-resistant bacteria, this observation was an understatement.

That homeopathy could be objectively dealt with in a standard allopathic medical publication — and this observer notes that *The Lancet* seems to have taken the lead in mold-breaking medical objectivity among the allopathic "learned journals" — shows that new thought is stirring.

As did the precedent-setting decision by insurance giant

Blue Cross of Washington and Alaska when, in 1994, it began a pilot project covering homeopathy, naturopathy and acupuncture for several thousand participants.

What may stand as the modern-era breakthrough thrust in which allopathy did its best to "test" homeopathy was reported December 10, 1994 — *The Lancet* again as the forum. When David Reilly *et al.*, Glasgow Royal Infirmary and University of Glasgow, published "Is evidence for homoeopathy reproducible?" the medical world was treated to a well-honed serving of truth being squeezed out through layers of cognitive dissonance and abstracted with some of the most agonizing semantics yet mounted against a seemingly unwanted reality — namely, that homeopathy "works."

Reilly *et al.*, conducted a "meta-analysis" of three trials involving the use of homeopathics against asthma in 28 patients. It may be said that the analysis measured "oral homoeopathic immunotherapy" in every conceivable "rigorously scientific" way — literally, up, down and sideways.

When all was said and done, the investigators were forced to admit that the results "strengthened the evidence that homoeopathy does more than placebo." Incredibly, the authors ended the "summary" portion of the article with a question, one reflecting negative cognitive dissonance: "Is the reproducibility of evidence in favour of homoeopathy proof of its activity or proof of the clinical trial's capacity to produce false-positive results?"

In the "discussion" portion of the study, after finding the undoubted evidence that homeopathic efficacy could plainly *not* be explained by the placebo effect (i.e., it's all in your head), the authors inscribed the following historic overview, reflective of the very honest, if allopathic, mind attempting to explain the inexplicable:

> *For today's science . . . the main barrier to homoeopathy is the issue of serially vibrated dilutions that lack any molecules at all of the original substance. Can water or alcohol of fixed*

biochemical composition encode differing biological information? Using current metaphors, does the chaos-inducing vibration, central to the production of a homoeopathic dilution, encourage biophysically different fractal-like patterns of the diluent critically dependent upon the starting conditions? Theoretical physicists seem more at ease with such ideas [emphasis mine] *than pharmacologists, considering the possibilities of isotopic stereodiversity, clathrates, or resonance and coherence within water as possible modes of transmission, while other workers are exploring the idea of* electromagnetic changes [emphasis mine]. *Nuclear magnetic resonance changes in homoeopathic dilutions have been reported and, if reproducible,* may be offering us a glimpse of a future territory [emphasis mine] . . . *Our results lead us to conclude that homoeopathy differs from placebo in an inexplicable but reproducible way.* (41a)

Degobbledegooked, the message here actually is clear — chaos-inducing vibrations, fractal-like patterns of the diluent and isotopic stereodiversity notwithstanding — damn it, homeopathy works and we just can't explain it, but it may involve higher physics.

The resurgence of homeopathy, the delineation of PNI, even renewed interest in radionics, speak to growing concepts of *energetic medicine* — using "vibrations," "resonances," "frequencies," various manifestations of subtle energy both in the diagnosis and management of disease.

Everything is energy

While the field is naturally wide-open to charlatanry, the idea of subtle energies, ever more in alignment with modern physics and increasingly removed from magic and superstition, can make at least a tangential case for some of the admittedly off-the-wall techniques and therapies advanced by "New Age" thinkers and the occultists of old:

If indeed everything is energy, or everything is at least an energetic vibration, then manipulations of such energy may somehow have a hand in healing. The therapeutic use of precious stones and quartz crystals, pillars of Western occultism and Eastern esotericism, thus may have some basis in reality: certain structures are better conductors and accumulators of energy than others. The use of colors, aromas, essences, light and even sound in therapy fall into a broad category of *energetic medicine*.

Understanding that everything is energy, and that there may be a subtle energy underlying all other expressions thereof, may explain a host of phenomena attributed to "touch" therapy and to the combination touch and visual gimmickry of the "faith healers" of the Philippines, some of whom have indeed provided some spectacular feats of apparent healing.

The same concept may bring some Western reasoning to the oft-demonstrated positive phenomena of accumulating energy in pyramidal shapes — "pyramid power" — an ancient demonstration of energy normally rejected in the West simply because it is not "plausible" under current concepts.

It is no longer necessary to be a dabbler in the occult or an exponent of an Eastern religious sect to become seriously interested in "frequency medicine," "directed energy" or "biomagnetism" — a peek at the shadows of scientific history in the West suggests that mankind has leapfrogged over some areas of science, leaving others in the darkness and forgotten or ignored, for a variety of reasons.

What some call bioelectrical therapy — the effect of energy fields on life — and/or "directed energy" (how to manipulate and direct energy for a given end above and beyond electricity and the known spectra of light and radiation) represents an aspect of healing which will play a profound role in the medicine of the 21st century.

The bridge uniting homeopathy and various forms of electromagnetism is increasingly evident in attempts to measure the frequencies and vibrations of subtle energies both for diagnostic and treatment purposes.

The therapeutic use of electromagnetic fields, electricity, bioelectricity, and magnetism is a composite new area drawing both on old-time remedies and high-tech science. Such approaches range from certain folk-medicine uses of magnets as cures to the quirky claims of radionics proponents claiming to heal at a distance.

Biophysics, magnets and oxidology

In the United States, some vital research has been attempted, at least anecdotally, to tie together what some of us have referred to as *oxidology* with magnetic-field therapy since, ultimately, the two areas are like peas in a biophysical pod.

Central to this new dimension of medicine is an understanding of the role of antioxidants and oxidative agents, the energy dynamics involved in the "catalysis" (accelerating a chemical reaction) of energy, alkaline-acid balance (pH), the seemingly universal role of calcium in metabolic function — and manipulating negative magnetic fields by the use of magnets.

Retiring in 1990 after 40 years of medical practice, an Oklahoma researcher, physician William H. Philpott MD, set himself the task — through the Bio-Electro-Magnetic Institute — to attempt to assemble, in FDA-approved ways, sufficiently scientific data to prove his decades of empirical evidence (also gleaned by others) that:

— A static magnetic field is an energy field; a negative magnetic field exposure increases molecular oxygen in humans; a negative magnetic field is the energy activator for the enzymes that release molecular oxygen from biological "reduced" substances; and such fields may heal inflammation, may act as antibiotics against bacteria, fungi, intestinal parasites, etc., may reduce toxins, decrease pain, normalize pH in cellular and body fluids to an alkaline state (which extensive observation from many angles equates with an absence of chronic degenerative conditions), encourage restorative sleep and in fact "govern biological healing in humans."[41b]

The utilization of magnets and of magnetic beds and other devices theoretically relieves the body of having to apply such a field to one of its own damaged areas.

Dr. Philpott has described cases of seeming control of numerous conditions, including advanced cancer, simply by the proper application of negative magnetic fields mediated through industrial magnets but strongly argues that hardcore data need to be established to buttress what appears to be abundant empirical evidence. His work, with considerable nods to the "Aharonov-Bohm" effect and the work of R.O. Becker MD,[41c,41d] also makes a case for helping maintain an alkaline medium nutritionally for the enhancement of overall health.

Hence, as the decade ends the areas of oxidology (stressing the central importance of oxygen metabolism to life and health) and of biophysics (particularly, magnetic energy applied to healing), together with renewed work in homeopathy, constitute trail-blazing events heading toward the medicine of the next century.

Rediscovering Tesla, Reich, Rife, Priore, et al.

Paralleling them has been a resurgence of interest in the work and theories of Nikola Tesla, the turn-of-the-century American inventor who is best known in the electrical orthodoxy as the developer of the alternating current motor and the high-frequency coil. Tesla was seeking nothing less than "wireless transmission of energy at a distance with no losses."

Modern reviewers of Tesla's work and theories alternately call him a madman and a genius, and by the middle of this century, most of his efforts had been ignored or forgotten — or, as Teslaites claim, stamped out by the energy monopolies which perceived a threat in his ideas. (What need would there be for human social organization if, for example, all the energy and sustenance one needed to survive could literally be plucked right out of the air?)

In the current era, in a West bedazzled by scientific gadgetry, various promoters utilizing "oscillating waves" and several forms of bioelectricity claim to be able to measure the electromagnetic fields of everything from the body itself to the minutest cell, and also claim they can interfere with these fields in such a way as to promote healing. There may be modern names for the techniques and their champions but they are echoes of the not-too-distant past.

The names of Wilhelm Reich, Royal R. Rife and Antoine Priore loom large in this appraisal.

The scientist and mystic Wilhelm Reich, an Austrian psychoanalyst, earlier in this century claimed an understanding of energy at variance with the theories of the day, and the discovery of what he called *bions*, minute particles of energy. He developed the concept of *orgone energy* (a kind of *prana* or *qi* definable as a combination of sexual energy and cosmic life force) and believed he had described the authentic relationship between physiological and mental disturbances. He developed "orgone energy accumulators" as treatment modalities and, naturally, ran very much afoul of federal authorities. While the imprisoned Reich faded from view and died, Alexander Lowen, who studied with him, though rejecting the orgone theory, developed the mind-body therapy called *bioenergetics*, now taught and practiced under various names in many countries.[42]

Royal R. Rife, a San Diego scientist, in the 1930s claimed both advanced microscopy so refined that activated viruses could actually be seen with the "Rife microscope," and the apparent ability to cure terminally ill cancer patients with a "ray tube" tuned to specific electronic frequencies which allegedly inhibited what he, and later others, believed to be "the cancer virus." Rife produced considerable controversy in his time, and proponents of his theories would claim, as did followers of Tesla and Reich, that vested interests were behind his harassment and the blocking of further research. But there are enough witnesses and background available for study to make the case that the inventor was doing serious work of considerable merit.[43]

(Reich's *bions* and Rife's "cancer virus" may possibly explain the visual evidence of particles of pure energy which take transitory, will-o'-the-wisp forms identifiable only in very high-resolution multi-phase microscopes, and which have haunted the fringes of both science in general and microscopy in particular for decades.

(A growing number of researchers have seen, or theorized, the presence of *pleomorphic* — that is, form-changing or "L-forms" — in the blood of diseased people and, allopathically, have tended to describe such now-you-see-it-now-you-don't bodies as *causes* of pathology.

(The speculated or visually inexplicable presence of tiny structures in the blood, seeming to appear and disappear, has given birth to several novel theories, aside from Wilhelm Reich's bions and Rife's "cancer virus."

(The late Dr. Virginia Livingston-Wheeler, continuing the work of several others, described a tiny particle she called *progenitor cryptocides* [ancestral hidden killer] as both the wellspring of disease and life.

(In later years, Canadian biologist Gaston Naessens, also updating the work of others, elaborated the theory of *somatids* — primitive life-forms beginning with minuscule spore-like structures — describing their pleomorphism as detectable through high-power microscopy and their relationship to disease. But somatids are also seemingly similar to, if not the same as, the *microzymas* described by France's Antoine Bechamp in the 19th century, and possibly the *protit*, a particle defined in this century by Germany's Guenther Enderlein.

(Involved in all such theories and research are the basic ideas of pleomorphism — even to the point of viruses and bacteria seemingly switching back and forth, with intermediate stops — and/or visual reflections of what some might call vibrational energy. They have had to be detected in powerful microscopes whose magnification/resolution powers are beyond the normal range — *incredibly* beyond them, skeptics would say — of most research microscopes.

(Our own research group also pioneered a high-resolution multiple-phase microscopy system which, particularly in dark-field, has visually, and at times transitorily, captured all manner of ill-defined and inexplicable bodies aswarm in the blood of diseased people. To a somatidist such structures are somatids; to followers of the "cancer microbe" theory they may be *progenitors* — who knows? Yet they are there, or at least are there part of the time. Understanding that a general rule in the development of radical scientific notions is that more often than not the genius is usually right, but for the wrong reason — and comes acropper because of theory when in fact it is *application*, as in medicine, which is important — the final explanation of what these infinitesimal forms are and what they are doing remains to be elucidated.)

In the 1960s, Antoine Priore, an Italian-born electrical genius who worked in France, demonstrated that he could overcome cancer with the "Priore ray," which allegedly altered magnetic fields.

The history of the harassment and persecution of Reich, Rife and Priore as well as the attacks on Tesla's theories is a lengthy, sad and at times disgusting accumulation of jealousy, perverted science and vested interests — of *scientism* hurled at unpopular proponents of unpopular beliefs under the guise of *science*, as occurred, on a lesser scale, with Immanuel Velikovsky (*IV*).

If Reich, Rife and Priore in general may have something in common besides a threat to vested energy interests and the politics which devolve therefrom, it would seem to be in their demonstration of the real nature of all matter: that it may be understood in electromagnetic terms; that all energy is, or ultimately is bound up in, electromagnetism; that both disease induction and healing may be understood from such a concept.

At the extreme end of this chain of thought is the obvious implication: if everything is energy and each individual could learn to harness it then there is suddenly an answer to problems of both energy in general and medicine in particular. Were even a small part of this true, then enormous industrial cartels — and dependence on government — would collapse.

But while Reich, Rife and Priore have been consigned to history's museum of interesting relics by the would-be rationalists of today's AIC, interest in electromagnetic fields and how they relate to health and healing keeps growing and flourishing.

Persons claiming to have "Rife instruments" and other "frequency machines" have peddled many a product to both the wary and unwary, and some of them, at least in some cases, and within a sea of hype and occasional outright charlatanry, seem to have "worked."

Interest in subtle energies and energy fields has also rekindled interest in applications of the known energies and hence reopened old debates.

In this vein there is renewed interest in the work of E. K. Knott, the probable father of ultraviolet irradiation of the blood.

In a provocative tome on a "trizoid" look at the American medical monolith, physician and cancer researcher Raymond K. Brown noted that Knott's UV approach, beginning in the 1920s, was demonstrated to be useful against viral and bacterial infections and inflammatory processes.

Wrote Brown:

For approximately twenty-five years, observations and results from several thousand patients were summarized and presented at medical meetings and in major medical journals; blood irradiation as a part of medical practice gradually died out when antibiotics and other products of modern technology appeared. Despite the formation of the Foundation for Irradiation, established by patients whose lives had been saved by the process and the physicians who had used it, irradiation of blood completely faded from the medical scene by the 1970s. At this time, the FDA was given the power to control all medical equipment and devices, so the possibility of a revival of blood irradiation in this country dissolved.[44]

Yet the AIDS plague has helped resuscitate it, and

scattered evidence suggests that UV treatment of blood is a useful way to rid it of pathogenic factors.

On both a terrifying yet scientifically absorbing scale, nuclear engineer and retired Army Lt. Col. Thomas E. Bearden has claimed that AIDS at the point of origin was actually a manmade disease "beamed into" the USA by Soviet scientists who, advancing the theories of Antoine Priore and others, had developed "phase conjugate, time-reversed scalar electromagnetic" weapons.[45]

Bearden, who updated the Priore work and similar research, in a 1993 open letter to the leaders of the American Foundation for AIDS Research, made both the astounding claim that by utilizing technological advances involving a new understanding of bioelectrical theory "the technical development of an AIDS cure should be possible in no more than three years" and that the former Soviets had used "microwave radiation" of US Embassy personnel in Moscow simply to see whether the Americans knew about Russian advances in the development of such weapons.

He also reprised the work in the former USSR of Vlail Kaznacheyev and associates who in 17,000 laboratory experiments were said to have shown that "essentially any kind of cellular death or disease pattern could be transmitted between cell cultures 'electromagnetically.'"

Wrote Bearden, whose 20-year Army career included specialization in air defense systems, tactical and technical intelligence, nuclear weapons, and research and development of Army missile systems:

> *The point here is that, from a fundamental physics viewpoint, it's just about all electromagnetics anyway, at the most fundamental level. But the quantum physicists are unaware of the earlier research work, and so are totally unaware that the physical structure, genetics, biochemistry, etc. of the living cell can in fact be directly engineered with the strange "new" kind of electromagnetics.*[46]

What is involved is a "'new', internal, hidden electromagnetics ... (a) fundamental extension to normal 'classical' electromagnetics that is of extraordinary importance to cellular healing," he wrote.

In his writings, Bearden has relayed the hitherto hidden history of competing theories of energy and the nature of matter, originating in the 19th century, indicating that many useful theories and approaches (particularly Priore's) were simply left unresolved or were squelched by establishment science.

If there is a "new, hidden electromagnetics" capable of uses far beyond the current understanding of physics, is the human mind closer to finding *prana* or *qi* in a demonstrable way? And, if so, are we nearing a "scientific breakthrough" which can explain the power of prayer and the capacity of healing through thought?

Bearden is not the only scientist associated directly or indirectly with the space program who has made contributions to a deeper understanding of energy and matter.

In 1968, Adrian V. Clark, a researcher associated with the Saturn V Moon Vehicle project of the National Aeronautics and Space Administration (NASA), adduced that the ultimate capability of man may be the controlling of matter through the energy of thought — that is, the "intellectual control of molecular motion."[47]

Clark was enamored of the suggestions of new concepts of energy and existence posed — as some investigators would have it — by the seemingly inexplicable phenomena attributed to unidentified flying objects (UFOs), perhaps the greatest unresolved scientific conundrum of the century, as well as by clues in the Bible as to the nature of energy and the universe.

Bearden, Clark and others are modern-era thinkers with credible backgrounds who understand energy and nature-of-matter concepts at variance with the scientific orthodoxy of our day — one, as we know from even recent history, susceptible of 180-degree turns and causing profound befuddlement. Cosmological concepts in general and quantum mechanics in particular are racing well ahead of Western rationalist science and have opened new vistas as to what may be the very nature of existence.

Toward the final link

In areas that seem less threatening and more comfortable to the ensconced orthodoxy, many scientific thinkers increasingly are describing the human body as a closed electrical system. There is, as some put it, truly a "body electric" or an "electro-vibratory body" which defines the physical aspect of the human and which, by definition, at some point impinges upon the subtle energies which in turn may be universal in nature.[48]

The link between body, mind, bioelectricity and subtle energy will eventually be sufficiently "quantified" to satisfy the proof requirements of the West while accommodating the intuitive truths of the East.

As this occurs, not only will the power of prayer be set forth in a comprehensible manner but it will become clear why meditation and simply thinking good thoughts — and the healing capacity of human touch — "work" in medicine.

The wheel will have come around full circle — the holistic paradigm which guided ancient medicine will have been restored in a new era. Mind-body-spirit will be seen as interdependent parts of a greater reality.

Perhaps by then it will be said that man better understands his relationship with God.

References

1. *The Choice*, XVIII: 2, 1992.
2. Baker, Elizabeth, *The UnMedical Miracle — Oxygen*. Indianola WA: Delwood Communications, 1992.
3. Bradford, RW, et al., *Exogenous Oxidative Mechanisms in Combating Infectious Diseases*. Chula Vista CA: The Bradford Foundation, 1986.
4. Culbert, ML, *AIDS: Hope, Hoax and Hoopla*, Chula Vista CA: The Bradford Foundation, 1990.
5. Kuhnau, WW, *Live Cell Therapy: My Life with a Medical Breakthrough*. Tijuana, Mexico: Artes Graficas, 1983.
6. Culbert, ML, *Live Cell Therapy for the 21st Century*. Chula Vista CA: The Bradford Foundation, 1994.
7. Bradford, RW, et al., *The Biochemical Basis of Live Cell Therapy*. Chula Vista CA: The Bradford Foundation, 1986.
8. Culbert, ML, *Live Cell, op. cit.*
9. Dossey, Larry, *Healing Words: The Power of Prayer and the Practice of Medicine*. New York: Harper, 1993.
10. Greengard, Samuel, "Doctor says prayer can be an essential part of cure." *American Medical News*, Dec. 20, 1993.
11. Siegel, Bernie, *Love, Medicine and Miracles*. New York: Harper and Row, 1986.

12. Greengard, *op. cit.*
13. Kent, Jaylene, *et al.*, "Unexpected recoveries: spontaneous remission and immune functioning." *Advances* (Institute for the Advancement of Health), VI:2, 1989.
14. Weinstock, Charles, "Recent progress in cancer psychobiology and psychiatry." *J. Am. Soc. Psychosom. Dent. & Med.* 24, 1977.
15. Rogers, MP, *et al.*, "The influence of the psyche and the brain on immunity and disease susceptibility: a critical review." *Psychosom. Med.* 41, 1979.
16. Holmes, TH, *et al.*, "Psychosocial and physiological studies of tuberculosis." *Psychosom. Med.* 19, 1957.
17. Dohrenwend, BS, and Dohrenwend, BP, eds., *Stressful Life Events; Their Nature and Effects.* New York: Wiley, 1974.
18. Minter, RE, and Kimball, CP, "Life events and illness onset: a review." *Psychosomatics* 19, 1978.
19. Kobasa, SC, "Stressful life events, personality and health: an inquiry into hardiness." *J. Pers. & Soc. Psychol.* 37, 1979.
20. Greer, S, and Pettingale, KW, "Psychological response to breast cancer: effect on outcome." *Lancet* 11, 1979.
21. Levy, SM, *Behavior and Cancer.* San Francisco: Jossey-Bass, 1985.
22. Cousins, Norman *Anatomy of an Illness.* New York: Norton, 1979.
23. Cousins, Norman, *The Healing Heart.* New York: Norton, 1983.
24. Regan, B, and Hershberg, C, *Spontaneous Remission: An Annotated Biography,* Sausalito CA: Institute of Noetic Sciences, 1993.
25. *Powers of Healing.* Alexandria VA: Time-Life Books, 1989.
26. Leshan, Lawrence, *You Can Fight for Your Life: Emotional Factors in the Causation of Cancer.* New York: Evans, 1977.
27. Grady, Denise, "AIDS survivors." *American Health,* September 1988.
28. Solomon, GE, *Psychoneuroimmunology.* New York: Academic Press, 1987.
29. Gelman, David, and Hager, Mary, "Body and Soul." *Newsweek,* Nov. 7, 1988.
30. Cited in Culbert, *AIDS, op. cit.*
31. *The Choice,* XIX: 3,4, 1993.
32. *Orange County Register,* in *The Choice,* XX:1, 1994.
33. Gordon, JS, "Healing with feeling." *The Washington Post,* August 29, 1993.
34. Simonton, Carl, *et al., Getting Well Again.* New York: Bantam, 1986.
35. Achterberg, Jeanne, *Imagery in Healing: Shamanism and Modern Medicine.* Boston: New Science Library, 1985.
36. Cited in *The Choice,* XIV: 3, 1988.
37. "Homeopathy: much ado about nothing?" *Consumer Reports,* March 1994.
38. *Ibid.*
39. *Ibid.*
40. Jacobs, J, *et al.*, "Treatment of acute childhood diarrhea with homeopathic medicine: a randomized clinical trial in Nicaragua." *Pediatrics* 93, 1994.
41. Berkowitz, CD, "Homoeopathy: keeping an open mind." *Lancet,* Sept. 10, 1994.
41a. Reilly, David, *et al.*, "Is evidence for homoeopathy reproducible?" *Lancet,* Dec. 10, 1994.
41b. Philpott, WH, *Cancer: the Magnetic/Oxygen Answer.* Choctaw OK, 1994.
41c. Aharonov, Y, and Bohm, D, "Significance of electromagnetic potentials in quantum theory." Cited in Philpott, *op. cit.*
41d. Becker, RO, and Seldon, G, *The Body Electric: Electro-Magnetism and the Foundation of Life.* New York: Morrow Co., 1986.
42. *Powers of Healing, op. cit.*
43. Lynes, Barry, *The Cancer Cure that Worked!* Toronto: Marcus Books, 1987.
44. Brown, RK, *AIDS, Cancer and the Medical Establishment.* New York: Speller, 1986.
45. Bearden, TE, *AIDS: Biological Warfare.* Greenville TX: Tesla Book Co. 1988. Also, Bearden, TE, "Soviet phase conjugate weapons (weapons that use time-reversed electromagnetic waves)." *Bulletin of the Committee to Restore the Constitution,* January 1988. Cited in Culbert, *AIDS, op. cit.*
46. Bearden, TE. Open letter to Elizabeth Taylor and Dr. Mathilde Krim. *Bulletin of the Committee to Restore the Constitution.* September 1993.
47. Clark, AV, *Cosmic Mysteries of the Universe.* West Nyack NY: Parker, 1968.
48. Beasley, Victor, *Your Electro-Vibratory Body.* Boulder Creek CO: University of the Trees Press, 1978.

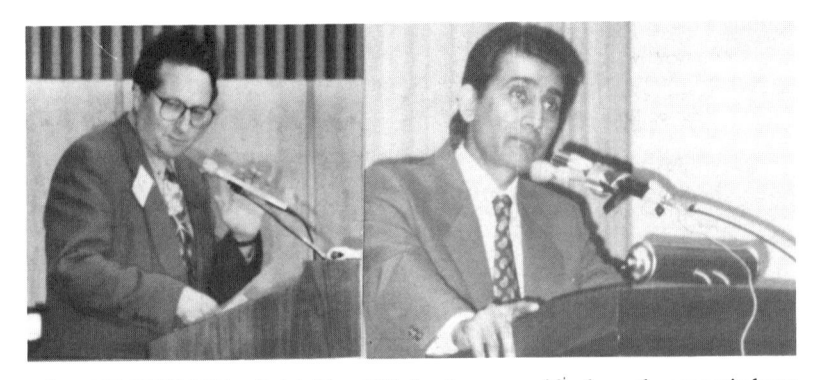

FOR NEW THOUGHT — Ralph Moss PhD, L, whose exposé books on the cancer industry have helped lead the fight for change. Columbia's Ali Majid MD, R, arguing strongly for a new medical evaluative model. — Mike Culbert photos

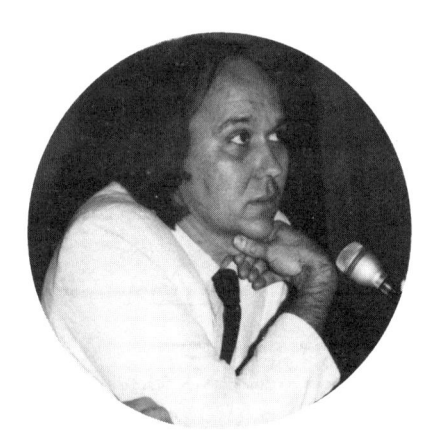

People Against Cancer's Frank Wiewel: spurring evaluation of "unorthodox" cancer treatments

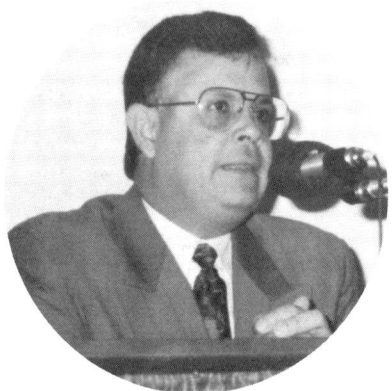

American Biologics-Mexico's Rodrigo Rodriguez MD: applying integrative protocols against disease

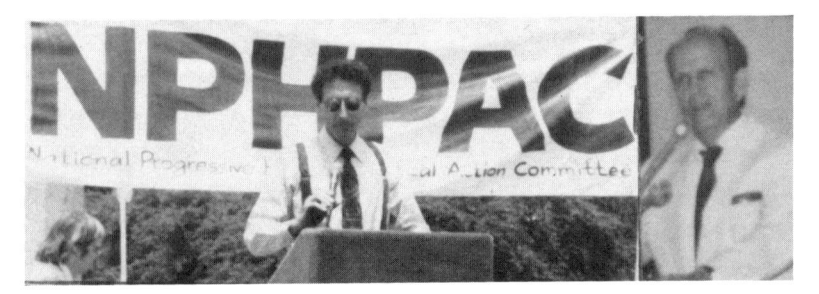

ACTIVISTS — New York radio commentator Gary Null, L, carries freedom-of-choice message to a Washington rally; at R, long-time lobbyist Clinton R. Miller, National Council for Improved Health (NCIH), makes a point. — Mike Culbert photos

618

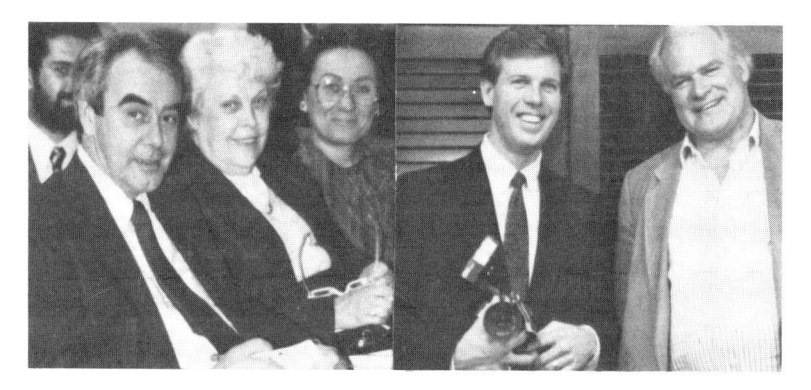

PIONEERS FOR CHANGE — Left photo, L to R, the late Bob DeBragga, who founded Project Cure; Marie Steinmeyer, president, IACVF; long-time health-rights activist Catherine Frompovich; right photo, L, freedom-of-choice advocate and attorney Mike Evers and, R, CANHELP's Patrick McGrady. — Mike Culbert photos

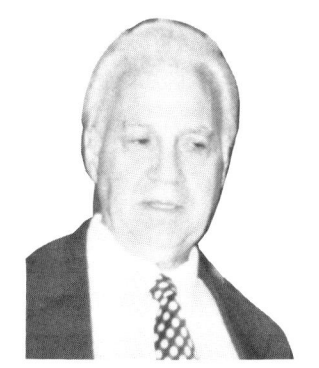

Former US Congressman and Staten Island Borough President Guy Molinari, who brought "alternatives" to congressional attention

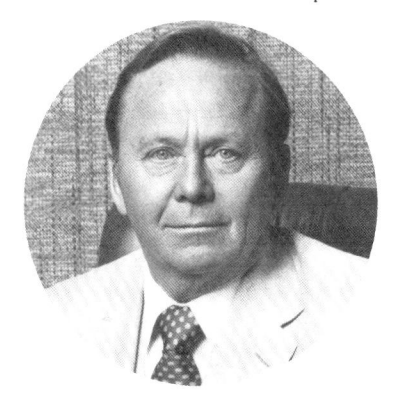

Dr. Robert W. Bradford, pioneer of oxidology, advanced medical microscopy, fighter for medical freedom of choice

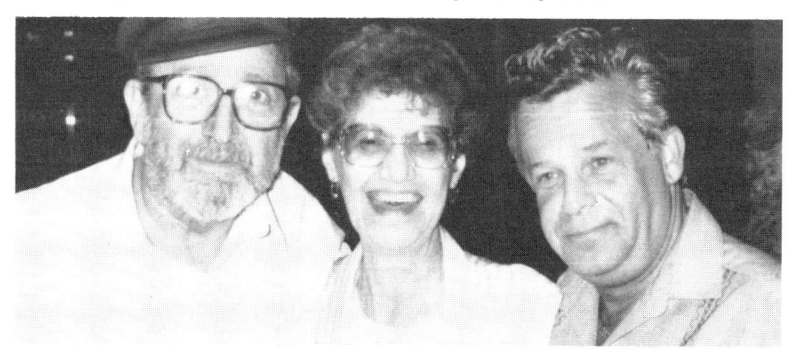

COMPARING NOTES — At L, Harold and Arline Brecher, key authors of chelation (and other) books; at R, medical writer/activist Michael L. Culbert, as the three met at pre-OAM meetings in Virginia. — Richard Cotten photos

VOLUME IV

APPENDIX A: Solving the healthcare crisis while rescuing liberty   **623**

APPENDIX B: The Committee for Freedom of Choice in Medicine Inc. plan for healthcare reform   **629**

    Addendum re: *Federal/State conspiracies against physicians, the healthfoods industry, and related matters*

APPENDIX C: Model state-level legislation for medical freedom of choice   **653**

APPENDIX D: Resources   **655**

INDEX   **669**

APPENDIX A

SOLVING THE HEALTHCARE CRISIS WHILE

RESCUING LIBERTY

An American challenge

In the final decade of this century, it is evident that the healthcare system of the United States is failing on various fronts:

— Despite its earlier success against infectious disease and the development of the most advanced biomedical high technology in the world, it seems utterly unable to curb the exponential growth of chronic diseases and multifactorial disorders, most of them the results of civilization. Such disorders now pose a threat to the survival of the species itself.

— Because of its mechanical successes in increasing overall life extension (if maintenance of one or more viable life systems is itself the extension of "life" rather than the prolongation of death) it has helped increase the numbers of people most apt to be affected by the chronic disorders of civilization.

— It is unable to evaluate new medical techniques and approaches because it is conceptually held hostage to an essentially unworkable paradigm — allopathic medicine — in which monotherapy, single causes, treatment by opposites and linear thought are the philosophical anchors. And the paradigm is, in turn, held hostage to vested economic interests.

— Increasing numbers of the population simply cannot afford the system even if they wish to utilize it.

Any number of politicians and social critics would have us believe that the answer is in the social distribution of the system, *not* in the philosophical essence of the system itself.

They hence have attempted to narrow the debate to being one of "universal healthcare" (socialized medicine) vs. private healthcare.

While this study has explained that what the United States currently has is a hybrid most classifiable as *fascist* medicine, it should be clear that the political issue of how healthcare is to be made available is separate and apart from the *nature* of medicine:

While it is certainly true that most civilized countries have a form of socialized medicine (though many, such as Germany, allow freedom of choice for other medical models not "covered" by the state), there is no correlation between the method of healthcare delivery and the implied goal of any system: delivery of good health.

No greater a model for socialized medicine existed than in the prior Soviet Union (and indeed, in all socialist-bloc states) — yet the rates of chronic, systemic diseases and metabolic disorders were as bad — and at times worse — in the USSR than in any Western nation.

As we have seen (*VII*), the United Kingdom's long-time flirtation with socialized medicine on a population base far inferior to that of the United States not only has failed to significantly curb degenerative diseases but has led to cries for reform there, including far more assent by the status quo to "complementary" therapies in that country than in ours.

Do not look to Canada

Americans who look to Canada should also be aware that, whatever the successes of Canada in redistributing the cost of medicine (while hiking taxes) so that it is of universal access, increasingly Canadian medics and citizens have opted out of the system:

— In 1994, most of the 23,000 doctors in Ontario, Canada's most populous province, took a one-week "vacation" without pay because the Canadian healthcare system could not afford to pay them for a full year.[1]

— In 1993, a record number of Canadian doctors — 650 — moved to the United States, while thousands of nursing graduates were said to be "flocking south" in search of greener fields. Why not? They had taken a 2 percent pay cut and hospital staffs faced reductions across the country.[2]

— More affluent Canadians, frustrated over long lines and long waits, routinely slip across the border for therapy in the USA. The Fraser Institute reported that 177,297 Canadians were on waiting lists for surgery in 1992, and that, as in Newfoundland, there were two-month waits for patients seeking

CAT scans and two-month delays for women needing "urgent" pap smears.[3]

In 1994, it was reported that a tenth of the 40,000 hospital beds in Toronto had been closed in the past three years due to funding shortages.[4]

Any governmental health system (as we have seen in Medicare and Medicaid in this country) faces the same problems:

— Availability and funding at the whim of master planners and politicians. In totalitarian societies, access to "free medicine" is a political function, so that dissidents (enemies of the state) may be denied such service.

— Increased demand (much of it from hypochondriacs and the chronically ill) will *always* exceed availability with the concomitant problems of ever-increasing waiting periods and rationed medical services.

— Caregivers will be either chronically overworked or even underworked, depending on where they are, with an increase in frustration and inattentiveness.

It cannot be stressed enough that international pharmaceutical interests, the motor of the allopathic paradigm, essentially do not care *what* the medical system is politically as long as it remains drug-dependent. The drug behemoths will be paid whether the payer is the patient, an insurance company or the government.

Comparing the United States with small, homogeneous countries in the distribution of healthcare services, as frequently done by proponents of socialized medicine, is a case of mixing apples and oranges.

Centralized planning, control and distribution are easier, even more effective, in small-population countries even if, over time, the same problems giant nation-states face with centralized planning will occur.

We would strongly argue that the urge to centralize control and planning, however seemingly rational and convenient it may seem for the short-term resolution of problems of social organization, is the central flaw in collective political thought which ineluctably leads to tyranny.

Liberty vs. central planning

This is because of the historically long observed phenomenon that there can be no effective central planning without an equal portion of central compliance — and that centralized compliance is the wellspring of political tyranny. The criminal actions of this nation's Food and Drug Administration (FDA) against "alternative" healers and their patients is a stark and unforgiving manifestation of this basic truth.

There are those who would argue that, by the end of the 20th century, it is somehow too late to argue about the relevance of giant government in the management and ultimate control of our lives (including all decisions on healthcare) — that the sands of time have irreversibly blown in the direction of gigantic governments, gigantic corporations, gigantic planning.

But some of us beg to differ. It is extremely unlikely that human liberty — assuming this to be a worthwhile goal at all — can flower in a collectivistic, big-government statist environment, no matter what the excuses or pretexts for such gargantuan governance are.

The framers of the American republic — frequently dismissed in the modern era as well-meaning gentleman agrarian aristocrats who could not foresee the eventual need for huge government to "manage" everything — were far shrewder than the historical revisionists give them credit for.

They fully understood the need not to further unleash the government and to put chains on the people but to free the people and place chains on the government. That — originally — was what this country was all about.

By the mid-1990s, as the nation remained in a raging debate over the healthcare crisis, at least several of the States had taken steps to attempt to impose healthcare reform within their borders — a decentralist move in keeping with the spirit of the US Constitution.

Others were moving to protect medical practitioners who

engaged in "alternative therapy" — a state-by-state effort redolent of that which in the 1970s and early 1980s had led to the "decriminalization" of laetrile in 24 states. (See *XII*).

That effort had demonstrated how a grass-roots, *decentralist* activity could rapidly outpace central planners and the central (federal) government. This constitutionally republicanist effort vindicated the wisdom of the Founding Fathers and proved to Americans that liberty in general was still rescuable.

In 1993, the Committee for Freedom of Choice in Medicine Inc. presented a conceptual program to the Clinton Administration as a model for an attempt at healthcare reform for earth's mightiest power within both the spirit and letter of the US Constitution.

The program (Appendix B) is a suggested mingling of federal and state actions to defang both governmental *and* private monopoly and to restore medical freedom of choice — with informed consent — for physician and patient, the single guiding doctrine of the Committee.

For if — in keeping with the spirit of the Constitution — the people and their healthcare practitioners (of *any* school) have access to freedom of choice in medicine the political barriers to medical reform will have ended and a free people can get about the business of a new paradigm:

The promotion of health.

References

1. Jacobson, Sherry, *The Dallas Morning News*. Feb. 27, 1994.
2. *Ibid.*
3. Lee, RW, "Should we copy Canada?" *The New American*. Nov. 1, 1993.
4. Jacobson, *op. cit.*

APPENDIX B

THE COMMITTEE FOR FREEDOM OF CHOICE IN MEDICINE INC. PLAN FOR HEALTHCARE REFORM

(Presented February 19, 1993, to the Presidential Task Force on Healthcare Reform)

Dear Chairperson Clinton:

The Committee for Freedom of Choice in Medicine, Inc. takes this opportunity to congratulate you on your appointment and to extend our best wishes as well as our ideas on the urgent need for healthcare reform in America.

You are aware of the healthcare crisis in this nation. Synthesizing our organization's views and suggestions on (a) the nature of this crisis and (b) how it may be managed and, hopefully, solved, we set forth the following:

THE PROBLEM(S): The extraordinarily high cost of medical care (to the extent that between 37 and 40 million Americans are unable to afford medical coverage) which will assume a constant-dollars total cost of $1 trillion by mid-decade and already consumes 15 percent of gross domestic product (GDP), while the existing medical structure is essentially a failure in coming to grips with the modern chronic killer diseases, now poised to destroy Western civilization.

GOALS: To solve the above while enhancing overall access by the public to achieving promotive health through the availability of options and choices within a political model which respects the virtues of Constitutional republicanism without enhancing the grasp and reach of government.

SOLUTIONS TO THE PROBLEM(S)

— Replacing the current allopathic paradigm with an integrative model in which all medical approaches are assured a level playing field.

— Decentralizing medical decision-making so that the States may assume greater burdens and their own innovations in the matter of licensure, surveillance, sanction and insurance. (President Clinton, at least rhetorically, has suggested this in terms of the diffusion of Medicare/Medicaid.)

— Dismantling the Food and Drug Administration (FDA) as currently constituted.

— Protecting consumer access to dietary and nutrient supplements as first-line preventive maintenance health options and allowing honest and accurate health claims to be made about them by producers and distributors.

— Providing tax incentives for corporate structures and companies to establish promotive-health programs and/or private group medical plans.

— Enhancing antitrust and racketeering enforcement against organizational and professional combines which seek to prevent the free interstate flow of medical information and/or to monopolize the medical marketplace for a single school of medical thought.

This endeavor implies a paradigm shift from emphasizing management of disease and the prolongation of death to encouraging promotive health. Politically, this means a vast decentralization on the federalist model, with the States assuming far more individual and creative responsibilities, the resurrection of an authentic free market of competitive medical ideas (thus an end to the Allopathic Industrial Complex/monopoly), a dismantling of the frequently corrupt Food and Drug Administration (FDA) or a rewriting of its enabling legislation to capture the original intent of establishing responsible surveillance over the purity (and labeling honesty) of foods and drugs.

Decentralizing medicine to the States and allowing States to assume many more of the functions of existing federal programs should vastly eliminate the bureaucratic paperwork gridlock at the top which is itself a significant contributor to our (currently) $900 billion healthcare tab. The overall economic goal: vast reduction in the cost of healthcare delivery.

Such a shift also implies empowering the general population (medical consumers) to make first-line or primary decisions on their health and well-being through access to a free market of medical practitioners of their choice as well as access to health-oriented products consisting of vitamins, minerals, amino acids, enzymes, herbs and/or any combination of the above, along with such parallel State-level developments as the legalization of midwifery and consumer-level nutritional counselors.

State-level legislative action (if necessary) should in effect persuade private insurers to provide fair and equal coverage of *all* forms of competitive medicine with the view in mind of vastly reducing the cost of medicine through free-market forces and hence lowering the cost of private medical insurance. Existing federal insurance schemes, however currently bloated and out of control (Medicare, Medicaid), should gradually be diffused in power, administration and authority to the States, with federal funds (matching or otherwise) available solely as safety-net operations for the most disadvantaged.

The IRS code should allow for tax incentives for companies and corporations for group private insurance plans.

Parallel to these developments, the nation's pharmaceutical industry should be congressionally investigated along the lines of domestic monopolism, restraint of trade, racketeering and, if necessary, legislatively trust-busted to allow for the competition of smaller firms involved in the research, development and distribution of medically oriented products. This investigation should look deeply into the international aspects of the major pharmaceutical companies with emphasis on monopolism, price-fixing, restraint of trade and racketeering, along with whatever conflict-of-interest relationships as may exist between pharmaceutical companies, the FDA and other federal and State governmental agencies.

Equal enforcement efforts should be mounted against any professional organization or combination of organizations, societies or individuals who or which are involved in restricting the free flow of information concerning medical products, medical theories and treatment practices for reasons of exclusion or monopoly, or who or which utilize positions of privilege to defame, malign, vilify or intimidate individuals, organizations or enterprises for reasons of exclusion or monopolism.

At the federal and State levels there should be an immediate end to the multi-agency harassment of medical practitioners and/or healthfoods and supplement companies who or which make honest claims on their products simply because the former may be practicing "non-mainstream" medicine or because the latter represent an economic threat to the allopathic industrial complex.

NATURE AND CAUSES OF THE PROBLEM(S)

The generic root of the problems lies in two of the great defining elements of human nature (greed and ego, with a greater proportion of the former than the latter) which devolve into these aspects:

— The primacy of a single model of medical thought, a paradigm which has guided American and therefore Western medicine for the better part of a century. This model, *allopathy* — which is usually what the existing American medical/pharmaceutical establishment actually means when it utilizes such terms as "mainstream", "orthodox", "conventional" and even "rigorously scientific" medicine, and even by use of the exclusive term "medicine" itself (the same establishment having also co-opted the term "physician" while indirectly attempting to appropriate "doctor") — has driven from the field all competitors in the ideological and conceptual marketplace except for those which have achieved partial rescue through legal action (chiropractic) and others which survive as allopathic hybrids (osteopathy).

So sweeping and total has been the genesis and nurturing of this paradigm that the majority of American medical practices/products consumers are not aware that there are other schools of legitimate medical thought. Allopathic medicine is that which is protected by sanction and licensure, with only trained allopaths accorded full access to patients and only allopaths bearing full hospital access. The allopathic model or paradigm is sustained and buttressed by the media and so interlocked with related vested interests that what is or is not "medicine" is often obscured in the public mind.

— The use or capture of this particular model of medical thought by international pharmaceutical interests. Extensive data detail the rise of drug-based medicine in this country (and elsewhere) as parallel to the enshrining of the allopathic model as the single healing paradigm to be accorded sanction and licensure in the United States. Several historical trends converged in the first two decades of the present century to allow the profit-driven pharmaceutical combines to utilize allopathy as a channel for their products (while, to be sure, assisting in notable victories over infectious disease) and to dominate "medical" education and "medical" literature. A huge role in this effort was played by the amassed-wealth foundations of several ultrawealthy families whose profits were protected by the tax-free foundation scheme while protected funds were deflected into such educational, research and propaganda measures as would build what is today the Allopathic Industrial Complex.

This complex (of interlocking pharmaceutical houses, research centers, universities, corporations, companies, hospitals, insurance plans, medications, drugs, hospital equipment, high-technology diagnostics) is so intertwined with corporate America (transportation, publishing, utilities, department stores, energy, etc., etc.) that lines of demarcation between the Allopathic Industrial Complex itself and its overlap with this broader complex, and the multitude of interests influenced by, or dependent upon it, may explain the seemingly ubiquitous presence of the allopathic medical paradigm and its seemingly wide acceptance by the consuming public.

— The American Medical Association (AMA), which actually grew out of mid-19th-century efforts to organize the "regulars" (that is, allopathic dispensers of minerals and surgery) against the "irregulars" (primarily the homeopaths, who represented both a conceptual and economic threat to the regulars), which has become the organized voice not of medicine itself but of allopathy, constituting in effect a labor union for allopathic physicians and an ongoing propaganda voice for the concept of "scientific medicine" (essentially an oxymoron, in that until this century medicine was essentially conceived of as an art rather than a science).

AMA is the education-orienting force of allopathy whose "seal of approval" on techniques, theories and products is the ever-present guiding hand of the medical establishment. Its ruthless efforts to suppress competitors only became fully public in the 1980s with the federal court victory by chiropractors against the AMA and its allies.

State medical boards, state "medical quality assurance" boards, state medical vigilance and punishment boards, are comprised in the main of AMA members. State-level AMAs constitute major political action committees (PACs) in every state and, in sum, constitute one of the major federal lobbying forces at the legislative level. It is perhaps more than symbolic that the *Journal* of the AMA is laden, cover to cover, with high-tech advertisements from the very international/pharmaceutical behemoths whose gargantuan profits depend on the primacy of the allopathic model.

— The Food and Drug Administration (FDA), an example of a good governmental idea gone woefully wrong. The "compliance" wing of this bloated federal satrapy has been used time and again in recent decades to suppress, harass, prosecute, persecute and intimidate the burgeoning healthfoods and supplements industries (which the Allopathic Industrial Complex regards as a major threat), as well as healthcare practitioners of all kinds (including progressive allopaths) who dare abandon the key elements of allopathy (surgery, radiation, toxic chemicals, invasive techniques, awesomely expensive diagnostics).

MDs, chiropractors, naturopaths, homeopaths, herbalists, Native American healers, acupuncturists, and even midwives have been among targets of the FDA and compliant State agencies involved in an ongoing conspiracy to punish medical rebels and protect the profits of the pharmaceutical industry. The attached litany of recent FDA-associated actions against individuals, companies and organizations constitutes a shameful and viciously tyrannical chapter in American history, and the most dispassionate review of FDA "compliance" behavior should indicate how far afield this bureaucracy-for-life has strayed from its original enabling legislation as a monitor of safety and purity in foods and drugs. As presently constituted, the FDA, compliance division, is little more than a police force for drug interests and, as recent history has shown, has often been corrupted.

CURRENT SITUATION

The above synthesis of the situation, and the out-of-control costs of delivering the allopathic medical product (with its attendant swollen prices in medicines, diagnostics, practices, etc.) would very likely be well tolerated by our people if in fact we were receiving value in kind. A synthesis of the current medical reality, however, discloses that we are not:

Despite the costliest medical establishment in the world, the United States has no cure for *most* of metastatic cancer, *all* of AIDS, and even much of that complex of conditions referred to as "heart disease", and is *24th* in infant mortality. It stands impuissant in the face of an ever-lengthening list of allegedly incurable maladies of the young and old: cystic fibrosis, muscular dystrophy, lupus, rheumatoid arthritis, multiple sclerosis, Parkinson's, Alzheimer's's, chronic fatigue, ALS, osteoporosis, and a veritable maze of conditions and metabolic disorders unknown earlier in this century.

Despite increases in overall life expectancy, allopathy's earlier triumphs over major infections and improvements in sophisticated diagnostic techniques, this nation has not a health-care delivery system so much as a death-prolonging "sick business". A few extra years of physical existence achieved by electronic hookup and stultifying drugs can only vaguely be defined as "life".

It is because so many Americans are increasingly informed of the above that they are turning — in droves, as recent information now proves — to so-called "alternative" or "unconventional" therapies. They first seek these out in the United States — that is, when their practitioner is not too afraid to provide them and who may risk his/her professional and social standing and medical license by so doing. Yet because the Allopathic Industrial Complex is so vast and nationwide in scope it is difficult to find healthcare givers in *any* State who are not in some way (be it statutorily or professionally) hamstrung in their efforts to provide more choices for our ever-sicker population (one member of which dies every 60 seconds from cancer).

With the compliant media also interlocked with the allopathic industrial complex and the allopathic model the only one seemingly operative at the conscious level in the minds of so many journalists, American medical consumers are often left either uninformed or ill-informed about available medical options and are, at the least, socially pressured into acceptance of the standard medical system even if it means certain death and suffering. Hence, should they be adequately informed and economically advantaged, they seek healthcare outside their home country. The Hobson's choice for an American with a life-threatening disorder who seeks "alternatives" to allopathy is simple: do without, attempt to go underground and locate a practitioner willing to place himself in jeopardy, or flee the country.

As these lines are written, no less than 30 clinics, hospitals and other operations claiming to offer "alternative medicine" and serving a clientele made up of up to 90% or more Americans now function in the area of Tijuana, Mexico, alone. This is a giant leap from a decade ago, when American medical and pharmaceutical front groups ("quackbusters") began their noisy if failing campaign to "alert" Americans to "quackery" and "quack clinics". While many of these operations are indeed suspect and some are outright frauds, in their totality they reflect the abject failure of American medicine against chronic degenerative disease. Studies continue to point out that Americans who seek "alternative" therapies either at home or abroad are, in the main, among the better-educated of our citizens.

There is no moral reason why an American citizen should have to leave this country to save his/her life! There is no *good* reason (though there are many *bad* ones) why an American with a life-threatening disease should have to face the prospect of being abandoned by this country and its medical establishment in an effort — however remote — to save his/her life.

SOLUTIONS: AN OVERVIEW

Approaches to this problem run the gamut of political theory, and it is not the Committee's position that any single individual or organization has a total solution. But we add here both suggestions and recommendations.

1. Socializing medicine (that is, establishing the federal government as a single payer) is not the solution if we are seeking promotive health for the general population. A socialist system might take the immediate sting out of medical costs for a majority of people, but history is eloquent in displaying how the costs of government in general rise when *any* presumed right is guaranteed and/or nurtured by the government. Western countries with socialist and semi-socialist systems have the same (and at times worse) rates of chronic disease as does the United States.

The role of the federal government in assuming medical care (if it be the nation's will that government should play any such role) should be, at best, what it often already is in several areas: safety net of last resort when all else fails. That is, neither the paying for nor setting forth the treatment parameters of healthcare should be mandated from top-down; rather they should rise, albeit disproportionately, from the ground up.

2. A free market in medicine is the proper goal of a republican society which also engages in competitive (rather than monopolist) capitalism. With the cancer and AIDS crises alone poised to wipe out not only American civilization but the Western gene pool itself, the times cry out not for more restrictive adherence to a set of postulates and doctrines which have plainly failed (as in allopathic medicine) but for the encouragement of the broadest possible field of options and ideas. If there is a federal role in this paradigm shift, it should be as a stated policy, not a new statute to be exercised by yet

another tax-enhancing bureaucracy. In the federalist mold, that of our Constitution, the manner in which a free market is approached should be at the State level.

WHAT THE STATES CAN DO

The States might undertake legislatively several changes:

1. It may not be necessary to license physicians at all. The licensure procedure itself is prone to corrupting influences.

2. But degrees from qualified (and state-licensed) medical schools (of all concepts) should be necessary for the practice of any form of medicine.

3. State legislation (as has already occurred in Alaska and Washington) should protect the right of *all* qualified practitioners to engage in putatively "unorthodox" or "non-mainstream" medical practices under the following qualifications:

   a. That the condition be life-threatening (though some States might waive this qualification).

   b. That the procedure, treatment or compound *itself* not be dangerous to the patient.

   c. That the practitioner discuss all known available options with the patient.

4. Existing medical insurance plans should not discriminate in reimbursing for medical services as long as the qualified practitioner and patient have made an informed-consent decision for the service.

5. There should be freedom on the part of all qualified practitioners of all schools of medicine to advertise for their services and freely compete for consumers within the statutory and regulatory confines of an orderly profession.

6. State medical boards of oversight, compliance/regulation, etc., should be composed of representatives of *all* forms of medicine practicing within that State.

Each State may view differently the issue of licensing midwives and allowing therapeutic abortions. The intent here is to decentralize medicine from its allopathic center to allow a broad range of options, which are both therapeutically and economically competitive. It is also assumed the States will continue to enforce statutes on the safety and purity of drugs, nutrients and medical equipment.

WHAT THE FEDERAL LEVEL CAN DO

At the federal level, real change could be accomplished swiftly in a single stroke (as suggested in 1992 at the "working group on unconventional medical practices" of the National Institutes of Health) by:

1. Removing the so-called Kefauver amendments ("efficacy clauses") of the Food, Drug and Cosmetic Act as amended in 1962. The language in the above equipped the FDA with enormous policing/compliance power, virtually all of it used *against* non-allopathic therapies and the healthfoods and supplements industries. The amendments allow the state to intervene in the doctor-patient relationship at precisely the point it should not: freedom of choice of both to reach an informed decision on therapy. Only the doctor and patient, working together, are in any real position to know what does or does not have "efficacy". In addition:

2. The food-purity aspects of the FDA might be transferred to the US Department of Agriculture.

And, however a new food and drug law is to be rewritten, it should be clear that:

3. No agency shall use the fact that a valid health claim is made on the label of a food, food supplement, nutrient, herbal or similar product as a pretext to attempt to monitor or control the same as a "drug".

4. Therapeutically high doses of vitamins, minerals, enzymes, amino acids, herbal compounds and similar products might be statutorily protected at both the federal and State levels by classifying them as "nutraceuticals", as suggested by several distinguished American researchers.

5. The primary federal research parameter for acceptance of a new drug, technique or practice should be one:

Disease-free survival time.

This does not preclude a reasonable review of foreign literature for non-American products seeking access to the American market, nor an end to limited testing on animals for toxicity of certain compounds. The reliance on animal test models and the numbing persistence of the monofactorial, randomized, placebo-controlled, double-blind cross-over approach may still have some merit in the toxicity assessments of single therapeutics but is essentially irrelevant in the development of multifactorial, natural therapies for individualized use in humans.

The presence of 17th-century "rigorously scientific" postulates for monopharmacy has been a major roadblock — together with the enormous costs of developing the same through FDA channels — in the elaboration both of new single compounds and certainly in the advent of individualized, multifactorial protocols against chronic disease.

The IRS code should be revised to allow for tax incentives for companies, corporations and other business structures and/or labor unions or any other business or professional or bureaucratic organization or combination to establish promotive-health programs for employees, members, associates or shareholders and/or to encourage such entities to provide, at least as partial payment, private-enterprise group medical coverage.

Such coverage should not discriminate on the basis of a given medical theory or school of thought and should include payment for the services of all recognized healthcare practitioners whose validity or certification may be determined by the individual States.

The IRS code should be changed, if necessary, to provide tax incentives for the elderly, the retired, or the elderly retired on fixed incomes, to seek out private medical insurance coverage (as a way to shift significant elements of the population off Medicare, Medicaid, etc.)

There should be an inducement at the federal level for insurance companies to explain billing procedures in a uniform way and to attempt as far as feasible to set fair, understandable, acceptable and provable rates for all those covered regardless of the State or Territory in which they live, notwithstanding the insurance company's conceivably legitimate explanation of why rates might have to vary from one locale to another.

The costs and administration of Medicare, Medicaid and any other similar federal program should be transferred increasingly and over time to the States on a State-by-State basis.

Coverage by Medicare, Medicaid or any other federal program should not discriminate on the basis of medical schools of thought and medical theories. Such programs should not discriminate in coverage between health practitioners as duly and separately certified, licensed or accepted based on the separate provisions of the States, Territories or the District of Columbia.

The Veterans Administration and/or any federal agency or department involved in healthcare delivery should not discriminate on the basis of medical schools of thought and medical theories.

It should be clear that the will of the nation is that no existing federal law, bureau or department has been or will be established to engage directly in the practice of medicine.

There should be a Congressional-level investigation of possible price-fixing activities and monopolism within the pharmaceutical industry, an overview of the domestic industry's links with international pharmaceutical conglomerates, and an investigation of the pharmaceutical industry's relations, particularly involving conflicts of interest and retirement policies, with federal and State governments, and of the lobbying efforts of AMA-aligned or AMA-directed State or federal level political action committees (PACs) in connection with attempts to establish, maintain or protect monopolies and/or hinder the free flow of medical information.

The federal government should not inhibit the importation into the USA from foreign sources by American patients of medicines, compounds and medical devices which may or may not be approved by federal or State statutes or regulations absent the finding that any such medicine, compound or device poses a direct, palpable danger to the patient or to society at large.

WHAT BOTH LEVELS CAN DO

Consumers (the general public) should be empowered to make medical decisions in no small part on their own and have access to nutritional therapies and products which credible scientific evidence suggests may assist them in the goal of promotive health, preventive medicine and at-home management of some disease conditions.

Insurance companies should be encouraged to provide coverage for *all* forms of medical endeavor based upon the certification, licensure or acceptance of any given school of medical thought in any State. Their guidelines at the federal level should be equally broad.

State and federal agencies should not be involved in the denial of medical options and choices either to consumers (the general public) or to healthcare providers, nor should any combination of State and federal agencies together or separately or in combination with professional and other organizations, individuals and combinations thereof seek to harass, prosecute, persecute, intimidate or undermine the legitimate interests of medical freedom of choice in options and the free market thereof or engage in any practice, tactic or endeavor which seeks to establish, empower, maintain or protect a medical monopoly for economic, ego, or any other reason.

State and federal law enforcement should investigate and prosecute any attempt by public or private agencies, bureaus, boards, professional groups or individuals who or which seek to establish, maintain or protect any form of medical-practice monopoly be it in services, techniques, equipment or products, or to slander, vilify or bring into public discredit the proponents, defenders, or owners or operators of "non-mainstream" medical centers, medical practices, medical techniques or products held not to or be part of allopathic services, techniques, equipment or products. Enforcement should be along the lines of investigating monopolism, trust-making, collusion, conspiracy, racketeering, and civil rights violations.

To the extent practicable, the practice of any form of

medicine should be separate from and distinct to the provision of goods and services which might be involved in this form of medicine.

Federal and state tax codes should be revised to allow for tax incentives for companies, corporations and other business structures and/or labor unions or any other business or professional or bureaucratic organization or other combination of citizens to establish promotive-health programs for employees, members, associates or shareholders and/or encourage such entities to provide, at least as partial payment, group medical coverage. Such coverage should not discriminate on the basis of a given medical theory or school of thought and should include payment for the services of all recognized healthcare practitioners whose validity or certification may be determined by the individual States. Nor should any such coverage be mandated or enforced as a requirement for employment, membership or association.

There should be a computer-based or other reliable tracking system so that a patient might know if a practitioner of any kind has undergone loss of insurance, legal problems, disciplinary problems, etc., so that a patient, particularly one with a life-threatening disorder or who is about to give birth in a hospital setting, would know the possible "negatives" about the practitioner into whose hands one is placing his/her body or life.

We believe that attempts to reform healthcare conceptually, economically and politically along the lines described above will result in a resurrection of medical freedom of choice for all Americans, a wholesale reduction in the runaway costs of the provision of medical goods and services, eventual victory over the killer diseases of the current era through unleashing the creative energies of the unfettered human mind operating in an essentially free marketplace of ideas, goods and services and research, and a reorienting of society toward promotive health rather than the management of death and disease.

With such a goal in mind, we reiterate our congratulations and best wishes to you in overseeing the considerable task with which you have been charged, and express our support and availability to discuss with you or work with you in the furtherance of these aims and objectives.

M.L. CULBERT,DSc, *chairman emeritus*
R.W. BRADFORD,DSc, *President-founder*

ADDENDUM TO STATEMENT TO CHAIRPERSON CLINTON RE: FEDERAL/STATE CONSPIRACIES AGAINST PHYSICIANS, THE HEALTHFOODS INDUSTRY, AND RELATED MATTERS

(Feb. 19, 1993)

The following is a condensed list of actions (legal, crypto-legal, questionable) conducted either by State agencies or State agencies in combination with federal agencies, and frequently with the at least indirect participation of local media, against selected targets (individuals, companies) who or which seem to represent either conceptual, ego or economic threats to the constellation of vested interests we define as the "allopathic industrial complex" in the United States.

The list is partial since there are indirect and anecdotal accounts of hundreds of other such actions, some almost certainly involving gross violations of civil rights.

The Jimmy Keller matter is deserving of particular attention since it is international in scope and may involve civil rights misbehavior and violations of international law on the part of US federal authorities.

By no means does this organization assume that all actions against all individuals and organizations or companies herein mentioned are utterly baseless; these are simply among the more brazen and well-known cases which are highly suggestive of an interstate conspiracy to intimidate practitioners of "non-mainstream" therapy and the burgeoning healthfoods and supplements industries, which represent major competition to the pharmaceutical synthetic drug conglomerate which is in de facto control of organized (allopathic) medicine. We do not presume the guilt or innocence on all counts or charges of any or all of the following:

MARYLAND (Jan. 16, 1993) — Maryland medical authorities suspend the medical license of Ahmad Shamim MD of Laurel following 10 years of harassment, criticism and intimidation due to this highly regarded physician's use of nutritional and metabolic therapies (including laetrile) against cancer. Dr Shamim has treated some of Maryland's longest-surviving cancer patients. During a recent round of state board activity against him (1991) reporter Jack Anderson — who brought his case to public attention — uncovered the figure of 1,500 MDs and other medical practitioners under some kind of state or federal harassment primarily due to their open espousal or use of "non-mainstream" (that is, non-allopathic or drug-based) medicine.

NEVADA (Nov. 2, 1992) — Vera Joan Allison ND, one of the best-known naturopaths in the USA as well as Nevada, is subjected to a 12-member federal/State/local raid on grounds of "practicing medicine without a license" (naturopathy laws were repealed in Nevada prior), "furnishing a dangerous drug without a prescription" and "possession of a dangerous drug" (a thyroid extract, the steroid progesterone, a brand of the commonly used chelating agent EDTA, a form of human growth hormone, and common solutions — such as heparin). Her records, equipment, supplies were seized as were her bank accounts, including one with which she paid the bills for her ailing 89-year-old mother. Doctor Allison, famed world-wide, was already widely known for championing the cause of laetrile and for using metabolic nutritional therapies on thousands of patients. Her case represents the possibility of federal/State bureaucracies biding their time until this visible champion of "non-mainstream" medicine could be "nailed." She faces the prospect of total economic destruction through the presumed usual tactic: legal and court costs.

WASHINGTON (May 6, 1992) — In a 14-hour raid at the Tahoma Clinic in Kent WA run by high-visibility metabolic practitioner Jonathan Wright MD (Harvard, Michigan), flak-jacketed police and federal agents kicked in doors, rushed in with drawn guns (thus terrorizing patients being treated), yanked out telephones, and seized records and equipment, while also raiding a nearby pharmacy associated with the clinic. The targets: injectable B vitamins, other non-toxic products and diagnostic devices. The raid was apparently in retaliation for Dr. Wright's suing the FDA to force it to return supplies of (non-contaminated) L-tryptophan (an amino acid) which it had seized the year before in the FDA's celebrated cost-to-coast crackdown on the natural product. Wright has been an honored, well-credentialed, widely-respected practitioner of "non-mainstream" medicine for 20 years. Thousands of his patients have rallied to his defense.

TEXAS (Feb. 4-7, 1992) — Whole Foods Market and Sun Harvest Farms, both major natural food supplements distributors, are subjected to inspections by officials of the Texas Division of Food and Drugs. Fifty-two products are embargoed at 11 stores, ranging from co-enzyme Q10 to guargum and various vitamin and herbal products.

TEXAS (Jan 29, 1992, and 9 years prior) — State of Texas seeks to enjoin famed emigre physician-biochemist Stanislaw Burzynski MD PhD from selling or distributing his antineoplaston anti-cancer compounds and attempts to have the existing stocks destroyed despite widespread evidence of their efficacy. This is part of a nearly decade-long battle between Burzynski and the FDA, which raided his clinic, confiscated patient records and, in tandem with insurance companies, involved the scientist in extensive, ongoing litigation.

FLORIDA (Feb. 1992) — Chiropractor Lawrence Hall DC enters Eglin Air Force Base to begin five years of federal detention on conviction of various Medicare and "mail fraud"-associated counts after years of federal harassment for his successful operation of several chiropractic-centered clinics in Florida. Part of the harassment may have been due to his contributing to a defense fund for a doctor under similar charges.

CALIFORNIA (ongoing) — Committee Vice President Bruce Halstead MD, a widely respected world researcher in herbs, marine biology and plant toxicology, remains on appeal from a 4-year prison term and involved in extensive legal maneuvers following his 1985 conviction on multiple state charges involving utilizing a Japanese herbal tea as an immune adjuvant therapy for cancer. Probable real reason for many years' harassment: Dr. Halstead's open advocacy of chelation therapy, laetrile, DMSO, herbal treatments, etc.

NORTH DAKOTA (ongoing) — Jimmy Keller remains in a federal prison as part of a 2-year sentence levied in Brownsville TX in December 1991. He had ostensibly been kidnapped by US officials in Mexico on a 1984 warrant charging him with "wire fraud" (using a telephone) when he operated a cancer clinic in Matamoros, Mexico. He was picked up in Tijuana, where he had broken no Mexican laws and was operating the St. Jude clinic. Sentencing on the old warrant followed testimony that Keller had helped many patients and never promised to cure anybody.

CALIFORNIA (May 1992 and year prior) — Biochemist Stephen Levine, operator of Nutricology/Allergy research, says he has spent $300,000 in legal bills in the past year to defend his companies against FDA claims of mail fraud and selling illegal drugs (nutritional supplements). Although Levine has won in US federal district court against the FDA several times, the agency continues to harass him.

IDAHO (Dec. 1991) — US Marshal's office and US Attorney's Office at the request of the FDA raid Thorne Research to seize six products, all of them vitamin and mineral supplements. The feds argued that claims were "implied" by the names on the labels.

CALIFORNIA, OREGON (ongoing since 1985) — Zane R. Gard MD, stripped of his license in 1991, is claiming various Constitutional violations by state medicrats in their ongoing attack on his professional standing. An expert in environmental toxins, he believes his lengthy litigation with the state has been due to his position on environmental medicine and espousal of metabolic therapies. Defense litigation brought him near financial ruin, he said.

NEVADA (ongoing) — Sports medicine expert Benjamin Zvenia ND is preparing for his third round of criminal charges on the same subject (practicing naturopathy in the State of Nevada) despite his reportedly good record in healing workers without the aid of harmful drugs and attaining "approved provider" status by the state and "approved affiliate physician" status by casinos.

OREGON (June 1992 and year prior) — Ken Scott, president of Highland Laboratories, says that since the October 1990 raid on his enterprise by the FDA he has spent $100,000 in legal fees and "we still do not have all of our equipment and supplies back. They've harassed and threatened our employees, defamed us personally and professionally — all for what crime? It's almost two years later, and they still haven't managed to charge us with a thing." FDA's excuse for the 24-agent raid: "label violations" on nutritional products.

ILLINOIS (1992, 1991) — Traco Laboratories has won three times in court against the FDA after the federal agency attempted to punish Traco for importations of black currant seed oil, arguing the same is a food additive and not a food and hence under FDA jurisdiction.

FLORIDA, ARIZONA (1992, 1991) — Life Extension Foundation/ Life Extension International are still involved in FDA litigation after beating the FDA in court over FDA-incited embargoes of LE nutritional products in Arizona by state authorities.

UTAH (April 5, 1991) — Pets Smell-Free (PSF) is awarded a summary judgment against the FDA, hence prohibiting FDA from destroying a quantity of a product it has seized and voiding an injunction against the product. The product is designed to stop odors from urine, feces, gas and bad breath in animals. Since it contains an antibiotic, the FDA considered it an "unapproved new drug." The federal judge agreed with PSF that a product to remove an offensive odor is not the treatment of a disease.

WASHINGTON, OREGON, UTAH (1991) — FDA raids are conducted against Vitacel-7 nutritional products at several different offices. Records, software and bank accounts are seized and employees intimidated. The final outcome of these raids is not known.

NEVADA (1990) — The outcome of two separate FDA-led raids of 13 and 16 hours respectively on the Century Clinic in Reno is not known. The Reno raid bore similarities to the Tahoma Clinic raid in 1992 and homeopathic medications and devices were among prime targets. Patients' entrance and egress were denied for many hours on both occasions. One patient has claimed intimidation at home by an FDA officer.

CALIFORNIA (1991) — Physician Valentine G. Birds MD says he has spent more than $80,000 in legal fees attempting to protect his medical license — suspended by the California Medical Board — against charges of dispensing an "illegal AIDS medication." While Dr. Birds favors metabolic and nutritional medical approaches, he states he did not dispense the drug in question.

CALIFORNIA (1990) — a 57-year-old woman, Mrs. Harrington-McGill, who operates a healthfood store for animals, is incarcerated in maximum security in a US federal detention facility following an ongoing battle with the FDA over labels for products for horses and dogs. She does 114 days' hard time in the company of hard-core criminals and almost dies of stroke.

Various of the above cases (Bruce Halstead, Harrington-McGill) and earlier cases involving Utah and California physicians driven from their practices and still practicing in Nevada under homeopathy statutes have brought forth testimony and anecdotes suggestive of an ongoing "hit list" of federal and state authorities against high-profile proponents of "non-mainstream" medicine.

Various "quackbuster" meetings since 1984 have brought together elements of the FDA (which has actually co-sponsored such meetings at taxpayer expense), US Post Office, other federal agencies, the insurance industry, state attorneys general and other policing authorities in league with allopathic medical groups to design media-oriented "anti-quackery" campaigns against all proponents, practitioners, devotees and supporters of "non-mainstream" medicine. At one point a federal grant was actually issued to an organization which was said to be "independent" but which in fact was designing a database to track "quackery" — meaning any dissent from the allopathic industrial complex. This operation was stopped.

In 1990-1991, the FDA, utilizing as a pretext the scattered deaths and poisoning due to one variety of improved L-tryptophan, an amino acid, decided to ban this useful nutrient from interstate commerce in the USA, thus depriving thousands of physicians and millions of patients of a substance useful in mitigating many forms of neurological distress (all the better, it was noted, for a spurt in sales of synthetic drugs inferentially linked to violence,suicide and serial killings). FDA statements suggested that all amino acids and most herbs might be either banned or brought under the "purview" of the FDA which in its entire history has never looked benignly on natural supplements. In fact, the FDA seemed to be finding in the L-tryptophan matter a way to circumvent the 1974 Proxmire Act, which had protected dietary supplements and related natural products from the grasp of the FDA.

The emerging pattern is that of a combined public-private conspiracy against "alternative" physicians, their patients, and providers of non-drug therapies, part of which surfaced in the 1980s litigation (*Wilk vs. AMA*) involving chiropractors and an earlier injunction by the Federal Trade Commission (FTC) against the AMA, *et al.* in which the AMA's long-standing conspiracy "to contain" and "to eliminate" the chiropractic profession was revealed.

These activities were paralleled in the 1970s and 1980s by the frenzied efforts of organized medicine to suppress laetrile, the movement for whose decriminalization provoked the mightiest challenge to monopoly medicine ever mounted in the USA. The effort to decriminalize laetrile led to the formation of the organization which has prepared this document and which can provide copious information on this earlier, shocking, tragic affair.

APPENDIX C
MODEL STATE-LEVEL LEGISLATION for MEDICAL FREEDOM OF CHOICE

1. Neither the State of _____ nor any agency, division, department or bureau thereof, shall interfere with the medical practices of any duly qualified practitioner of the medical arts because such practitioner engages in a form of the medical arts which may not be considered standard or orthodox practice by prevailing standard definitions *absent the finding* that any such practice represents a direct threat to the life or health of the patient.

2. Any duly qualified practitioner of the medical arts in _____ shall, at the request of a patient, provide information on optional treatments, or allow patient access to such information, particularly in those cases in which prevailing medical opinion has determined the patient to be in a "terminal," "incurable" or "end-state" condition.

3. Neither the State of _____ nor any agency, division, department or bureau thereof, shall interfere with the right of a duly qualified practitioner of the medical arts to receive into the state for his or her professional use any nutrient, herbal or other natural substance or combination of substances or any chemical substance or combination thereof or any device or technique which is not considered standard or orthodox practice for medical or diagnostic or evaluative use by prevailing standard definitions of orthodox medicine *absent the finding* that any such substance or combination of substances or device or technique represents a direct threat to the life or health of the patient.

4. Neither the State of _____ nor any agency, division, department or bureau thereof, shall interfere with the right of a duly qualified practitioner of the medical arts to counsel with, or provide information to, his or her patients concerning substances, therapies, devices or techniques which may not be considered standard practice by prevailing standard definitions, *absent the finding* that such counsel or information represents a direct threat to the life or health of the patient.

APPENDIX D

RESOURCES

SELECTED BIBLIOGRAPHY

(Recommended reading in aspects of medical history, medical politics and economics, iatrogenic medicine, metabolic and nutritional therapies, integrative treatments, medical futurism and novel theories)

Achterberg, Jeanne, *Imagery in Healing: Shamanism and Modern Medicine*. Boston: New Science Library, 1985.
Ackerknecht, E. K., *Therapeutics: From the Primitive to the 20th Century*. New York: Hafner, 1973.
Adams, Ruth, and Murray, Frank, *Megavitamin Therapy*. New York: Larchmont Books, 1975.
Airola, Paavo, *Hypoglycemia: A Better Approach*. Phoenix AZ: Health Plus, 1977.
Ali, Majid, *The Butterfly and Life Span Nutrition*. Bloomfield NJ: Institute of Preventive Medicine, 1992.
Ali, Majid, *The Canary and Chronic Fatigue*. Denville NJ: Life Span Press, 1994.
Ali, Majid, *The Cortical Monkey and Healing*. Bloomfield NJ: Institute of Preventive Medicine, 1990.
Allen, Gary, *The Rockefeller File*. Seal Beach CA: '76 Press, 1976.
Alternative Medicine. (The Goldberg Group) Puyallup WA: Future Medicine Publishing, 1993.
Andrews, L. B., *Deregulating Doctoring: Do Medical Licensing Laws Meet Today's Health Care Needs?* Emmaus PA: People's Medical Society, 1984.
Annis, E. R., *Code Blue — Health Care in Crisis*. Washington DC: Regnery Gateway, 1992.
Atkins, Robert, *Dr. Atkins' Health Revolution*. Boston: Houghton Mifflin, 1988.
Badgley, Lawrence, *Healing AIDS Naturally*. San Bruno CA: Human Energy Press, 1986.
Balch, James F. and Phyllis A., *Prescription for Nutritional Healing*. Garden City Park NY: Avery, 1990.
Beall, Morris A., *Super Drug Story*. Washington DC: Columbia Books, 1962.
Bearden, T.E., *AIDS: Biological Warfare*. Greenville TX: Tesla Book Co., 1988.

Beasley, Victor, *Your Electro-Vibratory Body*. Boulder Creek CO: University of the Trees Press, 1978.

Becker, R. O., and Seldon, G., *The Body Electric: Electro-Magnetism and the Foundation of Life*. New York: Morrow, 1986.

Bennett, J. T., and DiLorenzo, T. J., *Unhealthy Charities: Hazardous to Your Health and Wealth*. New York: Basic Books, 1994.

Berger, Stuart M., *What Your Doctor Didn't Learn in Medical School*. New York: Avon Books, 1989.

Berman, Edgar, *The Solid Gold Stethoscope*. New York: Macmillan, 1976.

Bland, Jeffrey, *Nutraerobics*. San Franciscoa: Harper & Row, 1983.

Bradford, Robert W., and Culbert, M. L., *Now That You Have Cancer*. Chula Vista CA: The Bradford Foundation, 1992.

Bradford, Robert W., et al., *Oxidology: The Study of Reactive Oxygen Toxic Species (ROTS) and Their Metabolism in Health and Disease*. Los Altos CA: The Bradford Foundation, 1983.

Bradford, Robert W., et al., *The Biochemical Basis of Live Cell Therapy*. Chula Vista CA: The Bradford Foundation, 1986.

Braverman, E. R., and Pfeiffer, C. C., *The Healing Nutrients Within*. New Canaan CT: Keats, 1987.

Brecher, Arline and Harold, *Forty Something Forever*. Herndon VA: Health Savers Press, 1992.

Brennan, R. O., *Nutrigenetics*. New York: M. Evans, 1975.

Brown, R. K., *AIDS, Cancer and the Medical Establishment*. New York: Speller, 1986.

Burk, Dean, *A Brief on Foods and Vitamins*. Sausalito CA: The McNaughton Foundation, 1975.

Caiazza, Stephen, *AIDS: One Doctor's Personal Struggle*. Highland Park: NJ, 1989.

Cameron, Ewan, and Pauling, Linus, *Vitamin C and Cancer*. Menlo Park CA: Linus Pauling Institute of Science and Medicine, 1979.

Cannon, Walter B., *The Wisdom of the Body*. New York: Norton, 1960.

Cantwell, Alan, *AIDS and the Doctors of Death*. Los Angeles, Aries Rising, 1988.

Carlson, Rick, *The End of Medicine*. New York: Wiley, 1975.

Carse, Mary, *Herbs of the Earth*. Hinesburg VT: Upper Access Publishers, 1989.

Carter, J. O., *Racketeering in Medicine*. Norfolk VA: Hampton Roads, 1992.

Carter, Richard, *The Doctor Business*. New York: Doubleday, 1985.

Carver, Cynthia, *Patient Beware*. Scarborough, Ontario, Prentice-Hall Canada, 1984.

Cassell, E. J., *The Healer's Art*. New York: Penguin, 1978.
Chaitow, Leon, and Martin, Simon, *A World without AIDS*. Great Britain: Thorsons Ltd., 1988.
Chang, S. T., *The Complete Book of Acupuncture*. Millbrae CA: Celestial Arts, 1976.
Cheraskin, E., *Psychodietetics*. New York: Bantam, 1974.
Cheraskin, E., and Ringsdorf, W. M., *New Hope for Incurable Diseases*. Hicksville NY: Exposition Press, 1971.
Cheraskin, Emanuel, et al., *The Vitamin C Connection*. New York: Harper and Row, 1983.
Chopra, Deepak, *Quantum Healing*. New York, Bantam, 1990.
Chopra, Deepak, *Unconditional Life*. New York: Bantam, 1991.
Christopher, John R., *School of Natural Healing*. Provo UT: BiWorld Publishers, 1976.
Cichoke, A. J., *New Hope for AIDS*. Portland OR: Seven C's Publishing, 1993.
Clark, Adrian V., *Cosmic Mysteries of the Universe*. West Nyack NY: Parker, 1968.
Cleave, T. L., *The Saccharine Disease*. New Canaan CT: Keats, 1974.
Corea, Gena, *The Hidden Malpractice*. New York: Harper and Row, 1985.
Coulter, Harris L., *AIDS and Syphilis: the Hidden Link*. Richmond CA: North Atlantic Books, 1987.
Coulter, Harris L., *Divided Legacy: the Conflict Between Homoeopathy and the American Medical Association*. Richmond CA: North Atlantic Books, 1973.
Cousins, Norman, *Anatomy of an Illness*. New York: Norton, 1979.
Cousins, Norman, *The Healing Heart*. New York: Norton, 1983.
Cranton, Elmer, and Brecher, Arline, *Bypassing Bypass*. Norfolk VA: Donning, 1989.
Crook, William G., *The Yeast Connection*. Jackson TN: Professional Books, 1984.
Culbert, Michael, *AIDS; Hope, Hoax and Hoopla*. Chula Vista CA: The Bradford Fundation, 1990.
Culbert, Michael, *AIDS: Terror, Truth and Triumph*. Chula Vista CA: The Bradford foundation, 1986.
Culbert, Michael, *CFS: Conquering the Crippler*. San Diego CA: C and C Communications, 1993.
Culbert, Michael, *Freedom from Cancer*. New York: Pocketbooks, 1977.
Culbert, Michael, *Live Cell Thrapy for the 21st Century*. Chula Vista CA: The Bradford Foundation, 1993.
Culbert, Michael, *Vitamin B17: Forbiden Weapon Against Cancer*. New Rochelle NY: Arlington House, 1974.

Culbert, Michael, *What the Medical Establishment Won't Tell You that Could Save Your Life*. Norfolk VA: Donning, 1983.
deGrazia, Alfred, ed., *The Velikovsky Affair (the Warfare of Science and Scientism)*. Hyde Park NY: University Books, 1966.
Davis, N. M., and Cohen, M. R., *Medication Errors: Causes and Prevention*. Philadelphia: George F. Stickley, 1981.
Dermer, G. B., *The Immortal Cell*. Garden City Park NY: Avery, 1994.
Diamantidis, Spiro, *Homoeopathic Medicine*. Athens: Medical Institute for Homoeopathic Research and Application, 1989.
Diet, Nutrition and Cancer. (National Research Council) Washington DC: National Academy Press, 1982.
Dohrenwend, B. S. and B. P., eds., *Stressful Life Events: Their Nature and Effects*. New York: Wiley, 1974.
Dossey, Larry, *Healing Words: the Power of Prayer and the Practice of Medicine*. New York: Harper, 1993.
Dossey, Larry, *Space, Time & Medicine*. Boston: Shambhala, 1982.
DuBois, J. E., *The Devil's Chemists*. Boston: Beacon, 1952.
Dubos, Rene, *The Mirage of Health*. New York: Harper, 1979.
Duffy, John, *The Healers: The Rise of the Medical Establishment*. New York: McGraw, 1976.
Dufty, William, *Sugar Blues*. Radnor PA: Chilton, 1975.
Epstein, Samuel, *The Politics of Cancer*. San Francisco: Sierra Club Books, 1978.
Ferguson, Wilburn, *The Jivaro and His Drugs*. Quito, Ecuador: Editorial Casa de la Cultura Ecuatoriana, 1957.
Fink, John, *Third Opinion*. Garden City Park NY: Avery, 1988.
Flynn, J. T., *God's Gold: the Story of Rockefeller and His Times*. New York: Harcourt Brace, 1932.
Forman, Brenda, *B-15: The 'Miracle' Vitamin*. New York: Grosset and Dunlap, 1979.
Fredericks, Carlton, *Breast Cancer and the Nutritional Approach*. New York: Grosset and Dunlap, 1977.
Fredericks, Carlton, *Eating Right for You*. New York: Grosset and Dunlap, 1972.
Fredericks, Carlton, *PsychoNutrition*. New York: Grosset and Dunlap, 1976.
Fredricks, Carlton, and Goodman, Herman, *Low Blood Sugar and You*. New York: Grosset and Dunlap, 1969.
Fredman, Steven, and Burger, Robert, *Forbidden Cures*. New York: Stein and Day, 1976.
Freese, A. S., *Managing Your Doctor*. New York: Stein and Day, 1975.
Fuchs, V. H., *Who Shall Live?* New York: Basic Books, 1974.
Garceau, Oliver, *The Political History of the American Medical Association*.

Cambridge MA: Harvard University Press, 1941.
Garrison, Omar, *The Dictocrats*. Chicago: Books for Today, 1970.
Gerson, Max, *A Cancer Therapy — Results of Fifty Cases*. New York: Whittier Books, 1958.
Gittleman, Ann Louise, *Super Nutrition for Women*. New York: Bantam, 1991.
Glasscheib, H. S., *The March of Medicine: Emergence and Triumph of Modern Medicine*. (tr. Savill) New York: Putnam, 1964.
Glassman, Judith, *The Cancer Survivors and How They Did It*. New York: Dial Press, 1981.
Gofman, J. W., and O'Connor, E., *X-rays: Health Effects of Common Exams*. San Francisco: Sierra Club Books, 1985.
Goulden, Joseph, *The Money Givers*. New York: Random House, 1971.
Greenberg, Kurt, ed., *Challenging Orthodoxy*. New Canaan CT: Keats, 1991.
Greenwald, Peter, ed., *Cancer, Diet and Nutrition*. Chicago: Marquis Who's Who, 1985.
Gregory, Scott, and Leonardo, Blanca, *They Conquered AIDS!* Palm Springs CA: Tree of Life Publications, 1989.
Griffin, G. E., *World without Cancer*. Westlake Village CA: American Media, 1974.
Griggs, Barbara, *Green Pharmacy*. New York: Viking Press, 1981.
Guinther, J., *The Malpractitioners*. New York: Doubleday, 1978.
Haggard, H. W., *Mystery, Magic and Medicine: the Rise of Medicine from Superstition to Science*. Garden City NY: Doubleday, Doran, 1933.
Halstead, Bruce, *Amygdalin Therapy*. Los Altos CA: Choice Publications, 1978.
Halstead, Bruce, *Metabolic Cancer Therapy*. Colton CA: Golden Quill, 1978.
Halstead, Bruce, *The DMSO Handbook*. Colton CA: Golden Quill, 1981.
Halstead, Bruce, *The Scientific Basis of EDTA Chelation Therapy*. Colton CA: Golden Quill, 1981.
Harmer, Ruth Mulvey, *American Medical Avarice*. New York: Abelard-Schuman, 1975.
Harper, Harold, and Culbert, M. L., *How You Can Beat the Killer Diseases*. New Rochelle NY: Arlington House, 1977.
Hausman, Patricia, *The Right Dose*. Emmaus PA: Rodale Press, 1987.
Hay, Louise, *You Can Heal Your Life, and Heal Your Body*. Santa Monica CA: Hay House, 1984.
Heimlich, Jane, *What Your Doctor Won't Tell You*. New York: HarperCollins, 1990.

Heinerman, John, *The Treatment of Cancer with Herbs.* Orem UT: BiWorld Publishers, 1980.
Hilfiker, David, *Healing the Wounds.* New York: Pantheon, 1985.
Hoffer, Abram, and Walker, Morton, *Orthomolecular Nutrition.* New Canaan CT: Keats, 1978.
Hoffman, W. H., *Using Energy to Heal..* (Privately published), 1979.
Hong-Yen Hsu and Preacher, W. G., *Chinese Herb Medicine and Therapy.* Nashville TN: Aurora Publishers, 1976.
Horne, Ross, *The Health Revolution.* Australia: Happy Landings Pty Ltd, 1989.
Houston, Robert G., *Repression and Reform in the Evaluation of Alternative Cancer Therapies.* Washington DC: Project Cure, 1989.
Hoxsey, Harry, *You Don't Have to Die.* 1956: reprinted by Nature Heals, Chapala, Mexico, 1977.
Huard, Pierre, and Wang, Ming, *Chinese Medicine.* New York: McGraw-Hill, 1972.
Hunt, Steven B., and Allen, James, *In Failing Health.* Skokie IL: National Textbooks Co., 1977.
Hur, Robin, *Food Reform: Our Desperate Need.* Austin TX: Heidelberg, 1975.
Illich, Ivan, *Medical Nemesis.* New York: Random House, 1976.
Inlander, C. B., et al., *Medicine on Trial.* New York: Pantheon Books, 1988.
Isaacs, James, and Lamb, John C., *Complementarity in Biology.* Baltimore: Johns Hopkins Press, 1969.
Jayasuriya, Anton, *Clinical Acupuncture*, 10th ed. Sri Lanka: Medicina Alternativa, 1985.
Jayasuriya, Anton, *Clinical Homeopathy*, 4th ed. Sri Lanka: Medicina Alternativa, 1985.
Jeffreys, Toni, *The Mile-High Staircase.* London: Hodder and Stoughton, 1982.
Jensen, Bernard, *Foods that Heal.* Garden City Park NY: Avery, 1988.
Jones, Rochelle, *The Supermeds.* New York: Macmillan, 1990.
Josephson, Matthew, *The Robber Barons.* New York: Harcourt Brace, 1934.
Kanfiran, M., *Homeopathy in America: the Rise and Fall of a Medical Heresy.* Baltimore: Johns Hopkins University Press, 1971.
Kaptchuk, T. J., *The Web that Has No Weaver: Understanding Chinese Medicine.* New York: Congdon and Weed, 1983.
Kaptchuk, T. J., and Croucher, Michael, *The Healing Arts.* New York: Summit, 1978.
Kiev, A., ed., *Magic, Faith and Healing.* New York: Macmillan, 1974.
Kittler, Glenn, D., *Laetrile — Control for Cancer.* New York: Paperback Library, 1963.

Klaw, Spencer, *The Great American Medical Show*. New York: Penguin, 1976.
Kloss, Jethro, *Back to Eden*. Santa Barbara CA: Lifeline Books, 1974.
Koch, W. F., *The Survival Factor in Neoplastic and Viral Diseases*. Detroit: Vanderkloot Press, 1961.
Kramer, C., *The Negligent Doctor*. New York: Crown, 1968.
Kuhnau, W. W., *Live-Cell Therapy: My Life with a Medical Breakthrough*. Tijuana BC, Mexico: Artes Graficas de Baja California, 1983. Rev. ed., 1992.
Kunin, R. A., *Mega-Nutrition*. New York: McGraw-Hill, 1980.
Kunnes, Richard, *Your Money or Your Life*. New York: Dodd, Mead, 1974.
Kushi, Michio, and Blauer, Steven, *The Macrobiotic Way*. Garden City Park NY: Avery, 1985.
Lambert, E. C., *Modern Medical Mistakes*. Bloomington IN: Indiana University Press, 1978.
Lambert, Samuel, and Goodwin, G. M., *Medical Leaders from Hippocrates to Osler*. Indianapolis: Bobbs-Merrill, 1929.
Lander, Louise, *Defective Medicine*. New York: Farrar, Straus, Giroux, 1978.
Lauritsen, John, *Poison by Prescription*. New York: Pagan Press, 1990.
Lauritsen, John, *The AIDS War: Propaganda, Profiteering and Genocide from the Medical-Industrial Complex*. New York: Pagan Press, 1993.
Lauritsen, John, and Wilson, Hank, *Death Rush: Poppers and AIDS*. New York: Pagan Press, 1986.
Lerner, Michael, *Choices in Healing*. Cambridge MA: MIT Press, 1994.
LeShan, Lawrence, *You Can Fight for Your Life: Emotional Factors in the Causation of Cancer*. New York: Evans, 1977.
Levy, S. M., *Behavior and Cancer*. San Francisco, Jossey-Bass, 1985.
Lisa, P. J., *Are You a Target for Elimination?* Huntington Beach CA: International Institute of Natural Health Sciences, 1985.
Lisa, P. J., *The Great Medical Monopoly Wars*. Huntington Beach CA: International Institute of Natural Health Sciences, 1986.
Livingston, Virginia: *Cancer: a New Breakthrough*. San Diego: Pruduction House, 1972.
Livingston, Virginia: *The Conquest of Cancer — Vaccines and Diet*. New York: Franklin Watts, 1984.
Longgood, William, *The Poisons in Your Food*. New York: Pyramid, 1960.
Lucas, Richard, *Nature's Medicines*. New York: Award Books, 1966.
Lucas, Scott, *The FDA*. Millbrae CA: Celestial Arts, 1978.
Lynes, Barry, *The Cancer Cure that Worked:* Toronto: Marcus Books, 1987.
Lynes, Barry, *The Healing of Cancer*. Toronto: Marcus Books, 1989.

Major, R. H., *A History of Medicine*. Springfield IL: Charles C. Thomas, 1954.

Manner, Harold, W., et al., *The Death of Cancer*. Evanston IL: Advanced Century, 1978.

Martin, Rose, *Fabian Freeway*. Belmont MA: Western Islands, 1966.

Martin, Wayne, *Medical Heroes and Heretics*. Old Greenwich CT: Devin-Adair, 1977.

McDonagh, E. W., *Chelation Can Cure*. Kansas City MO: Platinum Pen, 1983.

McGee, Charles, T., *Heart Frauds*. Coeur d'Alene ID: MediPress, 1993.

Melville, A., *Cured to Death: the Effects of Prescription Drugs*. New York: Stein and Day, 1982.

Mendelsohn, Robert S., *Confessions of a Medical Heretic*. New York: Warner, 1979.

Millman, Marcia, *The Unkindest Cut*. New York: Morrow, 1977.

Mindell, Earl, *Earl Mindell's Vitamin Bible*. New York: Rawson, Wade, 1980.

Montgomery, E. R., *The Story Behind Great Medical Discoveries*. New York: Dodd, Mead, 1945.

Moore, M. J., and Lynda, *The Complete Handbook of Holistic Health*. Englewood Cliffs NJ: Prentice-Hall, 1983.

Moore, Thomas, J., *Heart Failure*. New York: Random House, 1989.

Moss, Ralph W., *The Cancer Industry*. New York: Paragon House, 1991.

Moss, Raplh W., *The Cancer Syndrome*. New York: Grove Press, 1980.

Moyers, Bill, *Healing and the Mind*. New York: Doubleday, 1993.

Mullins, Eustace, *Murder by Injection*. Staunton VA: Council for Medical Research, 1988.

Murray, M. T., and Pizzorno, J. F., *An Encyclopedia of Natural Medicine*. Rocklin CA: Prime Publishing, 1990.

Needleman, Jacob, *The Way of the Physician*. San Francisco: Harper and Row, 1985.

Nichols, Joe D., *"Please, Doctor, DO Something!"* Dallas TX: Universal Media, 1992.

Nutrition Almanac (Nutrition Search, Inc.) New York: McGraw-Hill, 1984.

Ornish, Dean, *Dr. Dean Ornish's Program for Reversing Heart Disease*. New York: Random House, 1990.

Ornstein, Dolph, *Medicine Today, Healing Tomorrow*. Millbrae CA: Celestial Arts, 1976.

Ornstein, Robert, and Sobel, David, *The Healing Brain*. New York: Simon and Schuster, 1987.

Osler, Sir William, *The Evolution of Modern Medicine*. New Haven CT: Yale University Press, 1923.

Ostrom, Neenyah, *Fifty Things You Should Know About the Chronic Fatigue Syndrome Epidemic.* New York: St. Martin's Press, 1993.
Owen, Bob, *Roger's Recovery from AIDS.* Cannon Beach OR: DAVAR, 1987.
Passwater, Richard, *Cancer and Its Nutritional Therapies.* New Canaan CT: Keats, 1978.
Passwater, Richard, *Selenium as Food and Medicine.* New Canaan CT: Keats, 1980.
Passwater, Richard, *Supernutrition.* New York: Dial, 1975.
Passwater, Richard, *Supernutrition for Healthy Hearts.* New York: Dial, 1977.
Pauling, Linus, *How to Live Longer and Feel Better.* New York: Avon, 1987.
Pelletier, K. R., *Mind as Healer, Mind as Slayer.* New York: Delacorte Press, 1977.
Peltzman, Sam, *Regulation of Pharmaceutical Innovation: the 1962 Amendments.* Washington DC: American Enterprise Institute for Policy Research, 1974.
Pfeiffer, Carl, *Mental and Elemental Nutrients.* New Canaan CT: Keats, 1975.
Philpott, W. H., *Cancer: the Magnetic/Oxygen Answer.* Choctaw OK, 1994.
Philpott, W. H., and Kalita, D. W., *Brain Allergies: the Psycho-Nutrient Connection.* New Canaan CT: Keats, 1987.
Powers of Healing. Alexandria VA: Life-Time Books, 1989.
Preston, Thomas, *The Clay Pedestal.* Seattle: Madrona, 1981.
Price, Weston, *Nutrition and Physical Degeneration.* Santa Monica CA: Price Pottenger Foundation, 1945.
Rapp, Doris, *Is This Your Child?* New York: Morrow, 1991.
Rappoport, Jon, *AIDS, Inc.* San Bruno CA: Human Energy Press, 1988.
Rath, Matthias, *Eradicating Heart Disease.* San Francisco CA: Health Now, 1993.
Regan, B, and Hirshberg, C. *Spontaneous Remission: An Annotated Biography.* Sausalito CA: Institute of Noetic Sciences, 1993.
Riordan, H. D., *Medical Mavericks, vol. 1.* Wichita KS: Bio-Communications Press, 1988.
Richardson, J. A., and Griffin, P., *Laetrile Case Histories.* New York; Bantam, 1977.
Robertson, W. O., *Medical Malpractice: a Preventive Approach:* Seattle: University of Washington Press, 1985.
Roe, D. A., *Drug-Induced Nutritional Deficiencies.* Westport CT: Avi Publishing, 1976.

Root-Bernstein, Robert, *Rethinking AIDS: the Tragic Cost of Premature Consensus.* New York: Free Press, 1993.
Rosenbaum, M, and Susser, M, *Solving the Puzzle of Chronic Fatigue Syndrome.* Tacoma: Life Sciences Press, 1992.
Rosenberg, Harold, *The Doctor's Book of Vitamin Therapy.* New York: Berkley Windhover, 1974.
Ruesch, Hans, *Naked Empress.* Zurich: Buchverlag CIVIS, 1982.
Satillaro, Anthony, *Recalled by Life.* Boston: Houghton Mifflin, 1981.
Schauss, Alexander, *Diet, Crime and Delinquency.* Berkeley CA: Parker House, 1980.
Scheiber, S. C., and Doyle, B. B., *The Impaired Physician.* New York: Plenum Press, 1983.
Schneider, Robert, *When to say No to Surgery.* Englewood Cliffs NJ: Prentice-Hall, 1982.
Schrauzer, G., ed., *Inorganic and Nutritional Aspects of Cancer.* New York: Plenum, 1978.
Scott, C. J., and Hawk, J., eds., *Heal Thyself: the Health of Health Care Professionals.* New York: Brunner/Mazel, 1986.
Selye, Hans, *The Stress of Life.* New York: McGraw-Hill, 1956.
Sherman, Harold, *Your Power to Heal.* New York: Harper & Row, 1972.
Shilts, Randy, *And the Band Played On.* New York: St. Martin's Press, 1987.
Shute, Wilfred E., *Wilfred Shute's Complete Updated Vitamin E Book.* New Canaan CT: Keats, 1975.
Sidel, V. W., and R., *A Healthy State.* New York: Pantheon, 1983.
Siegel, Bernie, *Love, Medicine and Miracles.* New York: Harper and Row, 1986.
Simonton, Carl, et al., *Getting Well Again.* New York: Bantam, 1986.
Smith, Russell, *The Cholesterol Conspiracy.* St. Louis: Green, 1991.
Solomon, G. E., *Psychoneuroimmunology.* New York: Academic Press, 1987.
Starr, Paul, *The Social Transformation of American Medicine.* New York: Basic Books, 1982.
Stefansson, Vilhjalmur, *Cancer: Disease of Civilization.* New York: Hill and Wang, 1960.
Tansley, David V., *Radionics: Interface with the Ether-Fields.* London: Health Science Press, 1975.
Tilden, John H., *Toxemia: The Basic Cause of Disease.* Chicago: Natural Hygiene Press, 1974.
Trever, William, *In the Public Interest.* Los Angeles: Scriptures Unlimited, 1972.
Trowbridge, J. P., and Walker, Morton, *The Yeast Connection.* New York:

Bantam, 1986.
Venzmer, Gerhard, *Five Thousand Years of Medicine*. (tr. Koenig) New York: Taplinger, 1968.
Unconventional Cancer Therapies (H. Gelband, Project Director) Washington DC: US Congress, Office of Technology Assessment, 1990.
Vitamin A: Everyone's Basic Bodyguard. Emmaus PA: Rodale Press, 1972.
Vithoulkas, George, *Homeopathy: Medicine of the New Man*. New York: Arco Publishing, 1979.
Vithoulkas, George, *The Science of Homeopathy*. New York: Grove Press, 1980.
Vogel, Virgil, J., *American Indian Medicine*. New York: Ballantine, 1973.
Wade, Carlson, *Nature's Cures*. New York: Award Books, 1972.
Wade, Carlson, *The Rejuvenation Vitamin*. New York: Award Books, 1970.
Walker, Kenneth, *The Story of Medicine*. New York: Oxford University Press, 1954.
Walker, M. J., *Dirty Medicine*. London: Slingshot Publications, 1993.
Walker, Morton, *Chelation Therapy*. Atlanta GA: '76 Press, 1980.
Walker, Morton, *DMSO: The New Healing Power*. Old Greenwich CT: Devin-Adair, 1983.
Walker, Morton, *Total Health*. New York: Everest House, 1979.
Wallach, J. D., and Ma Lan, *Let's Play Doctor!* Alexandria VA: Lifestye Horizons, 1993.
Wallach, J. D., and Ma Lan, *Rare Earths*. Alexandria VA: Lifestyle Horizons, 1994.
Walters, Richard, *Options: The Alternative Cancer Therapy Book*. Garden City Park NY: Avery, 1993.
Weaver, Warren, *U.S. Philanthropic Organizations: Their History, Structure, Management and Record*. New York: Harper and Row, 1967.
Webster, James, *Vitamin C: The Protective Vitamin*. New York: Award Books, 1971.
Weill, Andrew, *Health and Healing*. Boston: Houghton Mifflin, 1983.
Weinberger, Stanley, *Healing Within*. Larkspur CA: Healing Within, 1993.
Weitz, Martin, *Health Shock*. Englewood Cliffs NJ: Prentice-Hall, 1982.
Werbach, Melvyn R., *Healing through Nutrition*. New York: HarperCollins, 1993.
Werbach, Melvyn R., *Nutritional Influences on Illness*. Tarzana CA: Third Line Press, 1987.
Wheelwright, E. C., *Medical Plants and Their History*. New York: Dover Books, 1974.
Wigmore, Ann, *Be Your Own Doctor: a Positive Guide to Natural Living*.

Garden City Park NY: Avery, 1982.
Wigmore, Ann, *The Hippocrates Diet and Health Program.* Garden City Park NY: Avery, 1984.
Wiles, Richard, et al., *Tap Water Blues: Herbicides in Drinking Water.* Washington DC: Environmental Working Group/ Physicians for Social Responsibility, 1984.
Williams, Roger J., *Nutrition Against Disease.* New York: Bantam, 1971.
Williams, Roger, J., *Physicians' Handbook of Nutritional Science.* Springfield: Charles C. Thomas, 1975.
Willner, Robert E., *Deadly Deception.* Peltec Publishing, 1994.
Wohl, Stanley, *The Medical Industrial Complex.* New York: Harmony Books, 1984.
Wolfe, Sydney, *Worst Pills/Best Pills.* Washington DC: Public Citizen Health Research Group, 1988.
Wright, Jonathan V., *Dr. Wright's Guide to Healing with Nutrition.* Emmaus PA: Rodale Press, 1989.
Yiamouyiannis, John, *Fluoride, the Aging Factor.* Delaware OH: Heaalth Action Press, 1983.
Yudkin, John, *Sweet and Dangerous.* New York: Bantam, 1972.

ORGANIZATIONS

Governmental

Office of Alternative Medicine (OAM)
National Institutes of Health
6120 Executive Boulevard,
Executive Plaza South, Suite 450
Rockville MD 20892-9904
Tel. (310) 402-2466
FAX (301) 402-4741

Research, information, referral, advocacy, supplements industry, patient services, etc.

American Assn. of Acupuncture and Oriental Medicine
433 Front St.
Catasauqua PA 18032

American Assn. of Naturopathic Physicians (AANP)
2366 Eastlake Ave. E., Suite 322
Seattle WA 98102
Tel. (206) 323-7610
FAX (206) 323-7612

American Chiropractic Assn.
1701 Clarendon blvd.
Arlington VA 22209
Tel. (703) 276-8800

American College for Advancement in Medicine (ACAM)
23121 Verdugo Drive, Suite 204
Laguna Hills CA 92653
Tel. (714) 583-7666
FAX (714) 455-9679

American Holistic Medical Assn. (AHMA)
4101 Lake Boone trail, Suite 201
Raleigh NC 27607
(919) 787-5146

American Naturopathic Medical Assn. (ANMA)
P O Box 96273
Las Vegas NV 89193
Tel. (702) 897-7053

American Preventive Medical Assn.
459 Walker Road
Great Falls VA 22066
Tels. (703) 759-0662
or (1-800) 230-2762

Ayurvedic Health Centers
RR 4, Box 603
Fairfield IA 52556
Tels. (515) 472-9580
(515) 472-8477

•

P O Box 344
Lancaster MA 01523
Tel. (508) 365-4549

•

17308 Sunset Blvd.
Pacific Palisades CA 90272
Tel. (310) 454-5531

•

4910 Massachusetts Ave., Suite 315
Washington DC 20016
Tel. (202) 244-2700

Bradford Research Institute
1180 Walnut Avenue
Chula Vista CA 91911
Tel. (619) 429-8200
or (1-800) 227-4458
FAX (619) 429-8004
(*Answers American Biologics*)

(The) Cancer Chronicles
161 West 61st St., Suite 5B
New York, NY 10023
Tel. (212) 974-7565
FAX (212) 765-4197

Cancer Control Society/Cancer Book House
2043 N. Berendo St.
Los Angeles CA 90027
Tel. (213) 663-7801

Cancer Support and Education
1035 Pine St.
Menlo Park CA 94025
Tel. (415) 327-6166

(The) Cancer Support Community
185 Lundys Lane
San Francisco CA 94110
Tel. (415) 929-7400

CANHELP
3100 Paradise Bay Road
Port Ludlow WA 98365-9771
Tel. (206) 437-2291

Center for Attitudinal Healing
33 Buchanan Drive
Sausalito CA 94965
Tel. (415) 331-6161

Center for Mind-Body Medicine
5225 Connecticut Ave., NW, Suite 414
Washington DC 20015

Citizens for Health
P O Box 1195
Tacoma WA 98401
Tel. (206) 922-2457
FAX (206) 922-7583

Collaborative Medicine Center
10 Willow, Suite 4
Mill Valley CA 94941
Tel. (415) 383-3197

Committee for Freedom of Choice in Medicine, Inc.
1180 Walnut Avenue
Chula Vista CA 91911
Tels. (619) 429-8200 and (1-800) 227-4458
FAX (619) 429-8004
(Answers American Biologics)
(*Publishes* The Choice)

Commonweal Cancer Help Program
P O Box 316
Bolinas CA 94924
Tel. (415) 868-0970

Corporate Angel Network (CAN)
Westchester County Airport
Building One
White Plains NY 10604
Tel. (914) 328-1313

Environmental Health Assn.
1800 Robertson Blvd., Suite 380
Los Angeles CA 90035
Tel. (310) 837-2048

Foundation for Homeopathic Education and Research
5916 Chabot Crest
Oakland CA 94618
Tel. (415) 649-8930

Herb Research Foundation
1007 Pearl St #200
Boulder CO 80302

International Assn. of Cancer Victors and Friends (IACVF)
7740 West Manchester Avenue
Playa del Rey CA 90293
Tel. (213) 822-5032

International Chiropractic Assn.
1110 N. Glebe Rd., Suite 1000
Arlington VA 22201
Tel. (703) 528-5000

International Foundation for Homeopathy
2366 Eastlake Avenue E., Suite 329
Seattle WA 98102
Tel. (206) 324-8230

Life Extension Foundation
2490 Griffin Rd.
Ft. Lauderdale FL 33012
Tel. (1-800) 841-5433
or
P O Box 229120
Tels. (305) 966-4886 and (1-800) 841-LIFE
•
Monterey Institute for the Study
of Alternative Healing Arts
(MISAHA)
400 Virgin Avenue
Monterey CA 93940
Tel./FAX (408) 646-8019
FAX (408) 646-0339

National Center for Homeopathy
801 N. Fairfax St., Suite 306
Alexandria VA 22314
Tel. (703) 548-7790
FAX (703) 548-7792

National Council for Improved Health (NCIH)
1555 West Seminole St.
San Marcos CA 92069
Tel. (619) 471-5090

National Health Federation
212 West Foothill Blvd.
Monrovia CA 91016

National Nutritional Foods Assn. (NNFA)
150 E. Paularino Ave. #285
Costa Mesa CA 92625
Tel. (714) 966-6632

Nutritional Health Alliance (NHA)
P O Box 25317
Washington DC 20007-8317

People Against Cancer
P O Box 10
Otho IA 50569-0010
Tel. (515) 972-4444
FAX (515) 972-4415
(*Publishes* Options *newsletter)*

Positive Alternative Therapies in
Healthcare, Inc. (PATH)
P O Box 651285
Miami FL 33265

Project Inform
1965 Market St #220
San Francisco CA 94103
Tel. US (1-800) 822-7422
Tel. CA (1-800) 334-7422
(Updated AIDS information)

Team Victory
Bethany Community Church
6240 S. Price Road
Tempe AZ 85283-3399

Wellspring Center for Life Enhancement
3 Otis St.
Watertown MA 02172
Tel. (617) 924-8515

Collegiate education

Bastyr University
144 NE 54th St.
Seattle WA 98105
Tel. (206) 523-9585
FAX (206) 527-4763

National College of Naturopathic Medicine
11231 SE Market St.
Portland OR 97216
Tel. (503) 255-4860

North American University
13402 N. Scottsdale Rd., Suite B-150
Scottsdale AZ 85254-4056
Tel. (602) 948-3353
FAX (602) 948-8150

Southwest College of Naturopathic Medicine
and Health Sciences
6535 East Osborn Rd., Suite 703
Scottsdale AZ 85251
Tel. (602) 990-7424
FAX (602) 990-0337

INDEX

Books One and Two

A

A Complaint Against Medical Tyranny as Practiced in the United States of America: American Medical Genocide 32
AARP *Bulletin* 253
Abbott Laboratories 164,181,243,264, 268,269,361
Abel, Ulrich 399
Abkhasians 440,558
Accreditation Council for Continuing Medical Education 264
ACE (adrenal cortical extract) 311-312
Achterberg, Jeanne 598
ACT-UP 218
acupressure 547,598
acupuncture 117,547,598
Adams, Samuel Hopkins 178
Ader, Robert 593
Adolph Coors Foundation 216
adrenal cortical extracat *see* ACE
Advisory Committee on Human Radiation experiments 415
African swine fever 505
African swine fever virus (ASFV) 503-506,530
Agency for Health Care Policy 85, 87
Agent Orange Syndrome 531
Aharanov-Bohm Effect 609
AIC (Allopathic Industrial Complex)
 — AIDS and, 27,256-257,475-476,566,518,522-523
 — anti-quackery and, 207
 — as gatekeeper of revealed truth 545
 —cancer and, 37,226,256,379,384
 — cognitive dissonance and, 141
 — defined, 77-78
 — deterioration of, 67
 — dietitians and, 563
 — dissidents of, 79-80
 — drug component of, 78
 — EDTA chelation therapy and, 360
 — emergence of 143,160,164,165, 168,170-180,185
 — food processing and, 560
 — greatest challenge to, 580
 — heart/circulatory disease and 357-358,327,329
 — hybrid seeds and, 552
 —insurance companies and, 197
 — international drug cartel and, 236-238
 — laetrile and, 436,437,442,443, 458,465,467,545
 — mental factors in, 592
 — New Medicine and, 580-581
 — nutrients and, 570-571
 — PACs and, 138
 — prayer and, 590-591,593
 — semantics and 68,136
 — synthetic chemical industry and, 247,
 — Vitamin B15 and, 442-443
AIDS (acquired immune deficiency syndrome)
 — Africa and, 473,491-495,502
 — AIC and, 475-476
 — AIDS in Africa Study Group and, 510
 — allopathic paradigm and, 484
 — ARC and, 498,504,525
 — as part of SID, 528
 — ASFV (African swine fever virus) and, 503-506
 — AZT (zidovudine, azidothymidine, Retrovir), and, 486,487,506,507-512
 — CD4 (T4) "helper" cells and, 476,479,483,510,512-513
 — CD8 (T8) "suppressor" cells, and, 479-480,513
 — CMV (cytomegalovirus) and,

485,487
— "co-factors" and, 485-506,499
— components of, 487
— Concorde AZT study and, 510
— conspiracy theories and, 501-507
— controversy over HIV discovery in, 490
— Cuba and, 487
— demographics of, 474-475
— didanosine (ddI, Videx) and, 506,508
— dissenters of HIV theory of, 483-484,485
— EBV (Epstein-Barr Virus) in, 485,487
— economics of, 474
— failing theories of, 513
— HHV-6 (human herpesvirus 6) and, 499-501, 504,506
— HIV antibody tests and, 478-479,494,497,513
— HIV, incidence of, in, 472, 473,475,499
— HIV, incubation period of, in, 497-498
— HIV-specific cytotoxic T-lymphocytes, and, 495
— HIV-2 and, 486
—HIVs, role in, 477,480,481, 482-487,490-491
— holistic/alternative treatment approach in, 514-518,521-524
— HTLV-III and, 482,490
— "inverted ratio" and, 479
— KS (Kaposi's sarcoma) and, 477-478,499
— mycoplasmas and, 486,499
— nucleoside analogue drugs and, 484
— oxidative agents and, 585
— PCP (*Pneumocystis carinii* pneumonia) and, 477,478,499,508,511
— Pediatric AIDS Clinical Trials Group Protocol 076 Study Group, and, 511-512
— Philippines and, 496-497
— protease inhibitors and, 486
— retroviruses and, 393,494
— selenium deficiency and, 517
— Solutein and, 523
— statistics of, 474-473
— stavudine (d4T, Zerit) and, 506
— syphilis and, 518-521
— Tenth International Conference on, 474,473
— Thailand and, 496-497
— varying definitions of, 476-477, 499
— Vitamin A deficiency and, 517
— Vitamin C and, 565
— zalcitabine (ddC, Hivid) and, 506,508
AIDS, Africa and Racism 492
AIDS and the Doctors of Death 502
"AIDS virus" *see* HIV
alachlor 551
alchemy 123,124,125
Alcoa Co. 181
Aldactone 249
Ali, Majid 581-582
Alivizatos, Hariton 428
Alliance for Aging Research 569
Allied Chemical 183
Allison, Joan Vera, 23-25
Allopathic Industrial Complex *see* AIC
allopathy (allopaths, allopathic medicine)
— AIDS and, 484,506-507
— AMA and, 138,159,227
— American apogee of 188-189

— as Western orthodox medicine 50,65,136-138
— cancer and 373
— Cartesian-Newtonian postulates and, 143
— challenged in the 20th century, 215
— derivation of term, 135-136
— failure of 542-543
— in 16th-century England, 145
— media and, 138-139
— osteopathy and, 222
— paradigm of, 131-132
— pharmaceutical expansion and, 161,189-190
— "scientific medicine" and, 161,170
— *scientism* of, 136
— threatened by "irregular" medicine in US, 151-157 (see also *AMA*)
Almy, Thomas 87
aloe vera, 575
Alpert, Susan, 409
alpha-2U-globulin 419
alpha-linoleic acid 365
alternative medicine *see* medicine
Alzheimer's disease 47,74,265,543, 549,568
AMA (American Medical Association)
— AIC and, 77,79
— American Political Action Committee (AMPAC) of, 227-228
— approval of deadly medicines by, 48
— as part of "healthcare delivery system" 44
— Bricker, John, and, 442
— business of, 234
— CCHI and, 207
— chiropractic and, 202-205,228
— cholesterol controversy and, 346-347
— citizen/docotor polls and, 67
— Code of Medical Ethics of, 142
— Committee on Quackery of, 205,207,211,212
— Council on Drugs of, 250,262
— Council on Medical Education of, 172
— Council on Pharmacy and Chemistry of, 261
— criticism from within of, 225
— Department of Investigation of, 205,207,211,212
— doctor benefits from membership in, 222-224
— drug industry and, 260-265
— early history of, 157-159,165-166,178,179-180
— ethics problems of, 232-239
— first 50 years of, 220
— Fishbein era of, 221
— Friedman critique of, 235
— Glyoxylide and, 447
— Group Health Insurance Assn. and, 228
— healthcare costs and, 73
— homeopathy and, 157-158
— internal debates of, 213
— laetrile and, 212,433,434, 452,458,460
— longevity rates of members of 549
— membership drop in, 232
— osteopathy and, 232
— "quackery" and, 204-219
— semantics and, 229
— socialized medicine and, 77, 186-187,188, 228-229
— structure of, 222
AMA Council on Pharmacy and Chemistry 539,545
AMA Drug Evaluations 262

Ambruster, Howard 282
American Assn. for Chronic Fatigue Syndrome Research 526
American Assn. for the Advancement of Science (AAAS) 424,433, 434,436
American Assn. for Labor Legislation 186
American Assn. of Poison Control Centers 291
American Biologics 465
American Biologics-Mexico SA Medical Center 37
American Cancer Society (ACS) 110, 111,174,207,267,374,376,377,378, 380,388,399,405,414-424,433, 434,444,452,458,460,539,573
American College of Obstetricians and Gynecologists 264
American College for Advancement in Medicine (ACAM), 363
American Council on Science and Health (ACSH), 216,320
American Dietetic Assn. 572
American Enterprise Institute for Public Policy Research 198
American Health Information Management Assn. 327
American Heart Assn. (AHA), 110,111,326,327,333,341,351, 355,359,419,424,580,590
American Home Products 183, 263,347
American Hospital Assn. 376
American I.G. Chemical 181
American Journal of the Medical Sciences 165
American Lancet 164
American Lung Assn. (ALA) 110, 111,419,424
American Medical Association *see* AMA
American Medical Avarice 49

American Medical News 94,202, 243,244,590
American Medical Services Inc. 232
American Medical Television 264
American Naturopathic Medical Assn. (ANMA) 548
American Nurses Assn. Committee on Impaired Nursing Practice 54
American Pharmaceutical Assn. 207
American Revolution 146
American School of Naturopathy 167
Ames, Bruce 418,425
Amstar 563
amygdalin *see* laetrile
amyotrophic lateral sclerosis (ALS) 568
Anaconda Co. 183
And the Band Played On 491
Anderson, Harold 283
Anderson, Jack, 89-90,209,255-256
anesthesia, deaths from 46
angiograms (arteriograms) 87,86,329-331
Annals of Internal Medicine 399
Annals of the Han Dynasty 121
Annis, Edward R., 98
antibiotic-resistant germs 58-59
antioxidants 366,567-570
Apollo 119
Arabs, ancient pharmacy and, 127
Archer Daniels Midland 216
Are You a Target for Elimination? 206
Aristotle 117,122
arrythmia 337
arteriograms *see* angiograms
arteriosclerosis *see* heart/circulatory disease
arthritis 47
Arthritis Foundation 207
Arthur, Patricia 202
Asclepius (Aesculapius) 119
Ashe, Arthur 509

Aslan, Ana 315
aspartame *see* Nutrasweet
aspirin 298,570
Association of American Medical Colleges 173
Astra AB 252
AT &T 183
Athotis, king of Egypt, 116
Atkins, Robert 29
atherosclerosis *see* heart/circulatory disease
Atlantic Monthly 345,355
atomic bomb 413,415
atrazine 551
attention deficit disorder (ADD) 531
Australia 533
autoimmune diseases 47,529
Avicenna 123
Ayerst Laboratories 299
Ayurvedic medicine 117,118,582,599
AZT (azidothymidine,zidovudine, Retrovir) 257-258,259 *see also* AIDS
azidothymidine *see* AZT

B

B vitamins 276,424,557,567
Bailar, John C. 371,382-383
BAITs (benzyl-aromatic-isothiocyanates) 467-468
Baker, Elizabeth 584
Baker, Harold 307
"balanced diet" 560-561
Balboa Naval Hospital 49
balloon angioplasty (PTCA) 334, 335,336
Barnes, Ernest G. 205
Bayh-Dole Act 108
Baylor College of Medicine Methodist Hospital 323
Beach, Wooster 134

Bealle, Morris 139,225-227,270-271
Beard, John 442
Bearden, Thomas 579,614-615
Beardsley, Tim 382
Beatrice Foods 563
Bechamp, Andre 611
Becker, R.O. 609
beclomethasone 294
Becton Dickinson 283
bed sores 59-80
Bedell, Berkley 540
Beldekas, John 503-504,505
Bendectin, 273
benign prostatic hypertrophy (BPH) 266
Bennett, James T. 110-111,420,421
benzaldehyde 468
benzodiazepine drugs 301-302
Benveniste, Jacques 601-603
beriberi 568
Berkeley Daily Gazette 453
Berkowitz, Carol D. 604
Berman, Edgar 49,114
Bernard, Claude 161-162
Berwick, Donald 88
beta-carotene 276,424,469,555,567, 568,570,573,576
bethanidine 294
Bethlehem Steel 183
Beverly Enterprises 196
B.F. Goodrich Co. 183
bioelectrical therapy 607
Bio-Electro-Magnetic Institute 608
bioenergetics 610
"biological" medicine 236
biological warfare 502
biomagnetism 607
bions 610
biophysics 609
biopsies 53
Birds, Valentine 26-27
bismuth 272
Bjork-Shiley heart valve 299

black currant seed oil 306
Black Death 123
Blair, Steven N., 359
Blalock, J. Edwin 594
Block, Gladys 574
Bluchel, Kurt 271
Blue Cross 51,95,187,188
Blue Cross/Blue Shield of New Hampshire 95
Blue Cross of Jamaica 95
Blue Cross of Maryland 95
Blue Cross of Washington DC 95
Blue Cross of Washington and Alaska 605
Blue Cross of West Virginia 95
blue-green algae 575
Blue Shield 95,187,188
Blumberg, Jeffrey 569,570
Bobst, Elmer and Mary, 422
Boerhaave, Herman 128,147
Bohanon, Luther 455-456
bonesetters 148
Borden Co. 181
Boston University School of Medicine 366
"botanic" doctors 148
Botanic Medical Board 151
bovine leukemia virus (BLV) 501
Bradford Research Institutes (BRI) 38,468,484,525,566,569
Bradford, Robert 435,454,455,457
Brassica 468
Braverman, Albert S. 371,348
Breast Cancer Prevention Trial 410
Brecher, Arline and Harold, 360,363
Brief, Ken 322
Brigham and Women's Hospital 66
Bristol Laboratories 338
Bristol Myers 181,398
Bristol-Myers Squibb 109,263,269, 299,506
Bristol Medical Journal 339,353,603
British medicine 144-146

British Research Council on Complementary Medicine 237-238
Broder, Samuel 398
Brook, Itzhak 508
Brown, June Gibbs 101
Brown, Raymond K. 613
Bruel & Kjaer Instruments 268
Bryden, James 202
bubonic plague *see* Black Death
Burk, Dean 433,438-439,451-453, 454,545,571
Burroughs Wellcome 257,258,259, 486,507,508,510,511
Bush, George 530
Burton IAT Therapy 215
Burton, Lawrence 429
Burzynski, Stanislaw 22-23
Bush administration 108,281
Business Week 87,193
Butz, Earl 556
Byrd, Randolph 590

C

caduceus 120
Caiazza, Stephen 518,520-521
Caisse, Rene 428
calcium 533,554,576
calcium channel blockers 337,339
California Board of Medicine 26,27
California Common Cause 228
California Medical Assn. 228
calomel 135,163
Cambridge University 349
Campbell Soup Co. 269
Canada, "quackbusters" in, 236
CanCell 409,522
Candida albicans 57,525
cancer
— AIDS Inc. and, 507
— animal testing and, 417-419
— big business of, 385-387

— Cancer Inc. and, 377,378,380, 385,386,391,397,409,423, 424,428,429,434,544,546
— CEA (carcinoembryonic antigen) test and, 388,407
— chemotherapy and, 386,387, 389,397-401
— Conquest of Cancer program and, 379,382,421,488,489
— control of, 427
— costs of, 376-377, 385
— diet and, 425-426,442,573-575
— genes and, 392-396
— Hemoccult test and, 406-407
— hormones and, 398,411,416-417
— industrial chemicals and, 401-402,411-412,416-417
— laetrile and, 433-470
— mammograms and, 383,384, 387-388,405-406
— mastectomies and, 372
— negative effects of standard therapies for, 390-391, 400-401
— nuclear radiation exposure and, 412-416
— nutrients and, 424
— oncogenes and, 392,393,394
— oncology and, 377,384
— Pap smear and, 383,388
— "primordial thesis" of, 395-396
— Proscar (finasteride) and, 410
— PSA (prostate-specific antigen) test and, 383,384,385,407-409
— radiation and, 386,387
— ROTS/free radicals and, 567
— spices/condiments and, 424
— "spontaneous remissions" and, 403-404
— statistics of, 374-375
— surgery and, 389
— survival rates in, 381-382
— Tamoxifen and, 410-411
— tobacco and, 388
— tumor obsession and, 399-400
— unitarianism and, 373
— "unproven remedies" for, 450-451
— viruses and, 392
"cancer virus" 610,611
Cantwell, Alan 502
carbenoxolone 294
cardiomyopathy 549
cardiovascular disease *see* heart/circulatory disease
Carnation Co. 181
Carnegie Foundation for the Advancement of Teaching 171,172
carotenids 367
carotid endarterectomy 82-83
Carpenter, Larry and Catherine, 30-31
Carter, H. Ballantine 408
Carter, James P. 218,360,363
Carter, Richard 224
Cartesian-Newtonian postulates 126, 128,143,389,599
Casdorph, Richard 360
Cason, James 463-464
cataract surgeries 81
Catholic Institute of International Relations 553
CD4 (T4) cells 476,479
CD8 (T8) cells 478-480
CDC *see* Centers for Disease Control and Prevention
CEA (carcinoembryonic antigen) *see* cancer
Ceclor 244
Cedars-Sinai Medical Center 351
cellular therapy *see* live cell therapy
Center for Mind-Body Studies 596
Center for Science in the Public Interest 216
Center for the Study of Drug

Development 295
Centers for Disease Control and Prevention (CDC) 62,63,259,291, 473,479,493,499,511,519-520,526
Central Intelligence Agency (CIA) 505
Century Clinic 11-12
cesarean operations ("c-sections") 80
CFS *see* chronic fatigue syndrome
Chandra, Rajit K. 576
chaparral 571
Chapman, Nathaniel 159
charitable organizations, 110-111
Charles II, 133-135
Chase Manhattan Bank 183
chelation therapy *see* heart/circulatory disease, EDTA
Chemie Grunenthal 272-273
"chemoprevention" 571
chemotherapy *see* cancer
chenodeoxychloric acid 294
"Chicago Four," the, 202
Children's Hospital (Orange CA) 400
Children's Hospital National Medical Center 84
China 117,118,121-122,558,598
China Medical Board 173
Chirimuuta, Rosalie 492
chiropractic 18,202-204,205,206,212
chlamydia 350
chloramphenicol (Chloromycetin) 262,283,300
chlorination 551
chlorozone 585
Chodak, Gerald 409
cholesterol 341-355 *see also* heart/circulatory disease
cholestyramine 345,346
"chondriana" 428
Chopra, Deepak 599
Chowka, Peter Barry 421
Christian Science 148, 149,166
Christianity, 122-123

chronic fatigue syndrome (CFS) 56,500,504,524-531
Church of Scientology 309
chymopapain 294
Ciba-Geigy 181,273-274,299,300,551
Ciba-Geigy Japan 274
Ciba Pharmaceuticals 283
CIGNA Co. 197
Circulation 323,353
Citizens Committee for Human Rights 310
Citizens for Health 305,555,556
Civil War 153,163
Clark, Adrian V. 615
Clarke, Norman E. 361,362
Classic of Internal Medicine 122
Cleave, T.L. 560
Clinoril 244
Clinton administration 76,228,242, 268,320,579
Clinton, Hillary Rodham 222
Clioquinol *see* Oxychinol
Clofibrate 300
CMV (cytomegalovirus) 350,485,500
Coalition for Equal Access to Medicines 268
Coca-Cola 216,563
Code of Hammurabi 116
cognitive dissonance 139-140,141
Cohen, Nicholas 593
Coleman, Vernon 201
Coley's toxins 446
Collagen Corporation 264
Columbia-Presbyterian Medical Center 478
Columbus, Christopher 139-140
Commercial Solvent Corp. 183
Committee for Freedom of Choice in Cancer Therapy 207,211,314,435, 436-438,454,455,456,458-459, 464,465
Committee for Freedom of Choice in Medicine 4,27,30,31-32,55,207,

210,374,475
Committee on Government Operations 257,258
Committee on the Costs of Medical Care (CCMC) 186-187
Common Catalog 554
Common Sense 347
Commmonwealth Fund 173,174
complementary medicine *see* medicine
computerized axial tomography (CAT) scan 85,89,90
Confessions of a Medical Heretic 50, 114,201,225
congestive heart failure *see* heart/circulatory disease
Congressional Budget Office 192
Congressional Record 302-303,447, 449
Connecticut State Medical Society 203
Conquest of Cancer program *see cancer*
Consumer Price Index (CPI) 243
Consumer Product Safety Commission 201
Consumer Reports 602-604
Consumers Union 198
Continental Can Co. 183,562
Contreras, Ernesto 453,455,462
Coordinating Council on Health Education (CCHI) 207,214
copper 576
Cornell University 558
Cornell University Medical College 189,241
coronary artery disease *see* heart/circulatory disease
Coronary Artery Surgery Study (CASS) 333
coronary bypass 83,331-334,335,336
Coronary Drug Project 346

Coronary Primary Prevention Trial (CPPT) 346
cosmic dualism 598
cortisone 311
Coulter, Harris 152,158,164,165,518
Council of Better Business Bureaus 207
Council on Foreign Relations (CFR) 184
Cousins, Norman 592
Cowles publishing 183
Cox News Service 411
Cranton, Elmer 360
Crichton, Michael 579
Crout, Richard 230,304
"Crusaders" (ABC-TV) 101
Cuba 487,503,505
Cullen, William 128
Curran, Helen 469
cyanazine 551

D

Dark Ages 123
Dartmouth Medical School 88
Dartmouth University 84,147
Data Control 183
Davis, Adelle 548
Davis, David A. 46
Davis, Devra Lee 376
Davis, Nathan Smith 158
"Day One" (ABC-TV) 508
DDT 189
Deaconess Hospital 358
Debendox 273
Declaration of Helsinki 32-33
Declaration of Independence 128
Defective Medicine 201
demerol 42
Department of Veterans Affairs (DVA) 103
Dermatron 12

Dermer, Gerald D. 371,393-394
Der Spiegel 399
DES (diethylstilbestrol) 299
Descartes, Rene 125-126
Des Moines Register 216
Detroit Medical Journal 164
Detroit Review of Medicine and Pharmacy 142
Devitt, James E. 427-428
diabetes 356,568 *see also* heart/circulatory disease
diagnostic-referral schemes 89-91
"diet and reinfarction trial" (DART) 366
Diet, Nutrition and Cancer 467
diet/nutritional revolution 543
dietary connections in health 558-560
dietary supplements *see* supplements industry
dimethyl sulfoxide *see* DMSO
DiLorenzo, Thomas J. 110-111, 420, 421
Dioxychlor 521,522,569,585
dipyridamole 60
Dirty Medicine 238
Disraeli, Benjamin 381
Distaval 273
Distillers Co. 273
DMSO (dimethyl sulfoxide) 303,315, 316-317
Dossey, Larry 113,589-590
Dow Chemical 181,554
Dow Chemical Canada 216
drug industry
— AMA and, 260-268
— as AIC component, 78
— early history of, in US, 163-165, 177-178
— earnings of top executives of, in US, 269-270
— costs of drug development and, 249-251
— generic drugs and, 281
— growth in the 1980s/1990s of, 198
— healthcare reform and, 242
— lobbying of physicians by, 230,263-265
— "me-too" drugs and, 247,248
— patent process of, in US, 254
— post-WWII expansion of, 189-190
— price comparisons with other countries of products of, 244,246
— profits of, 242-245
— threatened by supplements industry 47-48,215,571
— ties to Rockefeller-I.G. Farben combine of, 180-184
— worldwide cartel nature of, 270-272
Duesberg, Peter H. 393,471,483, 485,488,508,509
Duke University Center for Health Care Policy and Research 88
Duncan, Robert M. 314-315
Dupont 181
Dutch Consumers Union 239
Dutch Reformed Church 440
Dyazide 244

E

Eastern Virginia Medical School 590
Eastman Kodak 181
Eber Papyrus 117
Ebola hemorrhagic fever 483
echinacea 575
Eclectic Dispensatory 152
eclectic medicine 148,152,185
Eddy, David 88
Eddy, Mary Baker 148
Edison, Thomas Alva 539,580
Edlin, Gordon 71

EDTA *see* chelation therapy
Edwards, Charles C. 283
Egypt, medicine in ancient, 116
eicosapentaenoic acid 365
Einstein, Albert 129
Eisenberg, David 541
Eisenhower, Dwight D. 181
elderly, medical abuse of, 60-61
electromagnetic fields 532,608
Ellwood, Paul M. 83
Elting, L.S. 63
Eminase 252
Emory University 336
EMS (eiosinophilia-myalgia syndrome), 308-309
Enderlein, Guenther 611
endocrinological system 588
endoscopy 83
energetic medicine 606-608
Engleberg, Hyman 352
Enkaid 299,338
Enstrom, James E. 574
environmental chemicalization 532, 550-552
environmental illness ("e.i.") 529,531
Environmental Working Group of Physicians for Social Responsibility 550
Eraldin 272
Epstein-Barr Virus (EBV) 485,526
Epstein, Samuel 371,377,401-403, 410-411,413,415
Eskimos 440,558
essential fatty acids (EFA) 365, 366,564-565
Essex, Max 494
Essiac 428,522
estrogen *see* cancer, hormones and
European Union 559
evening primrose oil 306
Evers, Ray 313-315
Exxon 216

F

Fabian socialism 175
Faden, Ruth 415-416
faith healers of the Philippines 607
Faloon, William 15
Faltermayer, Edmund 82
Families USA Foundation (FUSAF) 244
Faulkner Breast Center 373
FDA (Food and Drug Administration)
— ACE (adrenal cortical extract) and, 211-212
— aging research and, 569
— AIC and, 78,164,289-290
— AIDS and, 293, 295,508-509, 523-524
— Aldactone and, 299
— Allison, Joan Vera, and, 23-24
— animals and, 320-321
— antibiotic levels and, 58
— arrhythmia drugs and, 338
— as murderer through drug industry policy of, 290-291
— as outgrowth of legislation 170
— beclomethasone and, 294
— benzodiazepine drugs and, 301-302
— bethanidine and, 294
— Bjork-Shiley heart valve and, 209
— bureaucracy of, 250
— Burzynski, Stanislaw, and, 22
— carbenoxolone and, 294
— CCHI and, 207
— Century Clinic and, 11-12
— chenodeoxychloric acid 294
— chloramphenicol (Chloromycetin) and, 283,300
— chymopapain and, 294
— Clofibrate and, 300
— costs of drug approval and, 295

688

— critique of employee behavior by officer of, 304-305
— cyclamates and, 305
— defibrillators and, 335
— DES (dimethylstilbestrol) and, 299
— difficulties in complying with drug-approval requirements of, 302-303
— DMSO and, 313,316-317
— drug-approval role of, 248-304, 297-298
— "drug lag" and, 294-295,297
— early history of, 164
— EDTA chelation therapy and, 294,313,361-362
— Enkaid and, 299
— Evers, Ray, and, 313-314
— Flagyl and, 299
— food labeling and, 319-320
— former officers of, in drug industry, 282-284
— Friedman attack on, 235
— GAO attack on drug-approval process of, 293
— GAO investigations of, 282,293, 317-318,320-321
— generic drug scandal and, 281
— Gerovital and, 315-316
— Glyoxylide and, 448
— Halcion and, 301
— Harrington-McGill, Gertrude (Sissy) and, 3-4
— heart scans and, 331
— Heritage Foundation and, 323
— HHS criticism of, 281
— Highland Laboratories and, 10-11
— House investigations of, 282
— IND and NDA machinery of, 286,293
— Kefauver Amendments and, 288-289

— Krebiozen and, 449
— lactulose and, 294
— laetrile and, 212,244,312-313, 433,434,452,455,456,458-459,460
— Librium and, 361
— Life Extension Foundation and, 14-15
— LSE Seronoa and, 310
— L-tryptophan and, 7-8, 308-309
— MER/29 and, 298
— methaqualone and, 298-299
— Michaelis, Steve, and, 314-315
— minoxodil and, 294
— monopoly power of, as discouragement for new drug development, 296
— NLEA and, 318-319
— NutraSweet (aspartame) and, 305-306
— Nutricology/Allergy Research Group and, 15-17
— nutritional supplements and, 546
— Oden, G. J., and, 30-31
— Orabilex and, 298
— oral diazoxide and, 294
— oral polio vaccine and, 298
— Orphan Drug Act and, 293
— OTA assessment of drug-approval policy of, 297
— part of healthcare delivery system, 44
— Peltzman critique of, 321-322
— Pets Smell-Free and, 21
— Phenacetin and, 300
— Phenformin and, 300
— power of, extended by FD&CA amendments, 192-193,288-289
— prescription-drug apparatus and, 286-287
— Proscar and, 310

689

- Proxmire Law and, 392
- Prozac and, 301
- PSA and, 268,409
- "quackbuster" conspiracy and, 210,213,217,218
- radionics and, 601
- saccharin and, 305
- scope of jurisdiction of, 289
- semantics and, 306-308
- Senate investigation of, 282
- silicone-gel breast implants and, 298
- sodium valproate and, 294
- supplements and, 214,284,291-292
- Tahoma Clinic and, 4-9,10
- tamoxifen and, 411
- taxol and, 109
- Thalidomide and, 272
- Traco Laboratories and, 306-307
- Valium and, 301
- verapimil and, 294
- Vitacel-7 and, 13-14
- vivisection and, 296
- Wiley, Harvey, and, 178-179-285

FDA Consumer 363
FDA Reports 291
Federal Trade Commission (FTC) 202,203-204,207,210,214
Feldene 244
Ferguson, Wilburn 118,450
fertilizers 550,552
fetal heartbeat monitor 85-86
fibromyalgia 56,525,529
Filipinos 558
Fine, Al 36-38,39,40
Fine, Marie 37
Firestone Rubber 181
Fishbein, Morris 221,222,226,229
Fitzgerald, Benedict F. Jr. 447,449, 450-451

Flagyl 299
flavones 468
flavonoids 366
Fletcher, Robert H. 388,407
Flexner, Abraham 172
Flexner Report 170,172-173,178
Flexner, Simon 172
Florida East Coast Railway 183
Florida Health Care Cost Containment Board 89
fluoridation 551
food additives 419
Food and Drug Administration *see* FDA
Food and Nutritional Board, National Research Council 561,562
Food Council (Netherlands) 239
Food, Drug and Cosmetic Act (FD&CA) 192,259,281,286,298, 304,311
Food Nutrition News 291
food preservatives 419
food processing industry 558,560-563
Ford Foundation 174
Ford, Gerald 503
Ford Motor Co. 181,183
Fortune 82,83,193,269
Foundation for Orthomolecular Education 238-239
Framingham Heart Study 346,356
Frederick II 271
Frederick Stearns Co. 164
free radicals 566,570,586
frequency machines 613
frequency medicine 607
Frey, Louis 433,453
Frick, M. Heiki 356
Friedman, Milton 235
Frost and Sullivan 386
FTC vs. the AMA 205-206
Fugh-Berman, Adrianne 410-411

G

Gaby, Alan R. 310
Galen 122,128,143,147
Gallegos, Julie 5
Gallo, Robert 486,490,499
Gallup polls 458
gammalinolenic acid *see* GLA
Gard, Zane R. 25-26
garlic 575
Garrison, Omar 282,283
G.D. Searle & Co. 299,305
gene p53 350
Genentech 252-253,339,340
generic drugs 281
genetics 392-393,394-396,582-584
General Accounting Office (GAO) 51,93,96,243,282,293,318,397,403
General Analine and Film 183
General Education Board 172,173
General Electric 181,183
General Foods 183,562
General Mills 181,216
General Motors 181,183,187
General Tire 181
Georgetown Medical School 596
Gerber Co. 563
Gerber, Michael 208
germ theory of disease 132,161-162
Germany, "alternative" medicine in, 236-237
Gerson, Max 446
Gerovital (GH3,procaine hydrochloride) 13,14,315-316,317
Getty Oil 183
Getzendanner, Susan 202
GH3 *see* Gerovital
ginkgo biloba 576
GLA (gammalinolenic acid) 306
Glaxo Inc. 243,263
Global Program on AIDS 472
glutathione 568

Glyoxylide 447-448
GMD (glucose metabolism dysfunction) 557
Goddard, James L. 283
Gofman, John W. 52,412-413
goldenseal 575
Goodyear Tire 181
Gordon, Garry F. 360
Gordon, James 596-597
Gori, Gio B. 563-564
Goteborg University 274
Gould, Jay M. 413-415
Goulden, Joseph 185
Graham, Sylvester 148
GRAS list 306
Grave's Disease 530
"Great Society" programs 97,186
Greco-Roman medicine, 122-123
Greece, medicine in ancient, 119-120
Greenwald, Peter 574
GRH (gonadotropin-releasing hormone) 415
Griffin, G.E., 183,282,438,454
Grossman, Karl 505
Gulf Oil 181
Gulf War Syndrome 504
GVH (graft-vs.-host disease) 500

H

Hahnemann, Samuel 149-150,600, 601
Halcion 301,309
Hall, Lawrence 1,17-19
Halstead, Bruce, 27,29,210-211, 220,360,508
Hamburg University 349
Hanford nuclear site 413
Hansson, Olle 274
Harkin, Tom 540
Harmer, Ruth Mulvey, 49,254-255, 261-262

Harper, Harold 301,306,557
Harrington-McGill, Gertrude (Sissy) 1,2-4
Harris polls 436,458
Hartford Insurance Co. 183
Harvard Community Health Plan 88
Harvard Medical School 60,66,89,541
Harvard Medical School Health Letter 276-277,576
Harvard University 54,62,147,336, 359,553,565
Harvard University Department of Nutrition 563
Harvard University School of Public Health 510,562,573
Harvey, Ken 57
Hatem, Joanne 65
Hayes, Woody 41
Hayward, Steven, 97-98,99
HBLV virus 501
Health Care Financing Administration (HCFA) 100,256
"healthcare delivery system," components of, 44
Health Council (Netherlands) 239
Health Information Designs Inc. 57, 247
Health Insurance Assn. of America 73
health maintenance organizations (HMOs) 193
Health Research Group 51
Healy, Bernadine 108
Hearst Corp. 183
heart and circulatory disease
— arteriosclerosis and, 326
— atherosclerosis and, 326,565
— big business of, 356-358
— cholesterol controversies and, 340-355
— components of, 326
— costs of, 327
— diabetes and, 326,356
— diagnostics for, 329-331
— dietary connections to, 365-368
— diets and, 358-359
— drugs and, 337-341,355
— EDTA chelation therapy and, 215,253,294,313-314,350-364
— exercise and, 358-359
— heart attack and, 327
— hypertension and, 337,338,568
— hypoglycemia and, 326
— mineral depletion and, 554-555
— review of, 327-328
— standard treatments for, 331-341
— triglycerides and, 355-356
heart attack *see* heart/circulatory disease
Heart-Diet Pilot Program 346
heart disease *see* heart/circulatory disease
Heart Failure 345
Heimlich, Jane 337,338,360
Heisenberg, Werner 129
Hellerstein, David 71
Helsinki University 356
hemicorporectomy 397
Hemoccult test *see* cancer
Henderson, Robert 335
Henry VIII 144,237
hepatitis B vaccine 502,503
herbalism 117-118
herbicides 419,450,551
herbs 575
Hering, Constantine 150
Heritage Foundation 98,192,322
Hewlett-Packard 183
HHV-6 virus 499-500,504,506,530
HHV-7 virus 501
Hicks, Jocelyn 84
Higgs, Robert 279
Highland Laboratories 10-12
Himmelstein, David 245

Hippocrates 117,119,120-121,122, 143,150,539
Hippocratic Oath 120
History of a Crime Against the Pure Food Law 285
HIV (HIV-1, HIV-2) *see* AIDS
Hodge, J.W. 201
Hoechst AG 252
Hoffman-LaRoche 181,275-276, 283,302
holism 113,547,582,584,597,616
Holmes, Oliver Wendell 113
Homeopathic Medical College 152
Homeopathic Yellow Fever Commission 153
homeopathy 130,135-136,148,149-156,160,161,185,215,599-606,609
homocysteine 350
Honolulu Star-Bulletin 372
Hospital Corporation of America 193,196,197
House Governmental Operations Subcommittee 93,107
House Ways and Means Committee 98
How We Die 58
Howard, Sir Albert 554
Hoxsey, Harry 221,226,447-448
Hoxsey herbals 447,448-449
HTLV-I 491
HTLV-III *see* AIDS
Huang Ti ("Yellow Emperor") 118, 112
Hullet, Stephen B. 340
Humana Corporation 193
"human intention factor" 598
Human Nutrition Report No.2, Benefits from Human Nutrition Research 556
Humphrey-Durham amendments 287
Hunzakuts 439-440,558
Hutt, Peter Barton 279
Huxley, Thomas 113

Hybritech Inc. 268,409
hydrogen peroxide 569,584
hydrogenation 564,565
hydrotherapy 149
hydroxyl radical 567
hypercholesterolemia 342
hypertension *see* heart/circulatory disease
Hypertension Detection and Followup Program 338
hypoglycemia 525,557 *see also* heart/circulatory disease
hysterectomies 48-49

I

IAT (immunoaugmentative therapy) 429
iatrogenic disease 45-49,55-56,63-64
IBM 183
Iceland 530-531,533
ICI Pharmaceuticals 268
idiopathic CD4 T-lymphocytopenia (ICL) 482
I.G. Farben 170,180-184,270,286
Illich, Ivan 49,50,198,241,302
imaging 597
"immortal cell lines" 394
immune dysregulation 528-531,593-594, *see also* AIDS, autoimmune disease, CFS
immunization *see* vaccines
immunotoxicology 566
Imperial Chemical Industries 268, 272,415
Incas 118
Inderal 244
India 117,599
"Indian doctors" 148
indoles 424,468
Inlander, Charles B., 42,57,64
Institute of Noetic Sciences 592

insurance (health)
— abuse of Medicare and Medicaid in, 100-101
— as contributor to healthcare cost crisis, 91-92
— Blue Cross/Blue Shield troubles of, 94-96
— federal components of, 97-101
— fight for survival of, 94
— fraudulent billings and, 93
— history of, 185-188
— vulnerability to fraud of, 93-94
— wastefulness of, 102
intensive-care medicine 43
interferons 387
interleukins 387
International Assn. for Enterostomal Therapy 59
International Chemical Industries 554
International Medical Commission of Lourdes (CMIL) 591
International Society for Individual Liberty 105
International Sugar Foundation 562
InterStudy 62,83
insecticides 550,552
In the Public Interest 204-205
"invasive" procedures 52-53
iodine 131,414,576
ipecac 197
Iraq 504
iron 576
Isoprinosine 258
isothiocyanates 424
IT & T 183
Ivy, Andrew C. 447,449

J

Jacob, Stanley 316
Jacobs, J. 604
Jastrow, Alan B. 427
Jefferson, Thomas 439
Jehovah's Witnesses 31
Jenner, Edward 151,162,163
Jenner, P. 568
Jensen, Lowell 16-17
Jivaro Indians 118,450
John Birch Society 437
Johns Hopkins Hospital 46
Johns Hopkins University 176,408, 415,517,576
Johnson & Johnson 196,197
Johnson, David 269
Johnson, Lyndon 97
Joint American Study Corporation (JASCO) 182
Joint Commission on Accreditation of Health Care Organization 88
Jones, Hardin B. 380
Jones, Rochelle 195
Journal of the American Medical Assn. (JAMA) 51,165,221,226,261, 275,291,329,333,354,388,427,545, 546,562
J.R. Reynolds 233

K

Kabi Pharmacia 252,268
Kaiser-Permanente 255
Kant, Immanuel 71
Kaposi, Moritz 519
Kaposi's sarcoma (KS) 500 *see also* AIDS
Kazman, Sam 322
Kaznacheyev, Vlail 614
Kefauver Amendments to FD&CA 288
Kefauver, Estes 288
Keller, Jimmy 19-21
Kellogg Foundation 173,174
Kellogg, M.W., Co. 181,347,562,563
Kennecott Copper 183

Kennedy, Edward M. 206,251-252
Kent, Saul 15,279
Kent WA police 6
Keshan Province, China 549
Kessler, David 279,310,320
Kittler, Glenn D., 438
Klaw, Spencer 56
Knight-Ridder 223,269,559
Knott, E.K. 613
Koch, Robert (and Vitacel-7) 13
Koch, Robert 130,131,161
Koch, William F. 447-448,585
Koop, C. Everett 107
Koppel, Ted 46
Krebiozen 447,448,449,450
Krebs, Ernst T. Jr. 438,440,442,455
Krebs, Ernst T. Sr. 24,438
Krimsky, Sheldon 76
Kuhnau, Wolfram 37
Kunnes, Richard 225
Kusserow, Richard P. 256,262
Kutz, Myer 169
Kyoto University 366

L

lactulose 294
laetrile 211-212,275,312,317,426, 433-445,446,449,451-469,543-544,567,584
"laetrile clinical trial" 464-466
"Lake Tahoe Syndrome" 525
Lambert, Edward L. 356
Lancet 365,372,398,405-406,427, 576,602,604,605-606
Lander, Louise 64,201
Lane, William 428
Largewhiskers, Thomas 578
L-arginine 20,21
Lasagna, Louis 297
Lasker, Albert 422
Laval University 367

"law of similars" 150
lead 523
Lederle Laboratories 181,299
Lee, Philip R. 87
Lemper, Paula 400
Leotrill 445
LeShan, Lawrence 593
Levin, Jeffrey S. 590
Levin, Lowell 46
Levin, Warren 29,208
Levine, Stephen 15-17,280-281
Levy, Jay 480
Levy, Stuart 58
Ley, Herbert 279
Life Extension Foundation 1,14-15, 30,279
Lilly, Eli, Co. 164,263,268,269-270, 309,409,554
Lincoln bacteriophage 446
linoleic acid 366
linolenic acid 366
Liotta, Lance 427
Lipid Research Clinics Coronary Primary Prevention Trial 351
lipoprotein (a) [Lp(a)] 349
Lisa, P. J., 206-207,210,213,216, 218,225
Lister, Joseph 162-163
live cell therapy 586-589
Livermore National Laboratory 412-413
Livingston-Wheeler, Virginia 611
Lo, Shyh-Ching 486,499
lobelia root 148
Loffler, Charles Lyman 226-227
London Daily Telegraph 237
London Observer 273
Lorgeril, Michel de, 365
Los Alamos nuclear site 416
Los Angeles Times 352
lovastatin (Mevacor) 345,347,355
Love, Susan 373
Lowen, Alexander 610

Loyola University 463
LSE Seronoa 310
L-tryptophan 7-8,280,308-311
Lundy, C.J. 349-350
lupus 529,543
Lust, Benedict 166-167
Lyme Disease 527
Lyon Diet Heart Study 365
LyphoMed 259
lysine 349,565

M

Macy Foundation 173,174
magnesium 554,555,557,576
magnetic-field therapy 608-609
magnetic resonance imaging (MRI) 85,89-90
mammograms *see* cancer
Mann, George B. 325
Manner, Harold 463
March of Dimes 174,419
Market for Cancer Therapy Products 386
Markle Foundation 173
Markle, G.E. 433
Marsa, Linda 26,110
Martin, John 530
Marzine 272
Massachusetts Medical Society 156-157
Matthiessen, Peter 237
Maya Indians 118
Mayo Clinic 46,235,406,435,459,467
McClellan, Mark 336
McDonagh, E. W. 360
McElroy, Carolyn J. 101
McGee, Charles T. 325,332,334,344, 351,363,560
McGill University 382
McIntosh, Henry 333-334
McKenna, Joan 518

McNaughton Foundation 438,439, 440,445,451
MDRs (minimum daily requirements) 561
media, as allopathic paradigm contributors, 138-139
Medicaid 76,97,98,99,101,104,171, 186,191-192,206,231,255,256,259, 268-269
Medical Age 16
medical-industrial complex (MIC) 193-197
Medical Nemesis 49,241,302
Medicare 76,84,97,98,99,100-101, 104,105,171,186,191-192,206,231, 232,255,259
Medicare Beneficiaries Defense Fund 100
Medicare Hsopital Insurance Trust Fund 99
medicine (*see also* AIC, allopathy, AMA)
— "alternative," "complementary" forms of, 547-548,598
— "alternative," startling growth in US of, 541-542
— ancient China and, 118,121-122
— ancient Egypt and, 116,118
— ancient Greece and, 117,119-120
— ancient Mesopotamia and, 116
— as religion and magic, 114-115,118-119
— Ayurvedic, 582,599
— British system of, 145
— Cartesian-Newtonian postulates and, 126
— Dark Ages and, 123
— Greco-Roman, 122
— in the Colonies, 146-147
— in 16th-century England, 148
— in 19th-century America, 143-160

696

— integrative concept of, 540-541
— need for new evaluative model in, 581
— new healing paradigm of in, 580
— pre-Columbian America and, 118
— prehistory of, 115-116
— rationalism in, 128-129
— shared human tradition of, 115
Medicine 165
"medicine men" 118
Medicine on Trial 53,201
Meditrends 376
"Mediterranean diet" 365
megavitamin therapy 546
Melmon, Kenneth L. 35
Memorial Sloan-Kettering Cancer Center 434,444,455,456
Memorial Sloan-Kettering Hospital 372
Mendelsohn, Robert S. 35,50,66,114, 201,225,227,274
mental depression 596
MER/29 298
Merck & Co. 164,243,268,269,271, 341,345
Merck Sharpe & Dohme 263,347
mercury 123,124,135,197
mercury amalgam fillings 529
Merrell Co. 164,273
Merrell (William S.) Co. 357
Merson, Michael 472
Mesue 123
metabolic therapy/therapists 275, 426-427,546-547
methaqualone 298-299
metolachlor 551
Metropolitan Life Insurance Co. 183-187
Meyers, Francis 367
Michaelis, Steve 313,314-315
Michigan Medical Society 157,159-160
Michigan State University 484
Middle Ages 144
Millerites 149
Millman, Marcia 35,49
minoxodil 294
misdiagnoses 66-67
Modell, Walter 189,241
Moertel, Charles G., 407,433,435,459
monoclonal antibodies 387
mononucleosis 525
Monroe County Medical Society 157
Monsanto Chemical 181,216,554
Montagnier, Luc 486,499
Moore, Thomas J. 325,345-347,355
Morehead, Penny 5
Mormons 149,558
Morse, M.Lee 247
Moss, Ralph 282,283,299,371,386, 387,444-445,456
Mossinghoff, Gerald J. 251-252
Mount Sinai Hospital 80
MRFIT (Multiple Risk Factor Intervention Trial) 338,346
Mulder, Daan 493
Mullis, Kary 471,483
multiple chemical sensitivity 531
multiple sclerosis 529,543
multivitamin therapy 575
Murphy, Marge 5
muscular dystrophy 587
Myers, Stephen A. 80

N

Nabisco 562
Naessens, Gaston 611
Naked Empress 169,201,225,271,296
Naprosyn 263
Nardil 42
National Academy of Sciences (NAS) 399, 467

National Advisory Council for Human Genome Research 395
National Aeronautics and Space Administration (NASA) 615
National Agricultural Chemical Assn. 216
National Breast Cancer Coalition 414
National Cancer Institute (NCI) 22, 109,257,258,378,383,388,394,397, 398,400,405,409,410,414,421,422, 424,433,439,445,465,482,486,488, 499,501,539,563,564,574
National Center for Health Statistics 291
National Cholesterol Education Program (NCEP) 346,354
National Foundation for Infantile Paralysis 174
National Health and Nutrition Survey 354
"national health fraud" conferences 216-218
National Health Service (UK) 237, 238
National Heart, Lung and Blood Institute 86,338,346,351,354
National Highway Traffic Safety Commission 291
National Institute of Allergy and Infectious Disease (NIAID) 258
National Institute of Medicine 88
National Institutes of Health (NIH) 77,107,108,190,302,380,395,517, 540,581,592
National Lead 183
National Medical Enterprises 196
National Medical Expenditure Survey 60,72
National Medical Liability Reform Coalition 73
National Nutritional Foods Assn. (NNFA) 290-291
National Registry of Myocardial Infarction 340
Nature 601-602
National Vaccine Information Center 65
naturopathy 166-167
necrotizing fasciitis 59
Nei Ching 118
Nelson, Gaylord 230
Nestle's 181
Nestor, John O. 305
Netherlands, supplements controversy in, 238-239
neuropeptides 594
neurosyphilis 519
neutraceuticals 568
Nevada Naturopathic Medical Assn. (NNMA) 24
New and Unofficial Remedies 261
New Deal, the 170,171
New England Journal of Medicine (NEJM) 45,46,104,351,352,397, 399,466,541,573,574
New Hampshire Medical Society 157
New Haven Medical Society 203
Newman, Thomas B. 340,354
New Medical Record 165
New Preparations 164,165
Newsday 505
Newsweek 58,59,594
Newton, Sir Isaac 125-126
New York Central Railway 183
New York College of Physicians and Surgeons 147
New York Empire Blue Cross/Blue Shield 94
New York Journal of Medicine 156,157
New York Native 504,528
New York State Journal of Medicine 544
New York Times 268-269,339
New York Times Magazine 320

698

New York Times News Service 558
New Zealand 533
niacin 576
Niehans, Paul 37,587,588
Nieper, Hans 12,30
Nieuwenhuis, R.A. 238-239
nitrilosides *see* laetrile
Nixon, Richard M. 379-488
North Carolina School of Medicine 367
Norton, Larry 372
nosocomial infections 62-63
NSAIDs 306
Nuclear Regulatory Commission (NRC) 414
Nuland, Sherman 58
Nureyev, Rudolph 509
NutraSweet 216,305-306
Nutricology/Allergy Research Group 15-17,281
Nutritional Labeling and Education Act of 1990 (NLEA) 291-292,318-319

oral polio vaccine 298
Orange County Register 245,263,269
organic farming 555
orgone energy 610
Ormont Drug and Chemical Co. 283
Ornish, Dean 358
Orphan Drug Act 293
orphan drugs 109
Orr, William 570
Oscar Mayer Co. 563
osteopathy 166,222
osteoporosis 47,543
Ostrom, Neenyah 504,528
OTA *see* Office of Technology Assessment
oxidation theory of arterial disease 567
oxidative (oxygen) therapy 584-586
oxidology 566-570,584,608,609
Oxychinol 273-274
ozone 522,569,585
ozone layer 532,584
Oyle, Irving 579

O

Oak Ridge nuclear site 413
O'Connor, Egan 52
Office of Alternative Medicine (OAM) 384,541,581,592-593,598
Office of Technology Assessment (OTA) 46,88,109,241,242,247-248,249-250,295,297,387
Ohio State University 41
O'Keefe, James 573
O'Leary, Dennis S. 88
Olin Corp. 183
omega-6 fatty acids 366
Omni magazine 76
oncogenes *see* cancer
oncology *see* cancer
Orabilex 298

P

Pacemakers 83,335
Paine, James C. 15
Pam 347
Pan American Railways 183
pangamic acid *see* Vitamin B15
Pap smear *see* cancer
Paracelsus 113,124-125,128,580
Paracetamol 272
paradigm capture 139
paradigm formation 115
Parke-Davis 164,262,283,300
Parkinson's disease 47,543,568,587,588
Parliament (British) 145
Pasteur Institute 486,489
Pasteur, Louis 130,131,161-162,163

Patterson, J. C. 349
Pauling, Limus 349,350,565
PCR (polymerase chain reaction) test) 483
Pear, Robert 269
Pediatrics 604
Pedigo, Michael 202
Pekkanen, John 91
pellagra 568
Peltzman, Sam 321-322
PEM (protein-energy malnutrition) 564
penicillin 189,519-520,521
Penn Central 183
pentamidine 257,259
People's Medical Society 63-64,201, 228
Pepper, Claude 214
PepsiCo Foundation 216
peripheral vascular disease *see* heart/circulatory disease
Persia, medicine in ancient, 121
pertussis vaccine 65
pesticides 419,550,551,552
Peterson, Erik 97-98,99
Peterson, J.C. 433
Pet Milk 181
Pets Smell-Free 21
Pfizer Pharmaceuticals 216,243
Pharmceutical Advertising Council 213
pharmaceutical industry *see* drug industry
Pharmaceutical Manufacturers Assn. (PMA) 242,243,249,251-252, 262,295
pharmacy, origins of, 123
Phenacetin 300
Phenformin 300
phenols 424,468
Philadelphia College of Physicians 165
Philip Morris 233

Philpott, William H. 608
physician, derivation of term, 144
Physician Insurers Assn. of America 48
Physician's Desk Reference 261-262
Pien Ts'io 121
Pisani, Joseph M. 283
Pittsburgh Glass 181
Plaxin 272
pleomorphism 611
Pliny the Elder 117
Plum Island 505
Pluto 119
Pneumocystis carinii pneumonia (PCP) 259
polio 174
polio vaccine 502
poppers 518
prana 599,615
Pravachol 341
Preludin 272
Premarin 244
President's Biomedical Research Panel 302
President's Cancer Board 382
Preston, Thomas 50-51,54-55,71,86
Price, Weston 560
primordial thesis *see* cancer
Priore, Antoine 610, 612,613,614
Procardia 244
Procardia AB 268
Procter and Gamble 181
progenitor cryptocides 611
progesterone 416 *see also* cancer, hormones and
Progessives 177,185
Project AIDS International 512-513
proline 349,565
Pronap 272
propoxyphene 60
Proscar 310 *see also* cancer
Prozac 301, 309-310
prostate, BPH and cancer of, 266-

268,310-311
protit 611
Providence Hospital 361
Proxmire Act 214
Proxmire, William 561-562
Prunasae 468
Pryor, David 255
PSA (prostate-specific antigen) test 266-267 *see also* cancer
psychoneuroendocrinology (PNE) 593
psychoneuroimmunology (PNI) 593-597
PTCA *see* balloon angioplasty
Public Citizen Health Research Group 61,80,223,263291
Pure Food and Drug Act 170,178,285
"pyramid power" 607

Q

qi 599,615
quack, derivation of term, 124
"quackbusters" 114,213-219,236-238,542,544,572,602,604
quacks 144
quacksalver 124
"quacks' charter," the 145,237
Queer Blood 502
quicksilver *see* mercury
quinine 197

R

Racketeering in Medicine 218
radiation 532 *see also* cancer
Radiation and Public Health Project 413
radionics, 20,21,601,606
Rall, David 551
RAND Corp. 48,59,62,83,85
Rath, Matthias 4,349,565

Rauscher, Frank 422
Rayfield, Allen E. 283
RCA 183
RDAs (recommended daily allowances) 560,561-562
Reader's Digest 91
refined carbohydrates 557,561
Reich, Charles 533, 534-535
Reich, Wilhelm 610,611,612,613
Reilly, David 605-606
Remington Arms 181
Renaissance 125,128,129,143
Republicans 153
Retrovir *see* AZT
retroviruses 393
Reunion Task Force 592
Revici, Emanuel 29,208
Rhazes 123
rheumatoid arthritis 529,543
Ribavirin 258
riboflavin 576
Richards, Alfred N. 271
Richards, Evelleen 169
Richardson, John A. 437,438,453-454,455,462
Richardson-Merrell 283
Richfield Oil 181
ricketts 568
Riegle, Donald 504
"Rife instruments" 429
"Rife microscope" 610
Rife, Royal R. 610,611,612,613
Riker Laboratories 338
RIMSO-50, 317
Ritalin 61
RN 55
Robinson, Mark 40
Robinson, Robert J. 283
Roche Holding Inc. 252
Roche Laboratories 506
Rockefeller Foundation 173
Rockefeller-I.G. Farben pact 181-182
Rockefeller Institute 271

Rockefeller Institute for Medical Research 171
Rockefeller, John D. 169,172
Rockefeller Power 169
Rockefeller, William Avery 172
Rockefeller, multiple corporate influences of, 182-184
Rodaquin 448
Roe, Robert A. 433,454
Roosevelt, Franklin D. 187
Root-Bernstein, Robert S. 471,484
root canals, 529-530
Rosaceae 468
Rosenthal, Benjamin S. 563
Ross-Loos 187
Rothenberg, Jo 55
Rothenberg, Michael B. 55
ROTS (reactive oxygen toxic species) 566-569
Royal Dutch Shell 554
Ruesch, Hans 169,225,271,272
Rush, Benjamin 128,147
Rutgers University 58,467
Rutherford, Glen L. 456,469

S

Sabin vaccine 174
Sacramento Bee 408
Sadusk, Joseph F. 283
Saint Bernadette 591
Saint Jude Clinic 19
salaries, medical, comparative 223-224
Salk vaccine 174
Salvoxyl-Wander Laboratories 272
Samuelson, Robert 75
Sammons, James H. 232
Sandoz 110,272
San Francisco Veterans Administration Hospital 330-331
San Jose Mercury News 85

Saturn V Moon Vehicle Project 615
saw palmetto berry 310
Schauss, Alexander 556
Scheele, Leonard 288
Schering Laboratories 268
Schering-Plough Corp. 268
Schmidt, Alexander McK. 300
Schondelmeyer, Stephen 253-254
Schoolman, Harold M. 71
Science 105,108,418,486,570
Scientific American 198,382
"scientific medicine" 114,126,128-129,141,143,161,171,176,185,190-191
"scientific method" 128,130
scientism 126-127,612
scleroderma 529,549
Scotland 559
Scott-Lucas Associates 263
Scripps Research Institute 109
scurvy 131,568
Seale, John 502
Sears 183
Seattle Computer Center 13
Seattle Post Intelligencer 5
Seattle Times 49
Second International Conference on Antioxidants in Disease Prevention 367
seeds 552-553
Seeds of Change 552,553
selenium 424,557
Seidl, L.G. 46
Semmelweiss, Ignasz 163
Senate Antitrust and Monopoly Subcommittee 288
Senate Committee on Labor and Human Resources 251
Senate Interstate and Foreign Commerce Committee 447
Senate Permanent Subcommittee on Investigations 94
Senate Select Committee on Aging

87,244,249
Senate Select Committee on Nutrition and Human Needs, Diet Related to Killer Diseases 556
Senate Select Committee on Small Business 198,230
Senate Subcommittee on Health 52,301
Seneca 205
714x 428
Serenoa repens 310
Seventh-Day Adventists 149,558
Shamim, Ahmad 208-209
shark cartilage 428
Sharpe & Dohme 164
Shaw, George Bernard 142,169
Shell Oil 181,183
Shen Nung 118
Shen Nung Pen Tsao Ching 118
Sherman Antitrust Act 229
Shilts, Randy 491
Shute brothers 349,350,548
sick building syndrome 531
SID (Syndrome of Immune Dysregulation) 528, 529,535
Sidel, V.M. and R. 35
Siegel, Bernie 590
silicone 531
silicone-gel breast implants 298
simazine 551
Simmons, George H. 220,222,229
Simonton, O. Carl 598
simvastatin (Zocor) 341
Sinclair Oil 181
Sinclair, Uptom 178
Sing, Charles 395
Sislowitz, Marcel J. 99
Sister Kenney 174
Sjogren's Syndrome 529
Skrabanek, Peter 351
Slaughter of the Innocent 225, 271,296
Sless, Rodger 14

Sloan Foundation 173,174
smallpox vaccine 502,503
Smith Barney, Harris Upham & Co. 254
Smith, Kline and French Laboratories 283
SmithKline Beecham 231,252
SMON (subacute myelo-optical neuropathy) 273-274
Social Security Act 187
Socialists 175,185
sodium valproate 294
Sohal, Rajindar 570
Soil Conservation Service, US Department of Agriculture 550
Solid Gold 3,4
Solomon, George 593-594
Solutein 523
somatids 611
Sonnabend, Joseph 485
Southern Pacific Railroad 183
"spontaneous remissions" 592
Squibb and Sons Pharmaceutical 181
Squibb, E.R. 164
Standard Oil 172,177,181,182,183
Stanford University 349,352,454
Staphylococcus aureus 58-59
Stark, Fortney H. 35
Starr, Paul 142,148
Sterling Drug 181,183
Sternglass, Ernest J. 413-415
steroids 300
Still, Andrew 166
Stone, Irwin 350
Strecker, Robert 501,502
Strecker, Ted 501
Streptokinase 252-253,339
stroke *see* heart/circulatory disease
strontium-90 414
St. Vincent's Hospital and Medical Center of New York 427
Subic Bay Naval Base 496
substance abuse, in medicine, 53-54

Sugar Association 562
Sugiura, Kanematsu 456
sulfanilamide 286
superoxide dismutase (SOD) 568
supplements industry 47-48, 571-573
surgery 51,55
"swine flu" 503
Swiss Medical Assn. 305
Symms, Steve 297,303
Synthroid 244
syphilis 123-124,162,518-521,525

T

tacrine 265
Tahoma Clinic 5
Takeda Pharmaceutical Co. 268
Tambocor 338
Tamoxifen *see* cancer
Tang, Yiwen 11
Taoism, 598
TAP Pharmaceuticals 268
Tapia, Roberto 37
Tap Water Blues 550-551
tax-free foundations 173-174,175-176
taxol 109
Taylor, Will 517-518
Teas, Jane 503,505
Temoshek, Lydia 593
Tesla, Nikola 609,610,612
Texaco 181
Thalidomide 272-273,288
The Antibiotic Paradox
The Associated Press 73
The Choice 3-4,11,12,13,18,24,26,36, 40,207,252-253,352,539
The Clay Pedestal 71
"The Club" *see* AIC
The Dictocrats 283
The Doctor Business 224
The Drug Story 226
The Great American Fraud 178

The Great Medical Monopoly Wars 266-267,218
The Impaired Physician 55
The Jungle 178
The Medical Industrial Complex 241
The Money Givers 185
The New American 104
The New Drug Story 226
The Physician Himself 142,155
The Politics of Cancer 401
The Politics of Therapeutic Evaluation: the Vitamin C and Cancer Controversy 169
The Proprietary Asssociation 283
Therapeutic Gazette 165
The Solid Gold Stethoscope 49,114
The Super Drug Story 139,270
The Supermeds 195
The Unkindest Cut 49
thiamine 576
thiocyanates 468
Thompson, Elizabeth 153
Thomson, Samuel 148
Thomsonianism 148,149,151,152
Thorup, Oscar 46
Tierra Marketing 14
"Tijuana Express" 68-69
Time magazine 244, 427
Tobey, Charles 446-447
tonsillectomies 81
topsoil deficiency problems 549-550
Townsend Letter for Doctors 310
T-PA (tissue plasminogen activator) 252-253,339
Traveler's Insurance Co. 183
Trever, William 204-206,225
triazines 550-551
triglycerides 355-356
Trimmer, R.W. 349
Trinity College 351
triparanol 357
trophoblastic thesis of cancer 443-444
Tso Yen 121

Tufts University 76,295,297
tumor necrosis factor (TNF) 387
TURP (transurethral resection of the prostate) 84

U

UFO (unidentified flying objects) 615
ulcers 256
ultraviolet irradiation of blood 613
UNICEF 48
Union Carbide 216
Union Oil 181
United Kingdom, "alternative medicine" in, 237-238
United Nations Center for Human Rights 32
United Nations Commission on Human Rights 512
United Press 226
"universal reactor syndrome" (URS) 56,528-529
University of Alabama 593
University of California 418
University of California-Berkeley 380,412,483
University of California-Berkeley School of Public Health 574
University of California-Davis 461
University of California-Los Angeles (UCLA) 349,593,595
University of California-San Francisco 354,593
University of California-San Francisco Medical School 589
University of Chicago 409
University of Connecticut 354
University of Georgia 517
University of Illinois School of Public Health 401
University of Massachusetts Medical School 263
University of Michigan 395
University of Minnesota 253,467
University of New Mexico 253,467
University of New York-Brooklyn 398
University of Pennsylvania 147
University of Pittsburgh 413
University of Rochester 593
University of Southern California 530
University of St. Louis School of Medicine 572
University of Toronto 405,409
Upjohn Co. 196,309
US Congress 377,401
US Constitution 176,177
US Court of Appeal 202
US Department of Agriculture 504, 505,561
US Department of Agriculture Human Nutrition Research Center 569
US Department of Commerce 72
US Department of Health and Human Services (HHS) 49,101,231-232, 237,256,281
US Department of Health, Education and Welfare 452
US Department of Justice 214,229, 447
US Department of Labor 243
US Department of Veterans Affairs 255
US Environmental Protection Agency (EPA) 419,550
US Navy 559
US Postal Service 207,210,214
US Public Health Service 65
US Rubber 181
US Steel 183
US Supreme Court 229,456,469
USA Today 372,401,541,573
Useful Drugs 261

V

vaccines 65
Valium 301-302
Van Atta, Dale 89-90, 255-256
Vance, Robert 208
Varner, Robert E. 313-314
Vascor heart valves 197
VDRL blood test 519
Vegalos, P. Roy 269
Velikovsky, Immanuel 126-127, 612
verapimil 294
Verdi, Tulio Suzzara 153
Vesalius 122, 143
Veterans Administration 77, 103, 332, 333
Vilcabamba Indians 439, 558
Vinuela, Eladio 506
viruses 392 *see also* cancer
vis medicatrix naturae 150, 600
Visna maedi virus (VMV) 501, 502
Vitacel-7 13
Vitamin A 276, 424, 367, 568, 574
Vitamin B6 276, 575
Vitamin B12 576
Vitamin B15 442
Vitamin B17 *see* laetrile
Vitamin C (ascorbic acid, ascorbate) 131, 349, 350, 424, 469, 521, 544, 553, 557, 565, 567, 568, 570, 573, 574, 576
Vitamin D 343, 533, 576
Vitamin E 253, 276, 367, 424, 548, 565, 567, 568, 570, 573
vivisection industry 296
Voltaire 71, 113
Voltaren 263

W

Walker, Martin J. 238
Walker, Morton 360
Wall Street Journal 252, 267-268, 341, 372, 420, 572
Wallach, Joel 548-549
Walter Reed Army/Navy Medical Hospital 104
Warburg, Otto 446
Warner Co. 164
Warner-Lambert 264, 265, 284
Washington, George 134
Washington Post 93, 387, 402-403, 602
Washington Times and Herald 226
Wasley, Terree P. 75
Wasson, John 408-409
water 550-551
Watkins, Kevin 553
Watts, Clyde 456
Waud, Douglas R. 263
Weill, Andrew 579
Weinstock, Charles 591-592
Weiss, Ted 93, 259
Weisse Magier 271
Welch, Henry 282
Wellcome PLC 252, 510
Wellness Watch 62
Wennberg, John 88-89
Western Michigan University 434
Western Union 183
Westinghouse 183
What Has Government Done to our Health Care? 75
wheat grass 575
Whelan, Elizabeth 320
Wilensky, Gail 100
Wiley, Harvey 178-179, 285
Wilk, Chester 202
Wilk vs. AMA 202
Willett, Walter 573
Williams, Roger J. 325, 548
Willner, Robert 499
Wilson, E. O. 553
Winthrop Laboratories 283
Wohl, Stanley 194, 196, 241

Wollstein, Jarret D. 75
Women's Health Network 410
Wood, Richard 269
Woolhandler, Steffi 60
World Health Organization (WHO)
210,300,327,472,501-502
World Without Cancer 183
Worlds in Collision 127
Worst Pills/Best Pills II 61,291
Wright, Jonathan 5,7,8-9,280
Wyden, Ron 108,109
Wythenshaw Hospital 336

X

Xanax 244, 309, 310
X- factor 589
X- rays 51- 52, 85

Y

Yale University 46, 254
Yamori, Yukio 366
Yankowitz, Morris 283
yin and *yang* 598
yoga 598
Young, Frank 281
Your Money or Your Life 225
Yu, V. L. 63

Z

Zantac 244, 263
Zeus 119
zidovudine *see* AZT
zinc 564
Zion, Libby 41-42
Zion, Sidney 41
Zutphen Elderly Study 366